Manufacturing Tibetan Medicine

Series: Epistemologies of Healing
General Editors: David Parkin and Elisabeth Hsu: both are at ISCA, Oxford

This series publishes monographs and edited volumes on indigenous (so-called traditional) medical knowledge and practice, alternative and complementary medicine, and ethnobiological studies that relate to health and illness. The emphasis of the series is on the way indigenous epistemologies inform healing, against a background of comparison with other practices, and in recognition of the fluidity between them.

Manufacturing Tibetan Medicine

The Creation of an Industry and the Moral Economy of Tibetanness

Martin Saxer

Berghahn Books
New York • Oxford

First published in 2013 by

Berghahn Books

www.berghahnbooks.com

©2013 Martin Saxer

Library of Congress Cataloging-in-Publication Data

Saxer, Martin, 1971-
  Manufacturing Tibetan medicine : the creation of an industry and the moral
economy of Tibetanness / Martin Saxer. – First edition.
      pages cm. – (Epistemologies of healing)
  Includes bibliographical references.
  ISBN 978-0-85745-772-1 (hardback : alk. paper) – ISBN 978-0-85745-775-2
(ebook)
  1. Medicine, Tibetan–China–Moral and ethical aspects. 2. Medicine,
Tibetan–Practice–China. I. Title.
  R603.T5S36 2013
  610.951–dc23

                                                                2012033461

British Library Cataloguing in Publication Data

A catalogue record for this book is available from the British Library

Printed in the United States on acid-free paper.

ISBN 978-0-85745-772-1 (hardback)
ISBN 978-0-85745-775-2 (ebook)

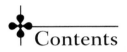

Contents

List of Figures

All images by the author, except Figure 3.3 by Kurt Fischer.

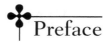

Preface

This is a study of an industry in the making. It explores the recent emergence of the industrial production of Tibetan medicines in the People's Republic of China (PRC) and its stake in shaping contemporary Tibet. While these developments are depicted as a big success by Chinese officialdom, they also meet with harsh criticism in Tibet. People complain that prices are on the rise while the quality of medicines is decreasing. Moreover, the industry, which relies extensively on wild herbs, is seen as a threat to the survival of several plant species. Industrialisation touches upon much more than technical strategies of manufacturing Tibetan drugs. What is at stake is a fundamental (re-)manufacturing of Tibetan medicine as a system of knowledge and practice.

Within a mere decade, hospital pharmacies throughout the Tibetan areas of China have been converted into pharmaceutical companies. In 2001, a new law declared so-called 'good manufacturing practices' (GMP) a compulsory requirement for the production of medicines. As a result, companies had to build new factories in order to comply with the regulations. Confronted with the logic of capital and profit, these companies now produce commodities for a nationwide market.

The emerging industry and its shiny new manufacturing plants captured my attention on a trip through Eastern Tibet in 2005. The brochures and products of the brand new factories, omnipresent in the pharmacies of the region, stood in stark contrast to the world of brown pills I was familiar with from the wards of Tibetan doctors. I decided to make the industrialisation of Tibetan medicine the topic of my PhD research, for which I carried out eighteen months of fieldwork between September 2007 and September 2009.

During these two years many parameters framing the industry underwent far-reaching changes. Some of them were triggered, directly or indirectly, by events. In 2007, for example, the former director of China's powerful State Food and Drug Administration (SFDA), Zheng Xiaoyu, was found guilty of corruption and sentenced to death. The trial revealed a scandal of epic proportions and its fall-out reached the Tibetan medicine industry in the form of a general tightening of regulations. Then, there was the widespread unrest that shattered Tibet in March 2008. The subsequent clampdown had serious implications for almost every aspect of life in Tibet, and the situation has remained tense ever since. While Tibetan medicine companies were largely left untouched (after all, Tibetan medicine has the status of being a 'pillar industry' in the region), the indirect effects of March 2008 are still unfolding. The cross-border trade in medicinal plants between Nepal and Tibet, for example, has since become much more restricted.

At the same time, drug regulations continue to change and new guidelines are issued frequently. Some of them, such as the GMP inspection checklist used by the SFDA (Kuwahara and Li 2008), define good practices for the supervision of good practices. Good practices are manufactured at an almost industrial pace in contemporary China. On 1 March 2011 a revised version of China's GMP standard came into effect. Existing factories have to comply with the revised regulations by the end of 2015. While the effects on the Tibetan medicine industry remain to be seen, the direction of the new provisions is crystal clear: they are meant to make Chinese drug production standards more compatible with the much stricter GMP standards of Europe, America and Japan.

The pace of development shows no signs of deceleration and the process of research, writing and publishing an academic book appears incredibly slow by comparison. By the time it will be read, factories may have changed hands and names, pressing problems will have found unexpected solutions, and other problems will have surfaced. Many of the stories I started to trace will be history. In short, this book is approaching a moving target.

What, then, one may ask, can an anthropological monograph documenting a brief period of time within a larger and ongoing transformation accomplish? I think the present case reveals a characteristic conjuncture of our times. There are three reasons why the processes I seek to understand and describe are relevant beyond the immediate context and time frame of the present case. First, the industry of

Tibetan medicine lies at the intersection of conflicting visions and agendas for Tibet. It serves as an allegorical figure of Tibet's rapid development and progress, its medicines are the target of a booming 'ethnicity industry', and the formulas serve as a showcase for the state's alleged efforts to protect Tibet's cultural heritage. The industrialisation of Tibetan medicine has emerged as an arena where these different visions and agendas clash and mingle. As such, it may facilitate new understandings of contemporary Tibet. Second, the speed and scope of the industry's creation are representative of similar ventures elsewhere in China, the Tibetan medicine industry exemplifies the Chinese party-state's strategies and style of planning as well as the tactical manoeuvring these plans encounter on the ground. And third, the attempt to make Tibetan medicine fit for global markets and consumers resonates with many similar endeavours around the globe. I hope that an ethnographic perspective on these ongoing developments will provide useful insights and enable a comparison with similar processes elsewhere.

My inquiry focuses on the companies producing Tibetan medicines, their tactics and strategies, their ethical reasoning and engagement in the market not only for pills and remedies but also for Tibetanness — a market, I argue, that bears the characteristics of a moral economy at large, enmeshed in the global political spectacle that surrounds the 'Tibet question' and China's rise as a world power. My basic thesis is that industrial production triggers an ongoing and profound transformation of the ways in which herbs are sourced, medicines are produced, packaged and sold, and Tibetan medicine as a system of knowledge and practice is perceived.

While this transformation evidently also affects medical practice, the views of doctors as well as patterns of consumption among Tibetan and Chinese patients lie beyond the topic of my inquiry. Such a study, although highly relevant to the present case, would require a different approach and a considerable amount of additional fieldwork. Furthermore, the voice of officials responsible for Tibetan medicine within the PRC's health bureaucracy is largely absent in my narrative. I had originally intended to interview officials in order to get a better understanding of their perspectives and reasoning. However, the unrest of March 2008 and the resulting situation made interviewing government officials a sensitive matter. As a result, I had to resort to the publications of news agencies, the statements and white papers of government offices, and what people involved in the industry told me as anecdotes. This unintended omission will have to be compensated for in future research.

Singapore, January 2012

✤ Acknowledgements

This book is the result of a journey on which I seldom travelled alone. It would not have been possible without the help and commitment of a great number of people. To list them all is beyond the space of these pages. A few stand out, however, and should be mentioned.

I owe my deepest gratitude to those who feature in this book with their real names or pseudonyms – Aku Jinpa, Rinchen Wangdu, Pema Gyatso, Tenpa Wangchug, Palden Dorji, Penba, Arjun and Raksha Deora, Ngawang Dawa, Jigme Phuntsog, and Lei Jufang. I would also like to express my thanks to Kalden Nyima, Ursula Rechbach, Kelsang Norbu, Tendor, Norbu, Nyima Norbu, Pema Tsamchoe, Rigzin, Thubten Kelsang, Tseten Dorji, Tsewang Rinchen, Tsewang Tanpa, Jampa and Jigme. They all spent their energy and patience introducing me to the subtleties of Tibetan medicine and contributed in one way or another to my stay in Lhasa.

I am also deeply indebted to the people who facilitated my research in Xining. Without the advice and help of Dhondup, Rinchen, Shawogyal, Thargo, Rinchen, Lobsang, Dugai Tserang, Huajor, Huasang, Lushamgyal and many others my work would not have been possible. In India, the same is true for Tenzin Thaye, Lobsang Tenzin Radko, Namgyal Tsering, Pema Gyatso, Tsering Thakchoe, Tsewang Gyatso, Tsultrim Kalsang, Wangdue, Tenzin Namdul, Naresh Mathu, the former director of Men-tsee-khang Dr Dawa and Dr Dawa from the Herbal Product and Research Department.

Indispensable for my research on plant trade in Kathmandu were Tsewang Lama, Brian Peniston, Carroll Dunham, Kesang Tseten, Karma Bhutia, Sherab Barma, Ibila, Tsebu, Tsewang Norbu (two different individuals of that name) and Gyan Man Singh. I will never forget the hospitality I encountered at Gyan Man Singh's herb store and his patience in answering my endless questions.

This book is based on my doctoral thesis at the University of Oxford. At Oxford, several people were instrumental in this project. Elisabeth Hsu and Charles Ramble were outstanding advisors and skilful navigators through the storms and calm of my time as a doctoral student. I am deeply grateful for their trust, expertise and humour, on which I relied throughout this rite of passage much more than they realised. David Parkin and David Gellner helped me see my work in the wider context of anthropology. Fernanda Pirie and Xiang Biao were critical and constructive readers at early stages of my work. Their input was crucial for this book and they have been a source of encouragement and advice on writing.

In many ways the journey that led to this book started long before I came to Oxford. In 2002 I met Barbara Gerke in Kalimpong, India. It was her enthusiasm that sparked my interest in Tibetan medicine. She has remained an inspiring friend over the years. It was Michael Oppitz who then encouraged me to apply to Oxford while I was his assistant at Zurich University. I am thankful to both of them.

A series of encounters with friends and fellow anthropologists, wanderers between the Himalayas and university libraries like myself, shaped my perspectives to a considerable degree. In Lhasa and Oxford, Kabir Heimsath has been enormously helpful, both as a source on all things Tibetan as well as a sharp and critical reader of my work in its early stages. So has Radhika Gupta, who took an interest in my work from early on. I look back on a series of inspiring conversations with her both in Delhi and Oxford. I have profited greatly from Theresia Hofer's knowledge about a different, non-industrial side of Sowa Rigpa as well as from her network of contacts in Lhasa. Stephan Kloos, whose simultaneous work on Tibetan medicine in exile revealed many parallels to my own, has generously shared his insights and contacts. Our meetings in Varanasi and Dharamsala stimulated my own inquiry. In Lhasa, Lobsang Yongdan and Alice Travers provided me with new perspectives on Tibetan history. My intellectual debts to these colleagues and friends are numerous and defy accounting. The same is true of the three anonymous reviewers who read my manuscript with much scrutiny and goodwill.

My view of Tibet was also shaped to a considerable degree by those Tibetans who accompanied me at different stages of this project. More teachers and friends than assistants and translators, Pema

Namgyal, Tashi Tsering, Penba Tashi, Pema Yangchen and Namlha were instrumental in my research.

Some of my debts are to institutions: Tibet University in Lhasa and the Qinghai Nationalities University in Xining provided me with backing during my time in Tibet. In terms of material support, I acknowledge the University of Oxford's Clarendon Bursary and Zurich University's *Forschungskredit*. The Society for South Asian Studies, Dr Peter Hauri and Kurt Fischer provided additional support.

Last but not least, I am grateful for the love and support of my family both in Switzerland and Russia. My mother, Rosmarie Saxer, and my parents-in-law Galina Orlova and Valerij Orlov, sheltered and supported my wife, daughter and me with all their love and energy. My daughter Alisa's smile helped me many times to gain distance and see things in perspective. And finally, Victoria, my wife, has travelled with me through the turmoils of these years. Her love for language has inspired me, her critical reading pushed me to re-think many notions taken for granted, her companionship gave me comfort, and her forbearance the freedom to bring this journey to a successful completion.

Notes on Transliteration and Transcription

Tibetan terms are italicised and rendered in a simple phonetic transcription. On first appearance, they are also given in their orthographic form, using the standard Wylie system of transliteration (Wylie 1959). Sowa Rigpa (*gso ba rig pa*), the Tibetan 'science of healing', is not italicised but treated as a name for a system of medical knowledge and practice, just like Ayurveda or TCM. The same is true for Sowa Rigpa's main text, the fourfold treatise known as the Gyüshi (*rgyud bzhi*) – it is capitalised but not italicised.

Phonetic transcription follows the THL simplified phonetic transcription of standard Tibetan (Germano and Tournadre 2003). This system employs umlauts for more precise phonetic rendering (Gyüshi instead of Gyushi, for instance). However, the proposed accentuated 'é' is replaced by a standard 'e', and 'g' is employed instead of 'k' (Gelugpa instead of Gelukpa). Furthermore, for names and places sometimes more familiar spellings are used, such as Shigatse instead of Zhikatsé.

Plural forms usually do not take a plural 's' (*amchi* refers to both singular and plural), unless a Tibetan or Sanskrit term is so common in English that it is not treated as a foreign word (four lamas, three Rinpoches, and two Buddhas, three thangkas, for example).

For Mandarin terms the most simple *pinyin* system is employed, without the use of diacritics or numerals to indicate tones.

✦ List of Abbreviations

CBD   Convention on Biological Diversity
CCP   Chinese Communist Party
CCTM   Central Committee for Tibetan Medicine (in India)
CITES   Convention on International Trade in Endangered Species of Wild Fauna and Flora
CMP   Chinese Medicine and Pharmacotherapy
CTIC   China Tibet Information Center
GAP   Good agricultural practices
GMP   Good manufacturing practices
GSP   Good supply practices
HAA   Himalayan Amchi Association
ICH   International Conference on Harmonisation of Technical Requirements for Registration of Pharmaceuticals for Human Use
ISO   International Organization for Standardization
NGO   Non-governmental Organisation
NITM   Bhutan's National Institute of Traditional Medicine in Thimphu
OTC   Over the counter
PLA   People's Liberation Army
PRC   People's Republic of China
PSB   Public Security Bureau
RCT   Randomised controlled trial, randomised clinical trial
SATCM   State Administration of Traditional Chinese Medicine
SFDA   State Food and Drug Administration
SIPO   State Intellectual Property Organisation
SOP   Standard operating procedure
TAR   Tibet Autonomous Region
TASS   Tibetan Academy of Social Sciences
TCM   Traditional Chinese medicine

THL	The Himalayan Library (www.thlib.org)
TMI	The Mountain Institute
TRIPS	Agreement on Trade Related Aspects of Intellectual Property Rights
UNESCO	United Nations Educational, Scientific and Cultural Organization
WHO	World Health Organization
WTO	World Trade Organization

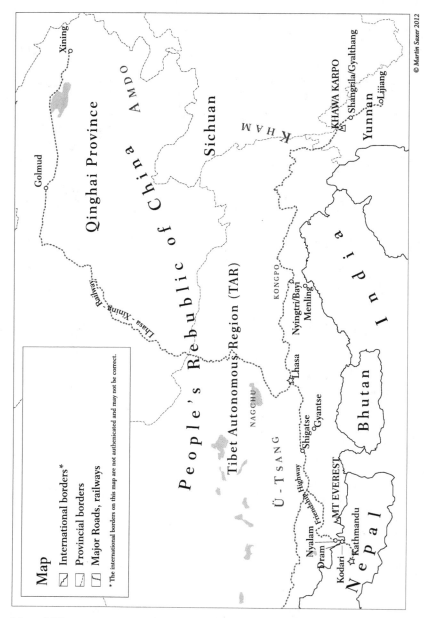

Map of Tibet.

Chapter 1
Introduction: Perspectives on Tibetan Medicine

Aku Jinpa

Aku Jinpa was sitting cross-legged on the bed of his simple study room. He was chanting. With his left hand he turned the pages of the Tibetan scripture that lay on the table in front of him, while his right hand rhythmically pulled the strings attached to two prayer wheels next to the table. To keep them turning seemed to require neither effort nor attention. Aku Jinpa, a man in his sixties with a big black moustache, wore a simple brown jacket. Nothing in his appearance betrayed the fact that he was one of the most famous Tibetan doctors in this part of Qinghai province, about a day's journey from its capital Xining. My friend and I had no appointment with him, but Aku Jinpa did not seem to be surprised to see us. We stood, smiling and a little bit shy, and watched him chant for a while until he stopped and offered us a seat.

I explained my reasons for our visit: that I was doing research on factories and the production of Tibetan medicine and that I kept hearing about him, his medicines and the school he had started a few years previously. Several people had told me I should visit him.

Aku Jinpa pointed to a picture on the wall showing an old monk and said: 'Yes, I established a private medical school. It was my lama's wish, so I built it'. My gaze was caught by a second photograph, depicting a large group of students in the courtyard of the new school compound still under construction, some of them in monk's robes and some in civilian clothing, their minds engrossed in the study of a text, either walking or standing, all keeping a distance from one another in order to focus on their task.

1

'Since it is a private school there is no support from the government. Therefore, I applied for the permit to establish this small factory and pharmacy. The factory and the pharmacy support the school', Aku Jinpa continued. The young woman who had shown us the way to his study opened the door and served us tea. I had trouble understanding Aku Jinpa's Amdo dialect but he seemed to be used to dealing with foreigners. He spoke slowly, making sure I understood and when I did not he paused to let my friend translate. As Aku Jinpa talked we drank tea.

> I am blessed with a beautiful culture. It should not be lost. So I just put a little effort into preserving this beautiful traditional culture. I don't know when I will die but all I want is to serve the Tibetans. That is my only wish in life.

> There was a businessman, a Chinese. He asked me if I wanted to work with him to build this school and I agreed. Then, he asked me, 'How are we going to divide the income?' And my answer was that there would be no income. So he asked how I could think of building a school that would not generate any income. And what is more, he asked what good it was if there was no income. My answer was that it was good for my Tibetan culture.

Aku Jinpa's argument, portraying Tibetan medicine as an antithesis of the world of Chinese business, echoed many similar conversations I had throughout my time in Tibet. Nonetheless, I was struck by the moral tone of his argument, linking religion and Tibetanness directly to the quality of the medicines produced:

> I actually don't have such a big medicine factory. I have applied for this factory permit and just got it this year. If it has a good reputation it is because it is traditional and if it is traditional you can never separate it from religion. Traditional Tibetan medicine is connected with religion and therefore you must be devout and you must have a pure heart. Apart from that, the herbs must be clean, and must be real. If these conditions are met your medicine will be good. So, generally speaking, there is not much to research on Tibetan medicine except these things.

Taking it as a hint at the relevance of my own research, I found myself looking for words to explain why I thought it was still important. I was about to say that, despite having my personal doubts about the recent industrialisation of Tibetan medicine, I saw its tremendous impact on the practice and future of Sowa Rigpa (*gso ba rig pa*),[1] and that I believed that these challenges and the ways people were facing them were a story worth telling. But before I was able to explain these things, we were interrupted by the arrival of an important Rinpoche, a close disciple of Aku Jinpa's teacher. His expensive Toyota Land Cruiser had just drawn into the courtyard and his entourage rushed in to announce his arrival. We all moved to the spacious living room in one of the adjacent buildings where tea was being served.

Rinpoche spoke some English and obviously had had his experiences with foreigners as well. In his questions I discerned a certain scepticism about me and my motivations. Many foreigners were coming to Tibet, some seeking Buddhist teaching and spiritual guidance, some coming with ties to NGOs, some with potential money from networks abroad, and some with the idea of helping to 'save' Tibet; some called themselves 'followers of Jesus', young American missionaries with monthly salaries from Christian companies back home, organising 'Christmas parties' in Starbucks-style coffee shops. Rinpoche was trying to fathom which category I belonged to. Working with foreigners, and especially foreign NGOs, had become much more sensitive since the violent uprisings throughout Tibet in March 2008. Aku Jinpa's new school and factory had finally been funded not by a Chinese business partner but an American NGO, now under tight supervision by the authorities and on the verge of losing its contract to work in the area.

Although foreign – mostly Western – agendas were often phrased in terms of 'development' and the 'preservation of Tibetan culture' – a phrasing almost identical to the official discourse of the Chinese party-state, and even the way Aku Jinpa himself had explained his mission, perspectives and meanings of these terms were highly contested. Western, Chinese and Tibetan ideas about what Tibet essentially was or should be were deeply entangled and often referred to each other as opposites while still using a similar language (cf. Barnett 2001b: 291). Aku Jinpa's pledge to preserve 'his beautiful culture' could be printed word for word in the annual report of a foreign NGO or a story by a government news agency about the achievements of a heroic Tibetan compatriot, despite the differences in meaning such a claim would convey. To navigate these straits wisely in the highly politicised space of contemporary Tibet was both a challenge and an important skill for those committed to furthering Tibetan medicine in contemporary China.

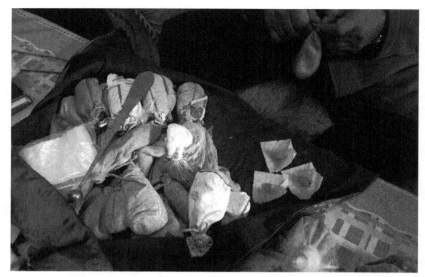

Figure 1.1: An *amchi*'s travelling pharmacy: powdered medicines are carried in leather bags.

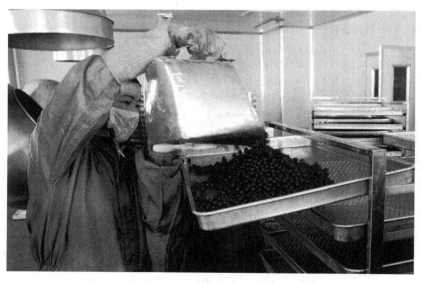

Figure 1.2: Freshly produced pills in a GMP manufacturing plant.

On our way to Aku Jinpa's home we had passed by the county's Tibetan hospital, where Aku Jinpa had held a leading position before he started his own enterprise. Adjacent to the hospital, amidst a fenced green and spacious lawn, contrasting sharply with the surrounding brownish grasslands of late October, stood a big, new, white Tibetan medicine factory, one of about two dozen recently constructed manufacturing plants on the Tibetan Plateau. In Xining, the capital of Qinghai province, people had spoken enthusiastically about the medicines produced by this factory, linking their quality directly to Aku Jinpa's knowledge and fame. As I learned now, Aku Jinpa no longer had anything to do with it and preferred not to talk about it. But the new pharmaceutical enterprise was still, by way of reputation and trust, related to and to some degree even dependent on Aku Jinpa's world of Buddhism and morality, a realm that has come to be seen as traditional and authentically Tibetan.

Aku Jinpa took us across the street to the new school compound. With a sense of pride he showed us his accomplishments. Construction work was in its very last stages and we were taken on a tour through the cold and empty buildings that would serve as dormitories, classrooms, a canteen and a small medicine factory. The buildings were made of concrete and featured a few superficial Tibetan architectural features, following the now dominant style of how Tibet is being reconstructed in a more contemporary way with a dash of tradition here and there. The look and feel of Aku Jinpa's new school compound tied in well with what official China would expect of such a site: Tibetan and yet part of modern China. Besides the intention that it be a realm of tradition, the compound was in some ways an aesthetic enterprise, presentable to its future students as well as the local government, American donors and guests such as Rinpoche, my Tibetan friend and me.

Finally, Aku Jinpa brought us to the roadside dispensary, which was already in operation and catering to the local residents. Without being ill or being subjected to any examination, my friend and I were both given medicines in ample quantities. The pills were packed in varicoloured composite plastic-aluminium pouches, indistinguishable from the commodities of big factories. They were given as presents rather than as remedies, endowed with Aku Jinpa's fame and status as a great Tibetan doctor of his time. He once more reminded me that only a Buddhist foundation would make my own project truly worthwhile, because only through Buddhism could Tibetan medicine really be understood and have a purpose. Despite Aku Jinpa's proselytising undertones, which for a second reminded me of the young Americans travelling with Jesus, I was moved by the commitment of this man and his calm and friendly charisma.

We were all invited to stay for dinner. Heaps of boiled mutton and yak were served, the traditional way to treat important guests. Rinpoche's initial reserve slowly gave way to a more sympathetic attitude, whether because of the questions I was putting to Aku Jinpa that might have convinced him of my sincerity, or simply because of my Oxford affiliation.

When we left Aku Jinpa's house it was already getting dark and the dogs started barking on the outskirts of the county town. It was a freezing cold October night. On the wide and well-paved road a nomad on a motorcycle was driving his yaks towards new pastures. Snow had fallen the day before.

Official Views

Aku Jinpa's decision to forgo the world of big factories is to be seen in relation to the highly visible presence they have gained in public and official discourse over the last few years, as the following passage from a report by the Tibet Information Centre, a government news agency, illustrates:

> The encouraging situation of [the] market economy and the favorable policy for developing the western part of China have supplied the industrialization of Tibetan medicines with good opportunities ... By the end of 2003, statistics showed that the annual output value of Tibetan medicines amounted to 1,000,000,000 yuan [US$146 million],[2] which is over 30 times more than that of 1996. These medicines are used not only in Tibetan-inhabited areas, but also in more than 600 hospitals of other places in the country. Some ... rare patent Tibetan medicines are sold in the sale[s] net of 30 provinces of the country, even [as] far away [as] Southeast Asia, South and North Americas. The industry of Tibetan medicines has achieved an average increase by 129% annually since 2000. (Huang 2006)

Despite all necessary scepticism about the reliability of such government statistics (to which I return in Chapter 2), it is safe to say that Tibetan medicine has gone through an unprecedented transformation. Within a mere decade a fully fledged pharmaceutical industry has been created on the Tibetan Plateau. It is with the creation of this industry that this book is concerned.

Leaving aside nuances and contradictions (which will make for the substance of this book) the story is quickly told. In 2001 China announced the instituting of a nationwide system of drug registration and the introduction of 'good manufacturing practices' (GMP), a compulsory quality standard for the production of all pharmaceuticals sold on the market, including Tibetan medicines. Both had been on the party-state's agenda for some time but gained importance in the process of China's WTO entry in the same year. Tight deadlines were set to comply with the new rules and regulations. By the end of 2004, all Tibetan medicine manufacturers had to pass GMP certification. The provisions made the construction of new factories necessary, and for this purpose substantial new investment was required. Contrary to the news report of the China Tibet Information Center quoted above, one can hardly speak of the 'encouraging situation of the market economy' or the 'favorable policy for developing the western part of China' as the driving forces behind these events. The construction of new and bigger factories was a direct reaction to the rules and deadlines set by the state.

These far-reaching and rapid developments are seen as a great success by the party-state. But this very positive image of the emerging industry contrasts with widespread scepticism, and not only by people like Aku Jinpa who have opted to dedicate their energy to endeavours outside mainstream industry. In fact, the vast majority of patients, doctors, factory workers and managers I talked to were far more outspoken than Aku Jinpa. Living in Tibet one simply cannot fail to hear ever-present concerns about the direction in which Tibetan medicine is heading.

The present situation was described to me by Rinchen Wangdu, a retired senior manager of one company, who was at ease with speaking out. His views are representative of those held by many.

Some young people trained in Western medicine are now in charge of managing Tibetan medicine within the government administration. But those who studied Tibetan medicine for thirty years cannot get into these government offices ... In the whole health bureau of the TAR [Tibet Autonomous Region], for example, there is not one single person who is knowledgeable about Tibetan medicine. So they don't take Tibetan medicine seriously. They think this is some kind of cultural thing ... They only follow the political orders from the central government. They force the Tibetan medicine factories to follow all these procedures and protocols, regardless of whether they are compatible with Tibetan medicine or not ... In order to survive, the factories have to distort the rules and regulations a little bit. This is really bad.

Rinchen Wangdu's remarks stand in sharp contrast with official pronouncements, which rave about the present as Tibetan medicine's 'best period of development in history' (CTIC 2006f), with ample funding for research (CTIC 2006e, 2008b) and higher patient numbers than ever before (IOSC 2008: 5). The difference between official pronouncements, Rinchen Wangdu's concerns and Aku Jinpa's moral reasoning point to the many layers of ambition, practice and discourse that shape the emerging industry.

The Topic of Inquiry

The perspectives outlined above entail two approaches to the topic of this book. On the one hand, the Tibetan medicine industry is seen as an industry, or more specifically a medicine industry, embedded in visions of modernity and larger development agendas. On the other hand, Tibetan medicine, including the production of pharmaceuticals, is seen as something distinctively Tibetan, as a locus of Tibetan identity and culture. These two angles will serve as a starting point for the following preliminary conceptualisation of the field.

Industrial Modernities

Industrialisation in Europe, America and elsewhere went hand in hand with far-reaching social change, for which the term 'modernity' has become a vague but powerful moniker. The transformation to industrial modernity was at the core of much of the classical scholarship in the social sciences. Industrialisation was analysed in terms of changing labour relations, the emergence of a working class, the accumulation of capital, and the fetishisation of commodities (Marx 1872). It was scrutinised in relation to the formation of bureaucracies and from the perspective of religious ethics particularly conducive to economic development (Weber 1947, 1986). Industrialisation was described as a history of mechanisation (Giedion 1975), or as the 'great transformation' in which local modes of production and consumption clashed with forms of the market economy (Polanyi 1957).

The insights of Marx, Weber, Polanyi, Giedion and many others whose work contributed to the understanding of industrial society stemmed from an analysis of Euro-American history. Early modernisation theories thereby often conceived of the Euro-American model as a great unifier that, by diffusion or natural evolution, would eventually lead to global convergence (cf. Rostow 1959). More recently, however, a number of authors have convincingly argued that different historical circumstances lead to multiple, plural or alternative modernities, entangled with but only partially resembling the Euro-American model.[3] In those states emerging from a communist revolution, for example, the grand project of industrialisation was conditioned by historical circumstances rather different from those in Europe and North America. These different 'entry points', as Goran Therborn (1995) argues, led to different routes to or through modernity.

In the Euro-American case, industry emerged simultaneously and interdependently with changing labour relations, the accumulation of capital, bureaucracies, technological developments, and new forms of statehood and governance. Yet, both Russia and China were largely agrarian societies at the time of their respective revolutions and, contrary to the vision of Marx and Engels, the revolutionary impetus did not come from a large, disenfranchised proletarian class. Many parameters on which Marxist analysis was based had to be rendered tangible in order to make communist ideology work in China (Lefort 1986: 205). As industry was largely absent, it had to be actively created together with extensive party bureaucracies to manage the planned economies. The notion of modernity thereby remained at the core of the communist project. However, communist ideology entailed its own vision of modernity: an industrial modernity without the flaws of its capitalist counterpart. In this sense, the *Communist Manifesto* (Marx and Engels 2002) can be seen as an essentially modern manifesto (Berman 1982: 87–90).

As the vanguard of communist modernity, industrial production acquired enormous symbolic meaning. Images of factories, power stations and industrialised agriculture appeared on stamps, banknotes and propaganda posters. Vladislav Todorov attributes industry in the Soviet Union with a largely aesthetic role: factories were not built to produce commodities, they were 'allegorical figures of industrialization', their essence was aesthetic rather than economic, and they resulted in 'a deficit of goods, but an overproduction of symbolic meanings' (Todorov 1995: 10). The production of symbolic meaning, I will argue, remains central to the Tibetan medicine industry. However, one can hardly speak of a 'deficit of goods', neither with regard to the Tibetan medicine industry nor to industry in the PRC in general.

While the disintegration of the Soviet Union led to a collapse of its industry, China embarked on a different route. With the advent of Deng Xiaoping's reform policies in the late 1970s and the subsequent proclamation of a 'socialist market economy', the style of government, bureaucracy and labour relations, and the role of capital, were reconfigured once again. This transformation was no longer exclusively conditioned by communist ideology as a critique of nineteenth-century European industrial modernity but also by the intention to actively learn from the contemporary Euro-American model of neoliberal governance and adapt it to Chinese conditions (Sigley 2006). The market and private entrepreneurship became cornerstones of Chinese economic and industrial policy. The rise of Chinese industry in the global economy and China's accession to the WTO in 2001 further amplified the entanglement of the party-state's policies with discourses and legal frameworks forged in the global arena. The resulting figuration (Houben and Schrempf 2008) or configuration (Randeria 2004) of modernity includes different layers, different visions of the modern, which at times stand in tension with one another.[4]

It is this context – a postsocialist industrial market society managed by a communist party – in which the Tibetan medicine industry was born. It was neither the outcome of the rise of a capitalist bourgeoisie and a free market nor a purely communist vision of industrial modernity. The agendas and policies that led to its creation were informed by both the party-state's belief in large-scale top-down planning, derived from decades of experience, as well as the more recent aspiration to learn from Euro-American approaches to industrial production, governance and the management of industries and markets.

An example of the latter are the policies that triggered the creation of a Tibetan medicine industry, namely the introduction of GMP and a system of drug regulation. These were directly inspired by Euro-American experiences with pharmaceutical industries and not the outcome of a communist modernisation project. GMP is part of what Kleinman and Petryna call the 'pharmaceutical nexus' (Petryna, Lakoff and Kleinman 2006), or, along similar lines, what Craig and Adams (2009) identify as 'Global Pharma', the dominant discourses about efficacy, scientific legitimacy and techniques of governance.[5] These discourses and techniques, embedded in national policies, play an important role in defining the space in which the industry operates. In this sense, GMP is a textbook example of what Ong and Collier describe as a 'global form', characterised by its capacity for 'decontextualization and recontextualization, abstractability and movement, across diverse social and cultural situations and spheres of life' (Ong and Collier 2005: 11).

The fact that global forms affect the local practice of medicine production is obvious and undeniable. Given the asymmetric power relations at work, this hardly comes as a surprise. However, it does not tell the full story. Recontextualisation – applying a global form to the context of a specific situation – is an unruly social process. When adapting ideas forged in the global arena to the conditions of the PRC, the party-state draws on its long experience in large-scale planning and a well-established apparatus to implement such plans. Generally, as Rinchen Wangdu's above statement bemoaning the lack of knowledge about Tibetan medicine in the health bureaucracy illustrates, the resulting approach tends to ignore local particularities.

In this respect, Rinchen Wangdu's assessment of the situation is reminiscent of the central argument of James Scott's enquiry into 'why certain schemes to improve the human condition have failed' (Scott 1998). Scott describes a variety of grand schemes, from the collectivisation of agriculture to the creation of planned cities like Chandigarh and Brasilia, which all have somehow failed their purpose. Scott notes that these failures are marked by a mix of four ingredients: a quest for legibility (the state's wish to make things countable and visible), a 'high-modernist ideology' (giving prominence to scientific development and planning), a strong state, and a weak civil society. Taken together, these are the recipe for disaster. He argues that high-modernist grand schemes tend to overlook practical, local knowledge (*mētis* in his terms); they hinder local microadaptation, tending to ignore social and environmental conditions and thereby create a gulf between the state's planning efforts and the realities on the ground.

11

The introduction of GMP for Tibetan medicine and a national-level system of drug registration can certainly be seen as a quest for legibility. Making Tibetan medicine a 'pillar industry' of the region's economic development bears the marks of high-modernist fervour. The People's Republic of China indeed seems like a strong state, at least at first sight. In addition, there are certainly angles from which Tibet can be seen as a weak civil society, and Scott's idea of how grand modernist schemes tend to ignore *mētis* accords with Rinchen Wangdu's complaints about the regulations of the central government, which give no regard to the peculiarities of Tibetan medicine. In short, the creation of a Tibetan medicine industry appears to be a good candidate for yet another well-intended 'scheme to improve the human condition' that is eventually bound to fail.

Thus, the notion of industry in the present case is linked to at least two layers of the modern project: global forms such as GMP (based on neoliberal ideas of governance) and high-modernist planning. While the content of GMP emphasises continuous self-assessment, management techniques and the internalisation of a philosophy of quality control, the way it is being implemented relies on grand-scheme, top-down planning, including tight deadlines and difficult-to-meet targets.

Scott's bold theory, together with the debate it has stirred (Gupta 1999; Rueschemeyer 1999; Wong 1999; Epp 2000), raises a series of questions pertaining to our case: Is the Chinese party-state really as strong or unified as imagined, and is Tibetan civil society really weak? And what happens to the party-state's modernist planning efforts when they become enmeshed in the preservation of cultural heritage?

This leads us to the second perspective on the Tibetan medicine industry, as represented by Aku Jinpa's endeavours.

Tibetanness and the Moral Space of Tradition

The Chinese Communist Party's view of religion and tradition has long been almost exclusively negative, seeing them as obstacles that needed to be overcome in order to establish a modern socialist society. However, this hostility towards religion and tradition, epitomised in the destruction of the 'four olds' (*si jiu*) – old customs, old culture, old habits, old ideas – during the Cultural Revolution, has since been overlaid by a more positive view of cultural heritage as something worth being preserved, documented and promoted. While a

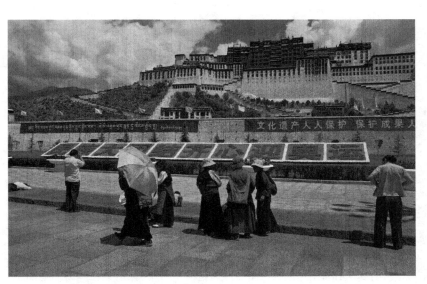

Figure 1.3: The Potala Palace in Lhasa, June 2008.

modernisation ethos remains the core of the party-state's Tibet policies, and the 'peaceful liberation' of Tibet from its feudal Buddhist past still plays an important role in the party-state's narrative of modernity (see, e.g., IOSC 2001; Yeh 2008), recent government white papers always emphasise both the achievements of modernisation as well as the efforts to preserve Tibet's cultural heritage, including Tibetan Buddhism (IOSC 2008, 2009a, 2009b).

Thus, the Tibetan medicine industry falls under both the state's quest to develop and modernise Tibet as well as the endeavour to preserve its cultural heritage. While at times the symbolic value of industry as an allegorical figure of modernisation is foregrounded, at other times Tibetan medicine is seen as 'some kind of cultural thing'. This, as Rinchen Wangdu complained, can mean it is not taken seriously. However, cultural heritage, along with its preservation, is also an important and legitimate space in which to make claims and be heard. It is this space that enables endeavours such as Aku Jinpa's school and pharmacy. Portraying his work as an effort to preserve 'beautiful Tibetan culture', Aku Jinpa employs the notion of cultural preservation as a legitimising framework for his efforts.

At the same time, the idea of cultural preservation provides the space in which the industrialisation of Tibetan medicine is criticised on moral grounds. In Aku Jinpa's view, there is a fundamental incompatibility between Chinese business culture (typified by the Chinese businessman asking how he intended to make his school profitable) and Sowa Rigpa's purpose to contribute to the benefit of all sentient beings. In order to be a good doctor or to make high-quality medicines, 'you must be devout and you must have a pure heart', Aku Jinpa emphasised. His statements mark a moral difference between 'authentic' Tibetanness and the world of Chinese business.

What is under attack in the party-state's rapid push to modernity is, in this sense, the moral foundation of the empirical world, the fact that religious ways of knowing are rendered invalid precisely because they are seen as corrupted by moral judgement (Craig 2007, 2010; Adams 2008: 111). In contrast to the world of industry, Aku Jinpa's project entails a vision of a local, Tibetan economy in which *amchi* (Tibetan doctors) trained in school would practice in the surrounding Tibetan areas, and the medicines produced would serve local doctors and patients.

The reasoning and efforts of Aku Jinpa and many other like-minded Tibetans evoke a vision of a moral economy which bears many similarities to the moral economies famously described by E.P. Thompson (1971) and James Scott (1976). Just as the outcry of the poor in Great Britain's eighteenth-century food riots was based on a popular consensus about certain capitalist practices being morally illegitimate (Thompson 1971: 79), Tibetan doctors brand the capitalist outlook of large factories as a moral problem. And just as the Southeast Asian peasantry responded to being incorporated in the more implacable forces of state rule and a larger market economy by revivifying moral understandings of minimal subsistence rights, Tibetans claim a moral right to Sowa Rigpa knowledge and low-cost, high-quality medicines.

Of course, the industrialisation of Tibetan medicine has not triggered an actual 'subsistence crisis' comparable to the food crises in Great Britain, Vietnam or Burma. What is at stake is not physical but rather cultural survival, for which Tibetan medicine has become an important realm. In the present case, the moral economy is similar in structure but different in form and scale from the classical cases of moral economies. The increasing pervasiveness of the market economy still creates friction and triggers resistance. Yet, the traded commodities are no longer exclusively material but also intangible. The result is a moral economy of cultural identity, a moral economy of Tibetanness.

The market for Tibetanness, however, is a global one. Consider the fact that, although targeted at the grassroots level and claiming a space for local modes of production, consumption and practice, Aku Jinpa's new school and factory compound was finally funded by an American NGO whose purpose is the preservation of Tibetan culture; in other words, the prevention of the 'cultural genocide' that his Holiness the Dalai Lama has proclaimed to be under way (Coonan 2008; Eimer and Chamberlain 2008). Aku Jinpa's endeavours are, willingly or not, enmeshed in the global political spectacle that surrounds moralised notions of 'saving Tibet' (McLagan 2002; Frangville 2009). The Tibetan medicine industry cannot operate outside this moral space of Tibetanness. Consider the fact that the medicines produced by the big, white GMP factory close to Aku Jinpa's premises were still linked to his reputation and fame, regardless of the fact that he no longer had any ties with it. Tibetanness plays a crucial part in the creation of a trusted brand.

The Industry as Assemblage

In summary, the conditions that frame the Tibetan medicine industry – as industry or medicine industry, and as the Tibetan medicine industry – can be described as an intersection where different figurations of modernity – modernist planning and neoliberal governance – meet with a moral economy of cultural identity. The companies at once have to deal with regulations and tight schedules that are difficult to meet; comply with ideals of scientific development and good governance; be economically successful; and engage in the moral economy of Tibetanness. The industry thereby aggregates a wide range of elements, ranging from herbs, machines, architectural arrangements and packaging materials to knowledge, technologies, laws, policies, consumer trust, Buddhist ethics and design preferences. To understand and describe this industrial assemblage is the aim of this book.

'Assemblage' – a term with several intellectual ancestors, including Michel Serres and Bruno Latour (1995), Paul Rabinow (2003) and Aihwa Ong and Stephen Collier (2005) – has a spatial as well as a temporal dimension. Michel Serres emphasises the latter. In his conversations with Bruno Latour on science, culture and time, the French author and philosopher argues that it is by assemblage that things are contemporary. 'Consider a late-model car', he suggests. 'It is a disparate aggregate of scientific and technical solutions dating from different periods' – some brand new, some ten years old, and the principle of the wheel going back to Neolithic times. 'The ensemble is only contemporary by assemblage, by its design, its finish, sometimes only by the slickness of the advertising surrounding it' (Serres and Latour 1995: 45). In the same way, the Tibetan medicine industry is contemporary insofar as it assembles concepts and technologies dating from different times. The notion of assemblage encourages a historical analysis of its elements to understand their present-day configuration.

The spatial dimension of an assemblage stems from the fact that its elements, the concepts as well as the technologies and materials, come from different places – in the present case: herbs from Nepal, ideas forged in a global arena, machines made in inland China. Just as the industry is contemporary by assemblage, it is territorial by assemblage (Ong and Collier 2005: 4). This stimulates an analysis of the spatial relations between the industry's locality and the origins of its elements.

The task at hand is therefore to locate the industry as an assemblage in time and space by exploring its layered histories and entangled spaces. Each of the following six principal chapters, around which this book is structured, approaches the industrial assemblage from a different angle and describes a set of its intertwined elements.

Chapter 2 looks into the history of Sowa Rigpa since the 1950s. The intervening period has seen the emergence of certain crucial parameters that have led to the subsequent industrialisation of Tibetan medicine. I will begin with an overview of the shifting political contexts Tibetan medicine has been faced with under Chinese rule and the different trajectories of Sowa Rigpa and traditional Chinese medicine (TCM) in the early decades of the People's Republic: while TCM, similar to Ayurveda, gained the support of a powerful nation-state, Tibetan medicine gradually lost its 'state' following the invasion of the People's Liberation Army in 1950/51. A second part of this chapter summarises the more recent events surrounding the transition from hospital pharmacies to factories producing medicines for a nationwide market and the political context in which this transition took place. The advent of the 'socialist market economy', privatisation efforts, the creation of binding pharmacopoeias, and a set of regulatory frameworks, including a system of drug registration, the new Drug Administration Law, and the introduction of 'good manufacturing practices' (GMP), will be scrutinised.

Chapter 3 takes a closer look at frequently voiced complaints about how these regulations interfere with traditional ways of producing Tibetan drugs. Relevant passages in the traditional texts are compared with corresponding articles in GMP, the Drug Administration Law and the Chinese pharmacopoeia. This textual comparison serves as a background for an ethnography of contemporary industrial production. We will see that GMP, taken literally, cannot be made responsible for the complaints and concerns so often voiced by the people working in the industry. Nevertheless, the actual implementation of GMP and its associated regulations had many unintended side effects. I will show that often, the way GMP was interpreted by the officials in charge contradicted the very spirit of the regulations themselves.

One of the most relevant impacts of industrialisation concerns the sourcing of medicinal plants, minerals and animal ingredients used in Sowa Rigpa, and the cultivation and collection of, and trade in, medicinal substances are the topic of Chapter 4. The rapidly growing amounts of ingredients needed to satisfy the demand of industrial production has led to a perceived decrease in quality and growing worries about the industry's sustainability. The factories had to adopt new sourcing strategies. Cultivation projects and their frequent failure will be discussed together with the broader issues of conservation and commercial trade. An account of a Tibetan plant trader's business trip to Nepal will provide an insight into the challenges of contemporary cross-border trade. The notion of 'border regimes' will be introduced in order to conceptualise the movements of herbs and traders across spatial as well as conceptual borders.

Chapters 3 and 4 form the ethnographic core of my inquiry into the 'manufacturing of Tibetan medicine' – understood in a literal sense, meaning the production of pharmaceuticals. Regulations, their sometimes paradoxical interpretation, the search for loopholes and the party-state's quest for legibility and control are highlighted. The subsequent chapters turn to the industry's role in the manufacturing or re-manufacturing of Tibetan medicine as a system of knowledge and practice.

Chapter 5 deals with the question of to whom Tibetan medicine belongs. Global debates about biopiracy and the protection of traditional knowledge found their ways into the PRC's traditional medicine strategies. The policies developed in this context have also become relevant for Tibetan medicine. Two cases are examined in this respect: China's administrative protection scheme for traditional medicine, which led to a legal dispute over the right to produce high-value 'precious pills', and the story of registering and patenting a lineage *amchi*'s secret formula. These accounts open questions of theoretical importance, namely, how knowledge is filtered and reshaped in the process of being subjected to intellectual property regimes. China's approaches to patents and administrative forms of knowledge protection thereby intersect with its apparatus of drug registration.

Chapter 6 looks into the visual, aesthetic and material side of the industry. The architectural arrangements and aesthetics of a manufacturing plant are explored in relation to the rituals of GMP production; the materials and design of packaging are examined for their capacity to render Tibetan medicines into a mobile, national commodity; and three advertising campaigns are analysed in terms of the visual themes they employ. Finally, the aesthetic endeavours of larger Tibetan medicine companies are inspected, including entry halls and exhibitions, a record-breaking museum, and a spiritual and aesthetic take on Tibetan spas.

Chapter 7 expands on the concept of moral economy, sketched out above. It shows how Tibetan medicine, its industry, and the visual, material, and aesthetic expressions of Tibetanness it produces, are embedded in a larger, state-sanctioned 'ethnicity economy' in the name of preservation and development of cultural heritage. On the one hand, 'cultural heritage' provides a legitimate framework for a variety of Tibetan initiatives. On the other hand, it ties Tibetanness to questions of morality and authenticity in new and burdened ways. The complex of 'authentic' Tibetanness, morality and economy oscillates between local, national and global spheres, and becomes intrinsically linked to the political spectacle of the 'Tibet question'. Companies try to balance Tibetan expectations of morality with the need to be economically successful and their role in the party-state's vision for a future Tibet.

In the Conclusion I come back to the notion of assemblage in order to bring the threads, disentangled and examined in groups over the preceding chapters, together again.

Language and Terminology

Before delving into the topic further, however, let me be clear about my usage of a few key terms. Language is a sensitive but highly relevant issue in the contested political space of contemporary Tibet. It starts with what I have so far referred to alternatively as Tibetan medicine and Sowa Rigpa. Chinese publications in English usually prefer 'Chinese Tibetan medicine' or 'Tibetan medicine of China', always educating the reader about the correct framework of interpretation. In Chinese, however, Tibetan medicine is usually just *zang yi*, a combination of the syllables *xi zang* (Tibet) and *yi* (medicine); *zhong guo* (China, literally 'middle kingdom' or 'central nation') is only added as emphasis in certain contexts. Pharmaceuticals are *yao*, a Tibetan medicine factory is therefore a *zang yao chang*. Sowa Rigpa as a system of knowledge falls under the category of so-called 'ethnic minority medicine' (*shaoshu minzu yixue*).

Chinese naming policies for Tibetan medicine are not the only ones entrenched in political agendas. In India, the question of adequate terminology sparked a heated debate at the Central Committee for Tibetan Medicine (CCTM). The CCTM was established in 2004 with the purpose of overseeing legal and political issues and giving a voice to the various medical traditions based on Sowa Rigpa, including Amchi medicine in Ladakh and Spiti and the Tibetan medicine practised by the Tibetans in exile. The Ladakhi doctors found fault with the word 'Tibetan' as they feared the dominance of exiled Tibetans, and applying for an official recognition of 'Tibetan' medicine in India seemed delicate, given the political sensibilities between India and China (Kloos 2010: 248–50). Finally an agreement was reached to use the term Sowa Rigpa (*gso ba rig pa*), literally 'the knowledge or the science of healing', one of the ten Tibetan classical sciences.

This decision also mirrors a trend in academia, where Sowa Rigpa has recently become the most accepted way of referring to Tibetan medicine. Using the term Sowa Rigpa aims at providing Tibetan medicine with a metonym for the various styles and schools of medicine based on the same texts and principles. Besides the fact that a genuine Tibetan term certainly has its advantages, it also promises to establish Sowa Rigpa as a field of inquiry, just as is the case with Ayurveda or TCM.

From my own experience, Sowa Rigpa is the common term used when speaking about medical knowledge or education in Tibet, but it is hardly ever used to mark a difference between Tibetan medicine and other medical traditions. When I used 'Sowa Rigpa' in conversation, Tibetans frequently asked me what kind of Sowa Rigpa I was referring to: Tibetan, Chinese, or Western? Moreover, nobody would speak about a Sowa Rigpa factory or the Sowa Rigpa industry. A Tibetan medicine factory is a *bömen sotra* (*bod sman bzo grwa*) – *bömen* literally meaning 'Tibetan medicine', and *sotra* a factory or workshop. Following this distinction, I will use the term Sowa Rigpa when emphasising the side of knowledge and tradition, and Tibetan medicine when dealing with the industry and its commodities: Tibetan medicines.

Another term that needs clarification at this early stage is 'Tibetan doctor'. A Tibetan doctor is often referred to as *amchi* (*am chi*). Amchi, originally a Mongolian term, is used in exile as well as in many parts of Tibet. However, in Amdo and Nagchu, for example, the term *menpa* (*sman pa*) – 'medicine person' – is more common and *amchi* is sometimes not even understood (Schrempf 2007: 91). I will use both terms, *amchi* and Tibetan doctor, interchangeably.

Finally, the usage of the terms 'Tibet' and 'China' are highly politicised and need clarification. 'Tibet' has been used as a synonym for Central and Western Tibet, the political heartland of the former Tibetan government and more or less the territory of the present-day Tibet Autonomous Region (TAR). It has also been used to denote all areas where Tibetans live, including the regions of Amdo and Kham, which now largely fall into the provinces Qinghai, Gansu, Sichuan and Yunnan.

There are good reasons to reserve the term 'Tibet' for the territory of the TAR (quite apart from the sensitivity of the Chinese leadership to any suggestion of a Greater Tibet that might include areas in contiguous provinces). Melvyn Goldstein (1994) argues that in 1949/50 even the Tibetan government used the term 'Tibet' to describe the territories under its direct control, which did not include most parts of Amdo and Kham. While some authors have chosen to follow Goldstein's argument or respect Chinese sensitivities, the term 'Tibet' will be used here to include all the areas inside the borders of the People's Republic of China where Tibetans live.

This decision is to be understood as a choice for simplicity, a way to avoid frequent repetitions of 'the TAR and the Tibetan counties and prefectures in Qinghai, Sichuan, Yunnan and Gansu', or the cumbersome 'ethnographic Tibet'. In addition, my vague usage of 'Tibet' is in accordance with the understanding of the majority of my interlocutors as well as the way Chinese travel agents in Beijing or Shanghai, for example, would advertise their Tibet tours, regardless of whether the destination lies inside the TAR or in adjacent provinces.

When Tibetans speak about the non-Tibetan regions of the PRC they use the term *gyanag* (*rgya nag*), which is usually translated as 'China'. When speaking Mandarin the terms *dalu* (mainland) or *neidi* (inland) are used. These terms primarily refer to the distinction between 'mainland China' and Taiwan, or 'inland China' and Hong Kong or Macau. In English, both terms are typically translated as mainland China. However, neither 'mainland China' nor 'inland China' is entirely appropriate to denote the difference between Tibet and the non-Tibetan regions of the PRC. As Tibet is on all counts more mainland than the 'mainland', I will use the less common term 'inland China' for this purpose.

Notes

1. Literally, the knowledge of healing; used here as a synonym for Tibetan medicine. A discussion of terminology will follow shortly.
2. As the euro and British pound have seen a sharp devaluation vis-à-vis the Chinese yuan over the last three years, figures will be given in US dollars (exchange rates as of June 2010).
3. The literature on alternative, plural and multiple modernities is vast. Important works include Therborn (1995), Ong (1996), Ong and Nonini (1997), Arnason (2000), Eisenstadt (2000), Kandiyoti (2000), Sahlins (2000), Wittrock (2000), Beck (2001), Conrad and Randeria (2002), Knauft (2002), Randeria (2002, 2004) and Houben and Schrempf (2008).
4. A case in point is Lisa Rofel's research on a silk factory in Hubei. She shows how the middle-aged women employees posit a nostalgic Maoist vision of modernity against a postsocialist version of the modern (Rofel 1997).
5. The term 'Global Pharma' is not meant to imply that large transnational pharmaceutical companies, the proponents of 'Big Pharma' (Law 2006), have started to take over the Tibetan medicine industry – something that has not happened for several reasons, as we will see.

Chapter 2
The Creation of an Industry

A comprehensive history of Sowa Rigpa in the twentieth century is yet to be written. Rather than taking on this greater task my aim here is to identify the forces that shaped the industrialisation of Tibetan medicine. Whereas the actual creation of the industry started only in the 1990s, earlier events in the history of Sowa Rigpa under communist rule set the basic conditions for its development.

In the first part of this chapter these basic conditions are discussed. I argue that the history of Sowa Rigpa in the People's Republic of China has to be understood in relation to the 'invention', standardisation, and institutionalisation of traditional Chinese medicine (TCM) in the late 1950s and early 1960s. On the one hand, Sowa Rigpa and TCM followed different trajectories; on the other hand, many of the regulations, institutions, and development paths framing TCM finally became also relevant for Tibetan medicine.

The second part of the chapter examines the actual creation of the Tibetan medicine industry, which took place in two stages roughly between 1995 and 2005. The first stage was conditioned by the proclamation of a 'socialist market economy'; the second stage was triggered by China's WTO accession and the introduction of 'good manufacturing practice' (GMP).

Sowa Rigpa and TCM: Different Trajectories

On the eve of Tibet's 'liberation' in 1950/51, Sowa Rigpa was in many ways in a better position than Chinese medicine. It was highly valued, practised in a variety of institutional settings and had close ties to the power centres of the Tibetan state, which had enjoyed de facto independence since the fall of the Manchu dynasty in 1911 (Shakabpa 1984: 246–59). Sowa Rigpa was taught in the medical faculties of several of the large monasteries. Of these monastic schools, the Chagpori (*lcags po ri*) in Lhasa and the medical college or *menpa dratsang* (*sman pa grwa tshang*) at Labrang monastery (*bla brang bkra shis 'khyil*) were among the most famous and respected (Gyatso 2004: 85). Being part of the monastic establishment in Tibet ensured Sowa Rigpa high status and influence.

Besides the monastic branch of Tibetan medicine, which mainly catered to the vast monk population,[1] a wide range of private practitioners offered their services throughout Tibet. The non-monastic sector of Sowa Rigpa was often linked to lineages of Tibetan physicians (*amchi*). It was common for such lineage-trained *amchi* to be associated with the Tibetan aristocracy and their landed estates. Privately trained *amchi* sometimes ran their own schools (Janes 1995: 12).

As an alternative to monastic training and private schools, the Mentsikhang (*sman rtsis khang*, literally 'the house of medicine and astrology'), was established in Lhasa in 1916. Khenrab Norbu, a highly renowned *amchi* from an important Lhasa lineage of Tibetan physicians, was appointed director. The Mentsikhang was an outcome of the thirteenth Dalai Lama's attempt to shift power away from the big monasteries towards the Kashag government (Goldstein and Rinpoche 1989). The army, monasteries and aristocratic families had to send quotas of students to the Mentsikhang, and trained *amchi* were sent back to needy communities and monasteries after completing their training (Shakabpa 1984: 258–59). Probably for the first time in Tibetan history a state-sponsored public healthcare system started to sprout (Janes 1995: 12).

Quite contrary to Tibetan medicine's strong standing and institutional basis, Chinese medicine was severely sidelined during the nationalist period (1928 to 1949). The ruling Chinese political and social circles considered scientific biomedicine far more advanced. In their view, it carried the promise that China would catch up with the rest of the world, which was considered an urgent necessity and the only way to restore China's political stature globally (Croizier 1976). There were even attempts to effectively outlaw Chinese medicine. In February 1929, the Ministry of Health brought forward a proposition titled 'The Abolition of Old-Style Medicine in Order to Clear Away Obstacles to Medicine and Public Health'. It was met with stiff resistance by doctors and pharmacists of Chinese medicine and finally the Ministry backed down. Yet, the difficult situation in which Chinese medicine found itself under the nationalist Guomindang government was to have a positive effect on its fate later on. The 1929 incident sparked the first professional association of Chinese physicians (Lei 2002).

During the civil war (1945 to 1949) the Chinese Communist Party (CCP) started embracing Chinese medicine for a number of reasons. Methods like acupuncture were seen as promising during times of war, especially considering the shortage of biomedical doctors. In the 1940s there were around 10,000 biomedical doctors in China and an estimated 500,000 practitioners of Chinese medicine (Taylor 2005: 34). These practitioners were reckoned as an important force in this context. However, traditional medicine did not easily conform to Mao's definition of the new democratic culture, which rested on the triad of unity, the new and science. While Mao recognised Chinese medicine's potential for the revolution he was also of the opinion that it had to become more 'scientific' in order to properly serve a new communist society. Consequently, Mao's proposed a unification of Chinese and Western medicines. There was no intention of maintaining Chinese medicine as a body of knowledge unto itself (ibid.: 35).

In short, on the eve of the Chinese invasion of Tibet in 1950/51, Sowa Rigpa was practised in a variety of settings and had the strong support of the Tibetan authorities. Its main state-run medical institution, the Mentsikhang in Lhasa, operated with student quotas and job assignments – features more in keeping with a socialist government than a decaying, theocratic state. At the same time, Chinese medicine was considered unfit for the socialist future of communist China, and despite its revolutionary potential it had much less institutional backing. The slogan 'Chinese medicine studies Western medicine' provides an apt description of the low status the CCP initially attributed to Chinese medicine (ibid.: 65, 71).

Interference and Non-interference

This situation, however, was radically reversed by subsequent events. In 1950, troops of the China's People's Liberation Army (PLA) moved into Eastern Tibet, and the Tibetans in turn vainly sought support from Great Britain, India and the USA. The USA demanded a clearer anti-communist attitude from Lhasa, but the Tibetan elite were divided into two camps. One favoured US-sponsored resistance against the PRC and the flight of the Dalai Lama to India; the other opted for cooperation with Chinese forces and the acceptance of the so-called 'Seventeen-point Agreement'. In Beijing, the Tibetan delegation signed the document in May 1951, albeit under enormous pressure and without the consent of the government in Lhasa (Shakya 1999: 33–91).

The Seventeen-point Agreement promised freedom of religion, acceptance of the existing Kashag government and far-reaching non-interference. No reforms would be implemented until Tibetans themselves demanded them. And most important for the ruling elite and the powerful monasteries, privileges of power and position were not to be touched. Mao opted to leave all feudal structures intact for the time being – quite contrary to his liberation propaganda. Mao knew how delicate a topic social change was, and his advice was simple: don't hurry (ibid.: 111). The Dalai Lama finally decided to support the Seventeen-point Agreement and stay in Tibet. The PLA's 'peaceful' takeover of Tibet was portrayed as a major victory in communist propaganda.

In accordance with the Seventeen-point Agreement, the communists did not interfere with existing institutions. The Mentsikhang in Lhasa was kept as a public facility under the rule of the Kashag. It was not incorporated into the Chinese health bureaucracy. The numerous private *amchi* and monastic colleges continued to operate without impediment. Naturally, the secular approach of the Mentsikhang appealed to the communists more than the private *amchi* and monastic institutions. Visiting Han experts were impressed by Tibetan medicine's integrity, scientific basis and socialist potential – much to the delight of the Mentsikhang's staff and students (Janes 1995: 16).

However, a very different situation was emerging in Eastern Tibet in the areas known as Kham and Amdo, now part of Sichuan, Yunnan, Qinghai and Gansu provinces. Unrestrained by the Seventeen-point Agreement, communist reform hit with full impact. The most incisive policy was certainly land reform and the collectivisation of agriculture. The monasteries were among the biggest land owners and it was only through their estates that they were able to feed thousands of monks. Collectivisation undermined the monasteries' power base (Shakya 1999: 139). Consequently, in Kham and Amdo where there was no such thing as a secular Mentsikhang, Sowa Rigpa's monastic support dwindled (Hua 2008: 95–99).

The importance of land reform and collectivisation can hardly be overstated. Shakya argues that 'the dissolution of the economic power base of the monasteries was the most significant social and political event in the history of Tibet since the introduction of Buddhism' (Shakya 1999: 254). Together with collectivisation, a campaign was launched against what was perceived as the old and unjust society. The monks and monasteries were its primary targets. Slogans like 'unhealthy customs' and 'feudal superstition' spread, and the monks were branded 'parasites on the peasant' (Janes 1995: 15).

In the mid 1950s Tibetan medicine found itself in a contradictory situation: while in Central Tibet it was left largely untouched under the Seventeen-point Agreement, and the Mentsikhang in Lhasa was even being lauded for its scientific basis and socialist potential, Sowa Rigpa was increasingly confronted with grim propaganda in Kham and Amdo. Coerced collectivisation and the first attempts at settling the Khampa nomads in Eastern Tibet triggered a series of violent incidents in Kham, which became known as the Kangding revolt (Shakya 1999: 140). The Lhasa government came under enormous pressure to deal with the rebellious Khampas. In the midst of this volatile political situation a spark was enough to cause widespread fire. A rumour that the Dalai Lama was to be abducted spread in Lhasa, and on 10 March 1959 thousands of people gathered in front of the Summer Palace in order to protect him. The crowd started attacking people they considered to be collaborators and the situation quickly spun out of control. The Lhasa uprising began, the PLA threatened to shell the Summer Palace, and the Dalai Lama fled to India (Shakya 1999: 186–211; Norbu 2001: 216).

The Lhasa uprising and the Dalai Lama's flight marked the beginning of a radical shift in Chinese policies towards Tibet, labelled the 'Democratic Reforms' in party speech. This shift also affected Tibetan medicine. Private training within lineages suffered greatly under the new regime, and the Chagpori medical school, destroyed during the revolt, was permanently closed. The Mentsikhang in Lhasa was brought under the direct control of the Lhasa city health bureau and hence the PRC's health bureaucracy. Recognised as a public hospital in 1961 and supplied with a modest annual budget, it remained the only stronghold of Sowa Rigpa in Tibet (Janes 1995: 17).

The Making of TCM

Within a decade, Sowa Rigpa had lost most of its state support and institutional backing. Only the Mentsikhang in Lhasa, its most secular institution, remained an approved and supported facility under the new regime. These developments stand in stark contrast to developments in Chinese medicine.

As mentioned above, Chinese medicine was not seen as fit enough for a socialist China at the outset. It had to catch up with Western medicine. Mao's vague instructions were interpreted by the Ministry of Health to mean that Chinese medicine had to be made 'scientific'. It was kept in name but most policies actually undermined it. In 1950/51 the Ministry of Health set up a qualification system, which required all Chinese medicine practitioners to take an examination. The vast majority of candidates were stripped of the right to practise legally as they failed the requisite examination (Taylor 2005: 37–40).

The Ministry's interpretation of Mao's vague instructions and the resulting policy came under attack in March 1953. In the subsequent turmoil the Ministry was blamed for failure and those responsible were purged. Their successors, anxious to avoid repeating the same mistakes, adopted a policy of supporting Chinese medicine, which went much further than Mao's idea of unifying Western and Chinese medicine. Mao himself may not have been convinced of the therapeutic viability of Chinese medicine but he had a habit of turning things around in a provocative way, never allowing the cadres to rest on their accomplishments. One of these turnarounds resulted in the slogan 'Doctors of Western Medicine Study Chinese Medicine'. The new programme, which began in 1954 and was meant to rid doctors trained in Western medicine of their arrogant bourgeois ideals, put Chinese doctors in the position of teachers of biomedical physicians for the very first time (ibid.: 40–43, 65, 71–73). Chinese medicine thus became part of the communist nation-building project. In February 1956, Zhou Enlai put forward a proposal to establish Chinese medicine academies. TCM was officially integrated into the state's higher education system. A process began that Taylor describes as the 'standardisation of TCM' (ibid.: 103–6, 111–31). It implied the writing of TCM textbooks and the institutionalisation of education and practice.

Elisabeth Hsu (2009b: 119) argues that the emergence of standardised and institutionalised TCM in the late 1950s and early 1960s can be seen as a veritable 'invention of tradition' in Hobsbawm and Ranger's sense (Hobsbawm and Ranger 1983): an invention marked by its rapid appearance (rather than its survival) and embedded in nationalist discourse. Between 1956 and 1960 twenty TCM colleges were established; in 1958 the first textbook was compiled, followed by a first full set of textbooks published in 1962 and a second set in 1964 (Hsu 2009).

Taylor emphasises the 'ad hoc processes by which TCM was formed' and argues 'that there was never a guarantee that it would all end in a TCM' (Taylor 2005: 110–11). But as shifting as the sands of party politics may have been, the outcome was that TCM was discovered as a medicine of revolution, gained ground in the People's Republic, and became part of the ongoing nation-building project. While it was thoroughly instituted and its education and practice acknowledged in standardised textbooks, colleges and clinics, Sowa Rigpa was losing much of its status.

The Tentative Integration of Sowa Rigpa

The party-state's approach to Tibetan medicine during the 1960s and early 1970s is best described as ambiguous. Tentative attempts at creating a new institutional basis for Tibetan medicine alternated with outright hostility. On the one hand, a technical secondary school for Tibetan medicine was established in Lhasa in the early 1960s, and in 1963 the government allowed a new class of forty-five students at the Mentsikhang (Hua 2008: 92). On the other hand, policies towards Central Tibet gradually became more restrictive around the same time. In 1962 the 'socialist education movement' started to be implemented. For the first time a Chinese campaign reached Tibet unaltered (Shakya 1999: 292). It aimed at an ideological purification and was in many ways a forerunner of events to come. In 1965 the Tibet Autonomous Region (TAR) was established and the exemptions granted under the Seventeen-point Agreement were formally brought to an end.

A year later the Cultural Revolution began. Tibetan medicine was quickly branded as part of the 'four olds' (old ideas, old culture, old customs, old habits), in spite of the Mentsikhang's full alignment with socialist ideology and the considerable number of patients treated. While the Mentsikhang was never officially shut down (Craig 2006: 90), Tibetan medicine was effectively delegitimised. The communes were no longer allowed to have any Tibetan medicine practitioners, possession of the Gyüshi (*rgyud bzhi*) – the paramount medical treatise of Sowa Rigpa – was forbidden (Janes 1995: 19), many *amchi* were killed, sent to prison camps or escaped to India and Nepal, and several well-known medical lineages were interrupted (Hofer 2009a: 181).

The turmoil and chaos of the Cultural Revolution and its aftermath (covering the years 1966 to 1976) also hit TCM: many doctors were persecuted, some even committed suicide, colleges were closed and the only remaining ideologically feasible approach were to further TCM's integration with Western medicine and scientific research (Croizier 1976: 351–52; Scheid 2001: 371). However, while certain aspects of Chinese medicine such as Qigong came under attack, no campaign was ever directly launched against TCM itself. In 1973, in the midst of the Cultural Revolution, China became a member of the WHO and received much international attention for its scientifically oriented TCM as well as its 'barefoot doctor' scheme. The training of barefoot doctors focused on delivering basic primary health care, but also included a minor and radically simplified TCM component (Hsu 2009: 11).

This focus on primary health care provided the framework under which Tibetan medicine slowly began to resurface in official agendas. In 1972, the Lhasa City Medical School trained a group of 181 students in basic Tibetan medicine. The students were later sent to different areas of the TAR (Hua 2008: 92). In 1974, several local programmes that aimed at combining Western and Tibetan medicine were established. Under the guidance of Jampa Trinley, a student of Mentsikhang founder Kenrab Norbu and at that time its director, a workshop was held in 1974 at which senior doctors met to 'recover, recollect and research what has been lost and disappeared during the Cultural Revolution' (Jampa Trinley 2004: 134, cited in Hofer 2009a: 182). New courses on Tibetan medicine for nurses and community health workers were set up in Lhasa and Shigatse. In this context, professors were granted permission again to lecture from the Gyüshi, although students were not allowed to study and memorise it. Textbooks devoid of Buddhist language were hastily prepared (Janes 1995: 20).

Textbooks and Standardised Practice

The issue of textbooks illustrates the different trajectories of TCM and Sowa Rigpa. Whereas the first TCM textbooks were heavily criticised by respected older Chinese physicians, a series of changes and republications, especially the renowned fifth edition of 1984/1985 (Hsu 2009a: 3, 7), finally led to a corpus of TCM textbooks that became the widely accepted basis of TCM education. The first attempt to convert Sowa Rigpa into textbook knowledge in the early 1970s was also almost uniformly considered a failure (Janes 1995: 20–21). But contrary to TCM, no attempt was made to continually improve Tibetan medicine textbooks. The ideological climate in which these textbooks were produced and the later official condemnation of the Cultural Revolution served as a pretext to abandon them as soon as possible. Sowa Rigpa education simply went back to the Gyüshi and its commentaries. Only recently have textbooks again acquired relevance in Sowa Rigpa education.

Textbook-based TCM education, the 'standardised mode of knowledge transmission' in Hsu's terms (Hsu 1999), also affected the practice of TCM. According to Judith Farquhar (1994) and Volker Scheid (2002), a clinical encounter in TCM is structured around a process called 'pattern differentiation' (*bianzheng lunzhi*), by which an initial description of a group of symptoms is understood as a pattern. A pattern is usually linked to a particular line of treatment and a basic formula. This formula is then further refined into an individual prescription: ingredients are added, left out or adjusted, until the final formula (*fang*) is chosen and administered (Farquhar 1994: 55–57).

This is certainly a blueprint of a clinical encounter and Hsu has remarked that Farquhar's account operates very much within the logic of a textbook so that it would be no surprise if it became part of the TCM curriculum one day (Hsu 1998: 163). What is important for my argument here is simply the fact that by linking a complex syndrome to both a standard treatment path and an individualised prescription, the concept of pattern differentiation has created a space in which TCM theory, medical practice and pharmaceutics interdependently form the nexus of contemporary TCM. The art of an able physician is reflected in the elegance, harmony and aesthetics of their formulas. The notion of pattern differentiation allows for a constant practice of this art, and much of the intellectual life of a TCM doctor revolves around the writing of prescriptions.

Scheid suggests that the pivotal importance of pattern differentiation emerged as such only during the communist period. It resonated with Mao's ideas of practice and made TCM appear systematic, scientific and open to modernisation while remaining fundamentally different from biomedicine. Only a treatment plan based on pattern differentiation and followed by treatment with an appropriate Chinese formula could be regarded as real TCM. As such, Chinese medicine 'could never be assimilated by (disease-based) Western medicine without, in the process, destroying its very nature and, by implication, the root of its efficacy' (Scheid 2002: 203, 209–16, 219).

In a similar way to TCM, Sowa Rigpa does not postulate a direct link between a symptom and a condition. Different patients may show different symptoms but still suffer from the same condition and a certain condition may have various symptoms. Tibetan medical theory suggests that a condition is caused by the rise of one or several of the three *nyepa* (*nyes pa*): *lung* (*rlung*), *tripa* (*mkhris pa*), and *beken* (*bad kan*) – literally wind, bile and phlegm. *Nyepa* means 'fault' but is often somewhat inaccurately translated as 'humour' in English (Gyatso 2006). The three *nyepa* are coupled with the Buddhist notion of the three poisons – attachment, anger and ignorance. The *nyepa* are also linked to the basic differentiation of hot and cold diseases: *tripa* is hot, *beken* is cold and *lung* can be either hot or cold. Furthermore, the *nyepa* are related to air, fire, earth, water and space – the five elements that make up the world.[2] Consequently, anything on this planet has medical value and authoritative texts such as the eighteenth-century *Crystal Rosary* (*shel phreng*) describe several thousand materials along with their tastes, properties and indications (De'umar Geshe Tenzin Phuntsog 1986). These materials are considered to be most effective when combined in multi-component formulations. Some of the most complex formulas consist of seventy or more ingredients (Dash 1988; Drungtso and Drungtso 2005). However, contrary to the case of TCM, in contemporary practice they are not frequently altered to suit the specific needs of a patient.

The Gyüshi mentions several forms of medicines, including powders, pills, decoctions, medicinal butters (or oils) and wines (Clark 1995: 187). Powders and decoctions can be combined into individualised formulations without much effort. The more complex man-

31

ufacturing processes of pills, butters and wines, however, prohibit such tailor-made formulations to a certain extent. While in local *amchi* practice powders remain widely used down to the present day (Besch 2006: 149), pills have become by far the most commonly used form of Tibetan medicine in Tibet as well as in exile (Samuel 2001). Individually compounded medicines therefore are an exception in contemporary Sowa Rigpa practice. This being said, Sowa Rigpa, just like TCM, also relies on individualised treatment plans, but contrary to TCM this is generally achieved by combining several ready-made compounds in a prescription; one compound is taken in the morning, one in the afternoon and one in the evening.

Herein lies a crucial difference between TCM and Sowa Rigpa. Leaving all diversity within both traditions aside, one can say that a standard clinical encounter in TCM results in an individual prescription that requires a patient to go to a pharmacy, buy herbs, and prepare decoctions at home. In Tibetan medicine, such a blueprint encounter results in the prescription of two to four different ready-made pills that the patient buys directly from the doctor or clinic and is instructed to take with hot water three times a day.

The point is that Tibetan medicine, with its focus on ready-made pills that usually require more complex manufacturing processes, is well suited to industrial production. By comparison, pattern differentiation and individual prescriptions are not compatible with large-scale industrial production. This is not to say that no industry for TCM pharmaceuticals exists[3] or that TCM relies solely on decoctions and individual prescriptions. But unlike Sowa Rigpa, TCM features a conceptual core, anchored in standardised, acknowledged textbooks, which gives preference to individualised formulations for which industrial production is not an option.

In summary, the point is that Sowa Rigpa and TCM followed different trajectories during the early decades of the People's Republic. Sowa Rigpa shifted from being a highly regarded science close to the power centres of the Tibetan state to a minor affair of a potentially troublesome minority at the periphery of the People's Republic. Thus, Sowa Rigpa was not part of the Communist nation-building project in the late 1950s and early 1960s. As a result, it was not faced with the same rigorous standardisation efforts as TCM and has not developed the same kind of institutional basis.

While this is seen in a positive light by many Tibetans and also contributes to Sowa Rigpa's contemporary appeal as 'authentic', 'unaltered' tradition, it puts Tibetan medicine in a vulnerable position. Decades later, when the push towards rapid industrialisation would finally demand thorough standardisation within an impossibly short time frame, no respected and well-established government offices were available to help negotiate exemptions from national laws and regulations, as was the case for TCM. In addition, as Tibetan medicine does not feature a recognised conceptual core that requires individualised formulations, its industrialisation has the potency to affect its entire practice in a particularly profound way.

From Pharmacy to Factory

Reform and Revival

During the 1980s, an unprecedented revival of Tibetan medicine took place in the PRC. With the deaths of Zhou Enlai and Mao Zedong in 1976, and Deng Xiaoping's rise to power in 1978, a period of reform and economic liberalisation began. The Cultural Revolution was labelled a 'lost decade', for which the leftist fraction of the communist party was made responsible.

The Deng Xiaoping leadership called for a new approach towards China's *minzu* or national minorities (Shakya 1999: 370). In 1979, Hu Yaobang openly acknowledged that the CCP had failed in Tibet and put the blame on the cadres there. In his speeches to the party elite, Hu Yaobang allegedly equated the first two decades of Chinese rule in Tibet with colonial occupation (Goldstein 1991: 141). A six-point policy was issued that promised the TAR full rights to exercise regional autonomy and included a tax exemption for three years (Goldstein 1999: 64). Together with the so-called 'household responsibility system', which replaced collectivised agriculture and entitled peasant families to the benefits of their produce (Yeh 2008), this tax exemption had a great impact on the rural population. The average annual income almost doubled between 1979 and 1981. Tibetans started wearing traditional clothes again, and many 'old ways', such as marriage practices and traditional social institutions, saw a revival. In addition, the number of Tibetans in the bureaucracy grew sharply (Shakya 1999: 382, 389–90). And being a rela-

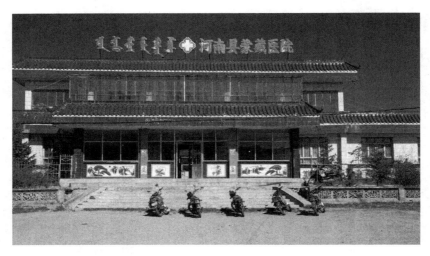

Figure 2.1: Tibetan and Mongolian Hospital in Henan (Qinghai province): patients from the nomadic areas park their motorbikes in front of the main entrance.

tively apolitical and safe arena, Tibetan medicine was singled out as especially worthy of development. It combined the benefits of providing the Chinese leadership with a means to demonstrate their respect for Tibetan culture with a cost-effective way to better medical care in Tibet, which was severely lagging behind the rest of the country (Janes 1995: 23).

In 1980, Sowa Rigpa training programmes were launched in Lhasa, Tsetang, Shigatse and Chamdo; in 1985 a department of Tibetan medicine was set up under the roof of Tibet University in Lhasa (Hua 2008: 93). Senior physicians who had practised before 1959 were recruited as teachers, and the Gyüshi replaced the unloved textbooks, despite the ambivalent feelings of the CCP elite. Janes describes how several young doctors assured him that they were again 'trained like the monks used to be trained' before the Chinese occupation (Janes 1995: 24).

Meanwhile, the Mentsikhang was granted tenfold state subsidies, and its status was lifted to a regional-level facility, just like the TAR People's Hospital in Lhasa. In 1985, an in-patient department with 150 beds was built. Between 1980 and 1990, the number of consultations per year rose from 32,400 to over 260,000. This undeniable success put the Mentsikhang in a position to consolidate its status: it became a branch of the TAR health bureau in 1985. In addition, a new factory for the production of Tibetan medicines was constructed to meet the hospital's rising demand. The factory produced 300 different medicines and is said to have reached an output of sixty tons per year (ibid.: 22).[4] An exhibition at the Mentsikhang factory in Lhasa (officially renamed the TAR Tibetan Medicine Factory) has a series of old machines on display, which vividly illustrate the transition from semi-manual to a mechanised production. After a decade of reform Tibetan medicine was, at least in terms of patient numbers, medicine production and institutional backing, stronger than ever before (ibid.: 32).

Apart from these developments in Lhasa, hospitals and production centres throughout Tibet were established during the 1980s (Arura 2006). In 1992, a Tibetan hospital was built in Beijing – the first of ten such hospitals in the major cities of inland China (Huang 2006). These new hospitals led to even higher patient numbers and a rising demand for Tibetan medicines. The larger hospitals established mechanised production centres to meet this increasing demand. These production centres can be seen as the first step towards the industrial production of Tibetan medicines. At first they did not operate as an actual industry producing commodities for a market; they were still tied to the hospitals for which they produced and functioned primarily as large-scale pharmacies. Yet, they would become the logical starting point for the industrialisation that was to follow.

The 'Socialist Market Economy'

A series of changes in China's economic and health policies prepared the ground for the transition from the prevailing factory-as-pharmacy model to an actual pharmaceutical industry. This transition started around 1995 and took place in two stages. During the first stage, roughly between the mid 1990s and the end of 2001, a series of profit-oriented Tibetan medicine companies producing for a wider market were established, a pharmacopoeia for Tibetan medicine was compiled, and a system of drug registration introduced. The second stage was triggered by the new Drug Administration Law in 2001, the introduction of GMP, and a new nationwide system of drug registration. The companies, which often were only a few years old, had to rebuild their manufacturing plants and attract substantial new investment.

The trend to establish profit-oriented businesses was fostered by the major shift in Chinese economic policy announced at the fourteenth Communist Party Congress in 1992. China embarked on the project of a 'socialist market economy', which envisioned 'capitalism with a Chinese face' and encouraged private entrepreneurship (Sigley 2006: 487). The situation in the TAR, however, was slightly different from the one in the rest of the country, including the Tibetan areas in other provinces. A series of demonstrations in Lhasa between 1987 and 1989 marked the end of the relatively open period of the early 1980s. The CCP elite considered the effort to win over the hearts and minds of Tibetans a failure. Hu Jintao, who was CCP Secretary of the TAR at that time, opted for a harder line. Martial law was proclaimed in 1989 and lifted only after thirteen months (Barnett 1996). Further unrest in Tibet in the early 1990s kept the security question high on the agenda of the Chinese party-state. These new protests, which were in part prompted by price rises (a consequence of deregulation), triggered a certain ambiguity among cadres in the TAR against the 'socialist market economy' (ibid.). However, the third National Forum on Work in Tibet, held

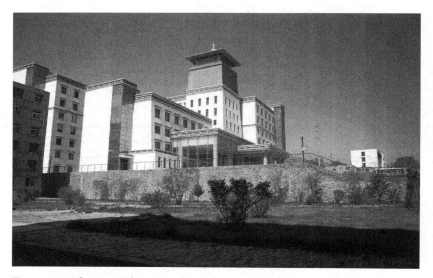

Figure 2.2: The new Tibetan medicine hospital in Xining, part of the Arura Group.

in Beijing in July 1994, explicitly reinforced the officially endowed strategy for the development of Tibet: economic growth and tighter integration with inland China.

The advent of the 'socialist market economy' in 1992 (delayed by a couple of years in the case of the TAR) had a profound effect on the state-run Tibetan medicine hospitals. According to Janes, state subsidies for the major Tibetan hospitals declined by as much as 50 per cent over the 1990s. At the same time, the hospitals were permitted and encouraged to establish businesses to generate profits and subsidise their activities, health policy was decentralised, and local authorities in counties and prefectures found themselves in the position of being able to make their own decisions over the allocation of limited budgets (Janes 2002: 271).

The 'socialist market economy' has to be seen in the light of the worldwide trend towards the implementation of neoliberal economic theory at that time. The rise of neoliberalism in the West since the Second World War, and especially since the 1973 oil crisis, was the source of inspiration for a 'market economy with a Chinese face'. Over the last fifteen years, the imperative to be economically successful, instead of dependent on the state, has become even more pronounced, not only in Sowa Rigpa but also in TCM. Hsu speaks of a shift from TCM to Chinese medicine and pharmacotherapy (CMP) (Hsu 2007, 2009a). Nationalist discourse, which had been a cornerstone of the creation of TCM, is thereby being substituted with an economic perspective that highlights global markets, capital and profit.

This is the context in which the founding of many Tibetan medicine companies took place. In fact, apart from a few companies – such as Cheezheng in Lanzhou (founded in 1993) and Jiumei Tibetan Medicine Co. Ltd. in Xining (1999) – most business-oriented Tibetan medicine factories were established from the nexus of a government-run hospital or medical college during the 1990s. This pattern can be seen in the company histories of the Deqin Shangri-la Tibetan Medicine Company in Zhongdian (Glover 2006: 46), Yumbhulhakang in Lokha, the Tibetan Medicine College Factory in Lhasa, the factory of the Tibetan and Mongolian hospital in Henan, the Arura Group in Xining, Shongpalhachu Tibetan Medicine Ltd. in Lhasa, and many others.

Founding Shongpalhachu

A good case in point to illustrate the transition to profit-oriented company is Shongpalhachu Tibetan Medicine Ltd., founded in 1996.

Shongpalhachu lies about 20 kilometres west of Lhasa. To get to the factory one follows the main road to the airport before branching off into a broad and peaceful valley flanked by rolling hills. Driving through the valley, one passes by the highly guarded freight yard, which has recently been constructed and serves as a terminus for the goods trains on the new railroad linking Tibet with inland China. A few kilometres further into the valley the road ends and a dirt track leads to Shongpalhachu.

Although situated close to Lhasa, the Shongpalhachu factory is related to the Mentsikhang in Nagchu, a county about 500 km north of Lhasa. The idea of establishing a for-profit company was born around 1994. A foreign donor approached the Nagchu Mentsikhang with a plan to contribute 400,000 yuan ($59,000) towards building a Sowa Rigpa school in Nagchu. 'Later, this plan was abandoned for various reasons', Tenpa Wangchuk, the current director of Shongpalhachu, explained to me:

> But the 400,000 yuan were still there. The foreign donor and members of the Nagchu Mentsikhang finally agreed to spend the money on the construction of a new Tibetan medicine factory ... But as Nagchu is not an ideal location for a Tibetan medicine factory, it was decided to build it near Lhasa. At that time, the total investment was about 2 million yuan [$293,000] including construction, machines, materials, labour, etc. Construction work started in April 1996, and on 20 September 1996 we produced our first medicine.

The history of Shongpalhachu clearly reflects the changes in China's economic policy and the pressure to establish economically successful companies from the nexus of state-owned institutions. However, this was not the only force at work. In the case of Shongpalhachu, the founders not only saw a new policy from above that needed to be implemented but also an opportunity to be seized. Establishing a relatively autonomous Tibetan medicine factory producing remedies for the benefit of patients, while at the same time being in line with official policy, was a promising prospect for a distinctively Tibetan endeavour after the troubled years of uprisings, repression and martial law.

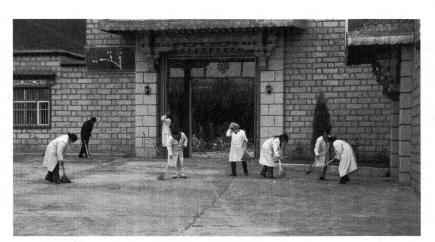

Figure 2.3: The end of the working day at Shongpalhachu.

Besides giving the factory its name, Shongpalhachu is also a pilgrimage site known for the healing properties of its water. Despite its proximity to the hustle and bustle of Lhasa, the place has a calm and relaxed atmosphere. Pema Gyatso, who was instrumental in the foundation of the company and has recently retired, explained to me how and why Shongpalhachu was chosen for the construction of the Nagchu Mentsikhang's factory. For half a year he had scouted for the ideal location in the vicinities of Lhasa. Apart from climate and transportation, the most important aspects, he pointed out, were the quality and availability of water as well as the way a certain place was meaningful in the Tibetan universe: 'It is not right to establish a factory on empty land devoid of any relevant history', he said. 'For Tibetans, traditionally, Tibetan medicine is linked to Tibetan culture'.

Of all the locations he had considered, Shongpalhachu met these criteria in an ideal way. It combined the availability of good water with the history of a sacred site linked to Guru Rinpoche, the famous eighth-century scholar and yogi who is regarded as central to the introduction of Buddhism in Tibet. The story goes that King Trisong Detsen, joined by 500 warriors on horseback, rode west from Lhasa in order to receive the famous yogi. They met Guru Rinpoche in Shongpalhachu. As no water was available in the vicinity, Trisong Detsen suggested that Guru Rinpoche ride back to Lhasa where arrangements for tea were already being made. But

Guru Rinpoche rammed his walking stick into the ground and water magically started to flow. He asked for a vessel, a *shongpa* (*gzhong pa*) in Tibetan, to collect the water. The place was named Shong-palhachu (*lha* meaning God and *chu* meaning water). Ever since, Shongpalhachu's water, warm in winter and cool in summer, has been praised for its healing qualities.

Pema Gyatso went on to mention that Shongpalhachu's suitability as a site for the new company was further enhanced by the fact that Yuthog Yonten Gonpo the Elder, one of the founding fathers of Tibetan medicine, was born in the region. In addition, there was a monastery nearby, which Tsongkhapa, the famous reformer and founder of the Gelugpa school of Tibetan Buddhism, had chosen as a pilgrimage site.

Besides being part of Tibet's sacred geography and offering the best possible water, Shongpalhachu was also known for the abundant medicinal herbs growing in the surrounding hills. Pema Gyatso recounted: 'many people were collecting herbs in the hills and they were happy to sell them to the factory. From the profits they made a living'. This, however, has changed: due to the size of the factory and its demand for higher volumes of medicinal ingredients, most of the herbs are now bought from other areas.

Pema Gyatso told me in great detail the story of how he found Shongpalhachu. I was dazzled by the amount of energy and care he had dedicated to the selection of the perfect site. At the same time, I remembered my visit to the factory a few days before. I had been shown the recently installed equipment used to purify Guru Rinpoche's holy water in accordance with current government regulations, and I wondered what the construction of the giant freight yard nearby meant for the sacredness of the place. But Pema Gyatso continued his account of Shongpalhachu's virtues and, with remarkable ease, he switched from the importance of sacred geography to more pragmatic aspects. He reiterated that Nagchu was not a very good environment for a Tibetan medicine factory.

[This is] due to the cold weather in Nagchu, the strong wind. People are not able to stay there for a long time and it is difficult to keep good relationships with the businessmen ... In order to reach beyond the regional level it is important to have good relations with those who are working in finance and business. Furthermore, in Nagchu it is difficult to get an idea about what is going on in the world and to understand the policies for

Tibetan Sowa Rigpa brought forward by the government. At that time, the government was adopting a policy of opening up towards the West. So I was thinking: if we build a factory here in Lhasa then we have good transportation facilities and it is easier to keep good relations with government offices. When you build a factory you need all the necessary permissions; we had to keep good relations with the regional authorities, including all levels of the Health Department and Health Research Office.

Balancing state policies and regulations, business interests and the will to maintain a sense of Tibetanness is not always as easy as this quote suggests. I will deal with this tightrope walk in more detail in the following chapters.

While Shongpalhachu was being planned and built, other far-reaching changes in government policy were already under way. The more Tibetan medicine companies were established, the more the emerging industry was faced with the government's quest to make it, in Scott's sense, 'legible' and thereby accessible to planning and control. One of the projects to achieve this goal was the compilation of a pharmacopoeia for Tibetan medicine and the introduction of a drug registration system.

Tibetan Drug Standards and Chinese Pharmacopoeia

In 1985, a full decade before Shongpalhachu was founded, the first version of China's Drug Administration Law stipulated that: 'The preparation of Chinese medicines shall be in accordance with the "Pharmacopoeia of the People's Republic of China", or in accordance with the "Preparation Standards" laid down by the department administering health in that province, autonomous region or municipality under the direct control of the Central Government' (Government of China 1984: article 6). However, in 1985 no suitable national standards for Tibetan formulas or raw materials existed. Therefore, the regulation of Tibetan medicine was left to the local authorities. Given the fact that hospitals and attached pharmacies were run by local authorities anyway, drug regulation was not a priority. Consequently, not much happened for a decade. Only in the mid 1990s, when the factories began producing commodities for the market, did this start to change. Along with the plans to establish a system of drug registration came the need for a comprehensive documentation of Tibetan formulas and raw materials. Standards for Tibetan medicine therefore had to be developed as quickly as possible.

Here, the fact that Tibetan medicine had so far not been subjected to the same standardisation efforts as TCM comes into play.
In September 1993, experts from the Tibetan areas, members of
the national Pharmacopoeia Commission, and representatives from
the department responsible for standardisation in the Ministry of
Health, gathered for an initial meeting. The meeting was held in
Lhasa and aimed at working towards a scientific standardisation of
Tibetan medicine (Arura 2006). Two years later, in 1995, the Ministry of Public Health published a set of drugs standards for Tibetan
Medicine (Ministry of Health 1995). The *Tibetan Drug Standards*,
as I will call them from here on, include monographs on the most
common ingredients of Tibetan medicine and over 200 Tibetan formulas. They also contain many mistakes, according to the general
consensus of Tibetan doctors and factory staff. Several people confirmed to me that some of the listed formulas posed a threat to patient safety. If one particular formula were followed, people could
die from the suggested dosage.

The *Tibetan Drug Standards* have to be seen in relation to the official *Pharmacopoeia of the People's Republic of China* (SPC 2005),
henceforth the *Chinese Pharmacopoeia*. Whereas the work on *Tibetan Drug Standards* only started in the mid 1990s, the compilation of the official, national *Chinese Pharmacopoeia* had begun in
November 1949. Only a month after the People's Republic of China
was proclaimed medical experts gathered in Beijing to start work on
official drug standards for the young state. The requirements specified by the Ministry of Health were clear: the *Chinese Pharmacopoeia* should be 'nationalistic, scientific and popular in nature' as
well as developed in 'conformity with the Chinese situation' (ibid.:
xi). An editorial commission was set up to tackle this challenging
task. It included eighty-four members grouped in eight panels. Each
panel was dedicated to particular aspects, ranging from nomenclature to units of measurements, monographs of formulas and raw
materials. Three years later, in 1953, the first edition of the *Chinese
Pharmacopoeia* was published.

Not everybody was satisfied with the first edition, however. In this
context of the standardisation of TCM that started in 1956, Minister
of Health Li Dequan pointed out that the first edition of the *Chinese
Pharmacopoeia* had one big flaw, namely, the absence of TCM. As a
result, eight senior Chinese doctors and three pharmacists were ap-

pointed to the Pharmacopoeia Commission in 1958. With their help, a largely expanded second edition was published in 1963. It comprised two volumes, the first being dedicated exclusively to TCM. It included monographs of 446 commonly-used medical materials and 197 formulas. The 1963 edition was followed by the revised and expanded 1977 edition. Since 1985, a new edition of the *Chinese Pharmacopoeia* has been published every five years (ibid.: xi–xviii).

When work on the *Tibetan Drug Standards* began in 1993, the *Chinese Pharmacopoeia* had already gone through four decades of revisions, to which hundreds of experts had dedicated their efforts. By contrast, the *Tibetan Drug Standards* were compiled within a very short time with considerably fewer resources and manpower. The result is regarded as unsatisfactory, to say the least, and all attempts to convince the authorities that a revision is urgently necessary have so far not been successful. The response has always been that the official *Chinese Pharmacopoeia* had absolute priority and that finally all Tibetan formulas would be included. However, the 2005 edition of the *Chinese Pharmacopoeia* only covers sixteen Tibetan formulas and a handful of raw materials.

In short, Tibetan medicine's late arrival on the stage of standardisation and its limited bargaining power as a peripheral minority medicine resulted in the hasty compilation of *Tibetan Drug Standards*, which, unlike the *Chinese Pharmacopoeia*, have not been subjected to continuous expansion and revision ever since. Based on these contested standards, the TAR government started to enforce drug registration around 1996. Registration numbers were given to the factories, which entitled them to produce and sell their products legally.

While some of the directors and managers argued that the system of drug registration was a major challenge for their companies, Shongpalhachu's Pema Gyatso mentioned laconically: 'At that time, it was somehow easy to get a registration number for a person who was good in dealing with the authorities in a polite and respectful way ... Nowadays, it is getting more and more difficult. There are always new rules'. Shongpalhachu's decision to build the factory close to Lhasa and the relevant government offices proved to be a wise decision.

The Introduction of Good Manufacturing Practice

By the turn of the millennium, the Ministry of Health decided it was time to move a step forward. A new version of the Drug Administration Law was drafted and came into effect in December 2001 (SFDA 2001). Article 9 entailed the following momentous stipulation: 'Drug manufacturers shall conduct production according to the Good Manufacturing Practice for Pharmaceutical Products ... formulated by the drug regulatory department under the State Council on the basis of this Law'.

'Good manufacturing practice' (GMP) covers various aspects of production, including personnel, facilities, equipment, material, hygiene, validation, documentation, production management, distribution standards, recall procedures and the handling of adverse reaction reports. The regulations, which will be discussed in more detail in the next chapter, date from 1998 and were based on an earlier version issued in 1992. Until 2001, however, GMP was not a binding standard and the companies that followed it were doing so proactively. The introduction of GMP marks the beginning of the second stage in the transformation from the factory-as-pharmacy model to a fully fledged industry.

The fact that GMP became an important priority for the Beijing government was related to China's aspirations regarding membership of the World Trade Organisation (WTO). The European Commission (EC) had complained that the Chinese (biomedical) pharmaceutical industry was able to produce pharmaceutical intermediates for about 50 per cent cheaper because they were not required to follow internationally acknowledged quality standards, namely GMP. The argument was that unfair competitive advantage had to be corrected. Acting on this suggestion, the WTO called for a level playing field (Scott 2004: 26).

It would, however, be short-sighted to view China's introduction of GMP simply as a result of growing international pressure. The new Drug Administration Law and GMP may have been triggered by China's entry into the WTO and, more generally, its efforts to gain respect in the international arena. But both the Drug Administration Law and GMP were also a logical continuation of Chinese policies towards traditional medicine and their emphasis on science and modernisation. GMP was an important milestone on this path.

It was given top priority, and it was directly supervised by the SFDA in Beijing. In early 2002, the SFDA announced that by June 2004 all factories had to pass GMP certification.[5] For the vast majority of Tibetan medicine companies, passing GMP certification meant building new manufacturing plants – less than ten years after the original factories had been established. The construction of new factories was the most immediate effect of GMP introduction. It had a series of consequences in terms of companies' ownership and outlook, as well as for relations between the new GMP plants and the hospitals from which they emerged. I will discuss each of these issues in turn.

Ownership and Investment

The construction of GMP-compliant factories required substantial new investment. Companies either had to take out a bank loan or approach a private investor.

While the advent of the 'socialist market economy' in 1992 had created opportunities for private entrepreneurship, it is important to note that most of the Tibetan medicine companies were still government-owned when GMP was introduced ten years later. Although Jiang Zemin had brought forward plans to privatise government companies already, at the fifteenth Communist Party Congress in September 1997, enterprises of strategic importance, among them pharmaceutical factories, were excluded. In 1999, the Party's Central Committee decided to abolish these restrictions. Finally, the tenth Five Year Plan announced in 2001 made privatisation a cornerstone of China's economic policy (Majumder 2003). This triggered a second wave of privatisation, which coincided with the need of the Tibetan medicine industry to attract new investment. The tenth Five Year Plan created favourable conditions to this end and helped the companies to negotiate bank loans. 'Of course, you don't get a loan from the banks just like this', Rinchen Wangdu, the now retired senior manager explained to me, 'but if the government tells them to give you a loan they will do it'.

The transition from hospital pharmacy to pharmaceutical factory and finally to private enterprise is well reflected in the history of the Arura Group in Xining, one of the major players in Qinghai province. Like most companies, Arura developed from the nexus of a government hospital, in this case the Qinghai Provincial Hospital of Tibetan Medicine in Xining. The hospital was founded in 1983 during the revival of Sowa Rigpa. In the early 1990s, the hospital started a production centre on the initiative of its newly appointed director, Dr Ao Tsochen, who was among the first to see the enormous market potential for Tibetan pharmaceuticals in the PRC. His idea was to propagate Tibetan medicine beyond the borders of the Tibetan inhabited areas. Arura was chosen as a brand name for the medicines manufactured by the hospital's production centre and sold on the market.[6] The production centre was regarded as a successful example of a government work unit (*danwei*) embarking on the path of the 'socialist market economy'.

From the very beginning, the hospital also had a research unit. Later on a college-level training facility was established in close connection with the hospital's work unit. The school is now part of the Qinghai University Medical College. After the Tibetan Medicine College in Lhasa, it is the second higher-education facility for aspiring Sowa Rigpa professionals. The hospital, production centre, research unit and college were merged into the Arura Group in 1999 – the medicine's brand now serving as the group's name.

At that time, the Arura Group was still a government-owned enterprise, and salaries were paid by the state. When restrictions on the privatisation of strategically important government enterprises were lifted, the Arura Group's production centre was turned into a private for-profit company under the name of Arura Tibetan Medicine Co. Ltd. 'There was a big push towards privatisation and the government really wanted us to do this', a senior manager told me. During the transition to GMP, a new manufacturing plant was built in 2003/4. The 'old' factory is now again catering for the needs of the hospital.

The role of private investors in the making of the industry is a topic of hot debate. A general sense that 'the Chinese are taking over' is prevalent among Tibetans in Tibet as well as in exile. The exile view goes a step further and portrays the recent developments as selling out Tibetan medicine to the Chinese (see Tashi Tsering 2005). Although I was not able to identify ownership for each and every company, my findings suggest a more complex picture.

In the case of Arura, the state currently owns 17 per cent of the company's shares. To the best of my knowledge, a part of the revenue from selling 83 per cent of the shares went into the construction of the new, well-equipped Tibetan hospital in Xining and another part was used for the newly established Tibetan Medicine Museum of China (which will be discussed in more detail in Chapter 6). Questions concerning to whom these shares were sold and who holds them now, however, are difficult to answer. As with any stock corporation, ownership is fluid. Given the demographic asymmetry between Tibetans and Han Chinese, a shift of ownership away from Tibetans is a reasonable guess.

Some private companies, however, remain or have become once again Tibetan-owned: Jiumei Tibetan Medicine Co. Ltd. in Xining, for example, is privately owned and managed by Jigme Phuntsog, a Tibetan monk turned businessman. Other examples include Shongpalhachu and the Tibetan medicine factory in Nyalam. In the case of the Nyalam factory, officially named God Monkey Medicine Industry Ltd. and known under the brand Qomolangma, ownership is shared between the workers (60 per cent), the current director (20 per cent) and the founder's family (20 per cent) – none of them is Chinese. Shongpalhachu is owned by a well-known Tibetan businessman (45 per cent) and the predominantly Tibetan members of staff (55 per cent). However, both factories took out substantial bank loans. Another example is Yarlung Tibetan Medicine (also known as Jinzhu Along), which has recently been acquired by a Tibetan businessman.

Furthermore, ownership is not directly correlated with control. A private company such as Arura, which is still part of the government-owned Arura Group, is certainly not under the control of private Chinese investors. Arura's board of directors is presided over by Ao Tsochen, a high-ranking Tibetan government official. By contrast, the Tibetan Medicine College Factory in Lhasa is owned by the government and has not been privatised. However, it has been leased out to a Chinese entrepreneur, who now runs its operations.

The fact is that the prospect of investing in the industry looked promising during the years of GMP introduction, even more so after the SARS crisis in 2003. The story of a Tibetan doctor in a SARS-free township of the otherwise heavily affected Guandong province using Tibetan incense as a protective measure against the disease triggered a veritable run on incense and other products from Tibet, including Tibetan precious pills and protective amulets (Craig 2003; Craig and Adams 2009). In view of this boom, potential investors were not too hard to find. Nevertheless, certain differences between the TAR and other Tibetan areas in the PRC are apparent.

Compared to other provinces, the drive towards the privatisation of government property has been less pronounced and set in later in the TAR. The work units, which have lost much of their position in inland China over the last two decades, are still prevalent and influential in the TAR.[7]

Remarkably, to the best of my knowledge no foreign investor bought shares in the industry. On the contrary, foreign money was no longer welcome, as Tenpa Wangchuk of Shongpalhachu recalls: 'In 2002, the government said that foreign supporters should not be involved in our factory and they were withdrawn from the Tibetan medicine council'. In 2005, the SFDA announced that foreign investment was officially banned in companies who produce 'prepared slices of Chinese crude drugs' or medicines based on secret formulas, such as some Tibetan precious pills (SFDA 2005b). However, I have no knowledge about how these provisions are implemented. While talk of joint ventures in the industry is again in the air, I doubt that such plans will materialise anytime soon.

Relations Between GMP Factories and Hospitals

More important than ownership is what new bank loans and private investors have meant for the companies' strategies. Regardless of its source, the investment required to build GMP-compliant factories changed the outlook and orientation of the industry to a considerable degree. Once the new factories were built, they needed to generate profit, grow and expand into the markets of inland China. This also affected relations between profit-oriented companies and medical institutions.

As many for-profit factories grew out of hospital pharmacies, they were often meant to serve a dual purpose during the first stage of the industry's creation: they had to produce medicines for the hospital to which they belonged and also manufacture commodities for the market. With the construction of new GMP-compliant factories, their orientation shifted towards the latter. The need to generate profit meant that production for an attached hospital became more and more of an impediment. From the perspective of the hospitals, the new orientation of 'their' factories was also considered less than ideal, and many doctors complained of a decrease in the quality of the medicines produced.

In this respect, it is important to emphasise that GMP applies to all drugs sold on the market but specifically exempts the medicines prepared by hospital pharmacies. GMP aims at regulating the pharmaceutical industry but not hospitals. The dual purpose of companies linked to a hospital meant that the problems associated with GMP were imported into the domain of medicines produced for the hospital's own use. On the contrary, TCM hospitals were less affected by GMP, as they continued to rely substantially on individually compounded formulations. The TCM lobby was strong enough to defend its territory in this respect, and the pharmacies catering for TCM patients are exempt from GMP. Even in Western countries, pharmacists have certain rights to prepare compounds outside the strict regulations of drug registration and GMP. It is therefore no surprise that the dual purpose of the hospital-derived Tibetan medicine companies created friction between the hospitals' interests and the factories' economic perspectives.

The Mentsikhang in Lhasa provides an apt example of this friction. With the construction of a new GMP plant, the Mentsikhang factory officially became the TAR Tibetan Medicine Factory. At the time of my research, the TAR Tibetan Medicine Factory still produced about 300 different types of medicines for the Mentsikhang's in- and out-patient departments, but only fifty-six of them had registration numbers and could legally be sold on the market. As the price of herbs and other raw materials has increased more rapidly than the government-controlled price of medicines over the last few years, the factory lost money with its operations for the hospital. The medicines produced for the market, on the other hand, are highly profitable as they are sold for a much higher price. Plans were afoot to build a new (non-GMP) Mentsikhang factory to meet the hospital's needs and enable the TAR Tibetan Medicine Factory to operate solely as a for-profit enterprise. The funds for the new hospital factory (as well as a new in-patient clinic and renovation works on the out-patient department) had already been granted I was ensured when I talked to several people at the Mentsikhang in 2008/9.

In some cases, the old pre-GMP factories, which were usually not destroyed because they had to operate until the new GMP plants were up and running, sometimes went back to producing non-GMP drugs for the attached hospital. The Deqin Shangri-la Tibetan Medicine Company's new factory in Zhongdian, for example, was initially meant to replace the local Tibetan hospital's factory. Later on, the old factory resumed operation as a producer of low-cost, high-quality supplies for the hospital (Glover 2006). The same is true for Arura's old factory attached to the hospital in Xining. In other cases, companies are using their old factory buildings for other ventures, such as the production of Tibetan incense, or simply as storerooms for herbs.

The SFDA and National Drug Registration

Besides declaring GMP a compulsory requirement for the production of pharmaceutical commodities, the 2001 Drug Administration Law also stipulated a new national system of drug registration. This had far-reaching implications for the whole pharmaceutical industry in China, including Tibetan medicine. After responsibility for the implementation of health policies was decentralised in the 1980s and 1990s, the nationalisation of drug registration was a move in the opposite direction. For the companies it implied a significant reconfiguration of their relations to the state and its authorities.

As mentioned above, drug registration was part of Beijing's agenda as early as the 1980s, and starting from 1995, when the *Tibetan Drug Standards* were published, it also became relevant for Tibetan medicine. However, the matter remained largely in the hands of the provincial authorities until the 2001 revision of the Drug Administration Law (SFDA 2001) specified that thenceforth the SFDA alone would be responsible for drug registration. The power to decide which factory was allowed to produce which drugs shifted from the provincial authorities to the SFDA in Beijing.

As we have seen, state-owned and semi-private companies usually emerged from the nexus of existing government-owned institutions. As such, they had close ties to a local (provincial, autonomous regional or prefectural) authority. By transferring the power of drug registration to the SFDA, the factories suddenly had to come to terms with an authority with which they no longer had any affinity. The SFDA, on the other hand, saw its power increase considerably. As the SFDA was now in charge of vital matters for the survival of the whole pharmaceutical industry in China, the companies had to find ways to establish friendly and good relations with it. As a result, the introduction of a centralised system of drug registration in 2002 became the stage for one of the largest corruption scandals in the People's Republic over the last decade.

The episode started with a series of incidents related to unsafe drugs. In two separate cases in 2006, eleven people died in Heilongjiang province and six in Anhui province. The authorities could no longer ignore the fact that there was a serious problem with the SFDA's role in these cases. SFDA officials had a habit of issuing drug registration numbers in return for gifts and payments, completely ignoring their responsibility to monitor drug safety. Furthermore, it was common practice that SFDA officials owned shares in the companies they were meant to supervise.

When the incidents became public and the scandal gained in coverage it finally reached Zheng Xiaoyu, who had been the SFDA's director since it was created in 1998. His name was closely linked to the introduction of GMP and the new system of drug registration. Zheng had already been removed from his post in 2005, but after the public outrage following the scandals in 2006 he was charged with 'dereliction of duty' and with taking bribes worth 6.49 million yuan ($950,000) from eight pharmaceutical companies in return for approving their products. On 29 May 2007, the First People's Intermediary Court in Beijing sentenced him to death and in July he was executed. His secretaries, wife and son were also convicted of being involved in the scheme. Other SFDA officials were urged to show remorse, and they subsequently turned in 2.6 million yuan ($380,000) they had received as 'presents'. Furthermore, they were ordered to divest themselves of the shares they held in pharmaceutical companies. New regulations of conduct were decreed, making it illegal for health officials to accept presents or services, or hold shares in the companies they were supervising.

Official China's strategy was clearly to contain the damage. The SFDA's spokeswoman Yan Jiangying said that 'this kind of serious case of law breaking by a small minority of corrupt elements ... really made us feel ashamed' (*China Daily* 2007a). A series of new health scandals since then suggests that the promised clean-up in the health bureaucracy has not had the intended effect. In 2008 alone, contaminated heparin, a widely used blood thinner, caused the death of eighty-one people (Alonso-Zaldivar 2008), and thousands of babies developed kidney stones after consuming milk powder contaminated with melamine (Langman 2009; Macartney and Yu 2009).

Rinchen Wangdu, my well-informed source on such matters, insisted that despite all these events officials still owned stocks in the companies they were supervising. This was also facilitated by the fact that they were not required to disclose their sources of income (cf. Qiu 2007: 636). The need to maintain good relations with all levels of authority was no less crucial than before, and the rules of the game had not changed. Building such relations still involved intermediaries, favours and expensive gifts. Rinchen Wangdu added that when he had held a senior position in the industry he had hardly been able to find time to do his job properly because of all the receptions and banquets he had had to attend. He detested them but considered them to be essential for success.

Gifts, favours and banquets are the ingredients of what is generally subsumed under the term *guanxi*, the art of social relations. *Guanxi* is considered to be different from *xinghui*, simple, straightforward corruption. While *xinghui* usually denotes a one-time exchange of money for a favour, *guanxi* is about building and maintaining long-term relations embedded in notions of friendship, support and loyalty. Mayfair Yang, whose work was the starting point for much of the *guanxi* scholarship of the last two decades (Yang 1988, 1989, 1994, 2002), remarks in an early article that the borders between *guanxi* and *xinghui* were sometimes blurred, but that 'the two are still conceptually distinguished by such things as cultural judgements of the level of instrumentalism, the form and art of gift giving (gifts or money, ordinary gifts or expensive gifts, temporal lengths of familiarity and repayment, and so forth), and whether the effects are considered ethical or unethical' (Yang 1989: 48). In the case of the SFDA scandal, the public's verdict on relations between pharmaceutical companies and the SFDA was clear: it came to be seen as a case of simple, large-scale, unethical corruption.

The Tibetan medicine industry was only a sideshow to these events; no Tibetan drug was involved in any major incident. However, the SFDA announced in 2002 that drugs registered at the provincial level needed to be re-certified according to central government standards. Re-certification (or re-registration) required following a complex protocol, which included scientific studies of the safety and efficacy of each product. The factories founded before 1997 were somewhat less affected by these changes, as the SFDA exempted all drugs registered locally before 1997 from the requirement to follow the protocol. These 'old drugs' were simply grandfathered into the new system. The factories that obtained the bulk of their registration numbers between 1997 and 2002, however, had to get their respective products re-registered.

The conditions mentioned in the protocol were simply impossible to meet, given the timeframe set by the SFDA. As a result, companies were faced with the choice either of losing their right to produce the medicines in question or of resorting to forgery, and presenting results of scientific studies that had never been carried out. When internal investigations into SFDA's practices began (years before Zheng's trial) inconsistencies in the research materials submitted by Tibetan medicine firms came to light. However, a pragmatic solution to the problem was apparently found, and to the best of my knowledge none of the factories I have been in contact with lost the right to produce any of their already registered products due to the investigation.[8] The status enjoyed by Tibetan medicine as a 'pillar industry', crucial for the development of the region, has probably helped in this case. Nevertheless, nationwide scandals continue to have an impact on the Tibetan medicine industry. Beijing's efforts to close loopholes and enforce stricter implementation of existing regulations have clearly become more pronounced over the past few years.

The Size of the Industry

During my research I made several attempts to compile a list of all the medicine factories in Tibet, including basic data about yearly output and revenue. Estimating the industry's size, however, proved much more complicated than I had assumed. The numbers I was given in interviews and collected from news reports, government statistics and factory websites were highly inconsistent.

The problem starts with a simple question: What counts as a Tibetan medicine factory? On the one hand, many smaller factories officially operating as hospital pharmacies, or even without a licence, still sell their products on the market regardless of the regulations that stipulate otherwise. These factories are usually not accounted for in published sources. On the other hand, government statistics on the industry usually include Chinese companies producing one or two medicines they chose to call Tibetan, Rinchen Wangdu insisted. These were not 'real' Tibetan medicine companies, he argued.

The next question is, accordingly: What counts as a Tibetan drug? Do all the popular products deriving from single herbs like *solomarpo* (*sro lo dmar po*, *Rhodiola*) or *yartsagunbu* (*dbyar rtswa dgun 'bu*, *Ophiocordyceps sinensis*) count as Tibetan remedies? And what about the raw Tibetan herbs many shops throughout Tibet sell to Chinese tourists? Finally, Rinchen Wangdu, frank as always, advised me not to trust the numbers the factory directors gave me, as everybody in the industry tended to under-report output and revenue numbers by 20 per cent or more for tax reasons and other benefits.

In the article mentioned in the introduction, Huang Fukai, president of the Tibetan hospital in Beijing, spoke of Tibetan medicine as a 1 billion yuan ($148 million) industry in 2003. Huang counted thirty-five Tibetan medicine companies and an additional eighteen TCM companies producing Tibetan medicines. As the process of GMP introduction was still under way, both GMP and non-GMP companies were included in his count. A report by the Tibet Justice Center (Tashi Tsering 2005), citing an unreferenced study, suggests that there are seventy-five companies dealing with Tibetan medicine on the Tibetan plateau, of which only thirty are run by Tibetans.

The factories I either visited personally, or at least had contact with, include nine inside and eight outside the TAR, counting only the GMP-certified ones that produce exclusively Tibetan medicines. But there are certainly more companies producing Tibetan medicine. In Xining alone, for example, seven such companies are said to exist, of which I only visited two. To make matters even more complex, I came across the products of companies that I have not been able to find, despite the address and phone numbers given on the packaging. These products were either fake or the companies had shut down or moved away.

A report by the China Tibet Information Center, a government news agency, states that seventeen Tibetan medicine companies produced goods to the value of 623 million yuan ($91 million) in 2006. It is unclear, however, which companies were included and whether the numbers only refer to the TAR or not. The same report mentions a total of nineteen Tibetan medicine companies in 'Tibet' (CTIC 2007c). A 2008 Xinhua News Agency report mentions an output value of 574 million yuan nationwide for 2007, which would be considerably less than in 2006. Nevertheless, a 1.7 per cent annual increase over the previous year's production is proclaimed (Xinhua 2008).

Furthermore, a *China Daily* report on Cheezheng, at the time of my research the biggest Tibetan medicine company, attributes an annual sales value of more than 400 million yuan to the company's line of products (*China Daily* 2008). As Cheezheng's patented pain-relief plaster accounts for most of the company's sales, this would mean that a substantial part of the industry's total output value is generated by one single product, which is by no means one of the well-known, traditional formulas.

The question of growth rates is also worth a second look. Huang stated in 2006 that the industry had grown by 129 per cent annually since 2000, and compared to 1996 its current output value had increased more than thirty times. In contrast, the Xinhua News Agency report cited above (Xinhua 2008) mentions a 1.7 per cent annual increase from 2006 to 2007. These numbers would suggest that growth was exponential at the outset and has since slowed down dramatically.

Regardless of the accuracy of these numbers, a certain deceleration in growth rates is corroborated by a set of unpublished statistical materials I managed to obtain for one province. These statistics are based on the data provided by seven factories and cover the period between 2004 and 2008. While some of the companies have seen stable double-digit growth rates during this period, others have seen their sales dwindle.

The published numbers, combined with these statistics and several anecdotal accounts about companies facing economic difficulties, make it reasonable to assume that the output value of Tibetan pharmaceuticals grew rapidly during the years of the industry's creation and that the industry has now entered a phase of consolidation.

Forces at Work

In conclusion, the conditions from which the industry emerged can be summarised as follows: The revival of Tibetan medicine during the 1980s led to rising patient numbers and an increase in demand for Tibetan medicines. The resulting mechanisation of production was a first step towards industrialisation.

The actual creation of the industry took place in two stages. First, the 'socialist market economy' proclaimed in 1992 endorsed the founding of business-oriented Tibetan medicine companies. On the one hand, the new economic policies were a challenge for Tibetan medicine because they implied decreasing state subsidies for hospitals and their production centres. On the other hand, the new freedoms that came along with the 'socialist market economy' were also taken as an opportunity for establishing companies with distinctively Tibetan outlooks. Such ventures were considered to increase the reach and fame of Sowa Rigpa in the PRC while still being in line with official development agendas. This is illustrated, for example, by Pema Gyatso's quest to root the Shongpalhachu factory in the universe of Tibetan Buddhist history as well as to position it favourably in the context of contemporary Tibet.

The second stage of the transformation from hospital pharmacy to industry was triggered by China's WTO membership, the 2001 revision of the Drug Administration Law, and the introduction of GMP. As GMP made the construction of new factories necessary, new investment had to be found, and a fully fledged pharmaceutical industry enmeshed in the logic of capital and markets emerged. These developments are seen as much more problematic than the construction of factories in the 1990s. They have led to increasing tensions between hospitals and factories, and the production of Tibetan pharmaceuticals is more and more confronted with legal frameworks developed without much 'sensibility' towards Sowa Rigpa (Adams, Schrempf and Craig 2010).

The reasons for this lie partly in Sowa Rigpa's marginal position in the PRC, partly in the enormous pace that marked the industry's creation and prevented a more gradual step-by-step approach, and partly in the fact that the rationales from which these legal frameworks stemmed were largely developed outside Tibet. These rationales emerged at the intersection of China's policies towards traditional medicine with the dominant perspectives in the global health arena, especially the World Health Organisation (see WHO 2002, 2003 2004, 2006a). While 'Global Pharma' may recognise the importance of traditional medicine, the consensus is that it needs to be aligned with notions of patient safety, efficacy and quality control.

In short, the forces shaping Tibetan medicine and its industry are increasingly forged in a global arena, adapted to suit the context of China, sometimes adjusted to the needs of TCM, and filtered to suit the special conditions of Tibet. In other words, the story told up to here is primarily one of global forms being recontextualised first in China and then in Tibet. These forces at work thereby refer to several modern rationales, ranging from neoliberalism to high-modernist planning and the occasional reminder of the security apparatus's claim for supremacy. Regardless of the flavour of such modern rationales, the power vectors undeniably point from the global via the national to the local level.

However, when the policies, laws and development agendas stemming from these positions are finally implemented on the ground, the conflicting figurations of the modern project encounter similarly conflicting visions of Tibetanness and morality. The state's instruments of governance inevitably face subtle and often morally underpinned forms of defiance and resistance.

The question is, then, how the legal frameworks designed to modernise and standardise traditional medicine are actually being implemented and how the factories are dealing with them on a day-to-day level. This next step of my inquiry leaves behind the bird's-eye view of the creation of the industry for a more ethnographic perspective on the practice of industrial production.

Notes

1. Around Lhasa, the two large monasteries of Drepung and Sera alone housed more than 15,000 monks in 1950 (Goldstein 1999: 5).
2. For an introduction to Sowa Rigpa's principles see e.g. Meyer 1981; Clark 1985; Donden 1986; Meyer 1992; Parfianovitch, Meyer and Dorje 1992; Clark 1995; Meyer 1995; Gyatso 2006.
3. In fact, the TCM industry is much larger than its Tibetan counterpart. According to a 2008 government white paper, 'the industrial output value of TCM reached 177.2 billion yuan [$25.9 billion], accounting for 26.53 percent of the total pharmaceutical industrial output value'(IOSC 2008). By comparison, the highest official figure for the industrial output of Tibetan medicine is one billion yuan ($146 million).
4. Sixty tons per year seems a rather high figure. Even if we estimate that 10 per cent of the production was sold to private *amchi*, the remaining 54 tons would still amount to more than 200 grammes of medicine handed out in each of the 260,000 consultations.
5. Apparently, the deadline was later extended to the end of 2004.
6. Arura *(a ru ra)* is the Tibetan name for *Terminalia chebula*, the myrobalan fruit – a crucial ingredient of many Tibetan formulas.
7. See You 1998 for an overview of privatisation and the changing function of the *danwei* in general, and Yeh 2008 for the persistence of forms of government enterprise in Tibet as compared to the Inland.

8. Many factories, however, lost the right to produce some of the high-value Precious Pills under the new SFDA regime. The consequences of national level drug registration for the question of intellectual property rights will be discussed in Chapter 5.

Chapter 3
Manufacturing Good Practice

> GMP for Tibetan medicine is like putting a goat's head on a sheep's body.
>
> —Private *amchi*, Xining

Talking to Tibetan doctors, pharmacists and factory staff one quickly notes that GMP ('good manufacturing practice') stands for much more than just a set of rules and regulations. It has become a symbol of the entire industrialisation of Tibetan medicine. In this context, the phrase *ra mgo lug la sbyar ba* (literally 'to stick a goat's head on a sheep') is sometimes used in relation to GMP (see, for example, Kalden Nyima 2006: 366). It is a reference to the Tibetan expression *ra ma lug*, rather like the English 'neither fish nor fowl', meaning neither here nor there, a mixture, often uncomfortable, of different things. The metaphor mirrors the strong notion that GMP is fundamentally incompatible with the traditional way of making Tibetan medicine.

Among the large majority of my interlocutors a considerable amount of scepticism regarding recent developments prevailed. This general scepticism is well documented in the contemporary academic literature on Sowa Rigpa in Tibet (Janes 1999, 2002; Adams 2002, 2004; Craig and Adams 2009; Hofer 2009a, 2009b; Craig 2010, 2011). During conversations with Tibetan medicine professionals, GMP was frequently depicted as good for hygiene and management but as something imported from the West and therefore inherently foreign to Sowa Rigpa. A majority of the people I talked to held this opinion. Rinchen Wangdu, for example, made clear at the very beginning of our first conversation: 'First, I want to say that GMP was not something that came from the factories or the Tibetan doctors, but from the government. At that time we were totally against this GMP thing'.

For analytic purposes, the goat-headed sheep image can be seen as describing two intertwined conflicts: First, the substitution of heads stands for a clash between GMP and Tibetan Sowa Rigpa as two incompatible systems of knowledge, two rationalities rooted in different epistemologies. In this conflict of knowledge systems, Sowa Rigpa is being devalued and superseded by GMP. Second, the goat's head as an unsuitable replacement also implies a conflict at the level of practice: GMP interferes with the well-established body of best practice in Tibetan pharmacy.

My aim is to analyse these two alleged conflicts in more detail. To do so, I will compare the regulations with the relevant passages of the traditional texts and analyse if and how they actually affect the practice of making Tibetan medicines. Laws, policies, machines, techniques, factory architecture, different forms of knowledge and practices are the intertwined elements of the industrial assemblage examined in this chapter.[1]

GMP in China

To some degree, the idea that GMP 'comes from the West' is certainly correct. GMP's historical roots go back to the US government's Pure Food and Drug Act of 1906.[2] However, it is important to note that GMP is neither a Western nor an international standard. Contrary to the ISO standards for quality control, for example, there is no international organisation that monitors or defines it. The WHO has published a set of GMP guidelines and recommendations (WHO 2005b, 2006, 2007), but they do not form a standard as such. GMP is a national affair; implementation and supervision of GMP are the sole responsibility of the respective national authorities. As a consequence, there is considerable variety among the GMP standards of different countries. It took Japan, Europe and the USA a full decade to harmonise and mutually recognise their respective GMPs (ICH n.d.).

Compared to the harmonised GMPs of Europe, America and Japan, the current Chinese version is much briefer and in many aspects much less specific. The Chinese GMP, however, has to be understood in relation to the entire framework of the PRC's drug regulations, including the Drug Administration Law, the *Chinese Pharmacopoeia* and various decrees and guidelines.[3]

A good starting point to get an impression of the style, scope and interdependence of the regulations in this framework is Article 9 of the Chinese GMP. It says of the production premises that they 'shall be designed in such a way as to allow production to take place in a logical sequence corresponding to the required sequence of operations and to meet the requisite cleanliness classifications' (Kuwahara and Li 2007: 49). This simple and reasonable statement is further elaborated in Article 23, which stipulates a strict separation of production areas from those where pre-processing of herbal and animal raw materials takes place. Furthermore, appropriate ventilation and dust collection for the slicing and crushing of ingredients is listed as a requirement (ibid.: 76). With regard to the 'requisite cleanliness' mentioned in Article 9 we need to turn to Article 16 (ibid.: 68), which defines a 'static pressure differential' of more than 10 Pa between clean and unclassified areas. What 'clean area' means is broadly defined in Article 85 (ibid.: 13), which further refers to Article 1 of Annex 2, where four cleanliness classes including their respective maximum numbers of particles and micro-organisms per cubic metre of air are given (ibid.: 228). In order to find out which of these cleanliness classes is applicable one needs to look into the requirements for each formula as defined by the *Chinese Pharmacopoeia* (SPC 2005).

The goat's head, I am tempted to say, is not an easy one to understand. The jungle of interconnected regulations requires guidance and opens a considerable space for interpretation (for example, when a Tibetan formula is not mentioned in the *Chinese Pharmacopoeia* and therefore not associated with a cleanliness class). There should be no doubt, however, with whom the power of interpretation rests. Article 87 of the Chinese GMP explicitly states: 'These provisions are subject to interpretation by the State Food and Drug Administration [of China]' (Kuwahara and Li 2007: 213) – an article with far reaching consequences, as we shall see.

In the case of the brief foray into the regulation jungle outlined above, the simple result was that in order to produce Tibetan medicines according to GMP guidelines, a factory especially designed and constructed for this purpose became mandatory – with sealed windows and doors, an internal air pressure slightly higher than outside, equipped with the necessary machines to ensure and monitor its cleanliness, and an architectural design that allows for a strict separation of the different steps of production.

It is no secret that GMP's primary focus is on the production of biomedical pharmaceuticals. In fact, Tibetan medicine is not mentioned once, neither in the GMP nor in the Drug Administration Law. However, considerable space in both the Drug Administration Law and GMP is dedicated to traditional Chinese medicine (TCM). The Chinese GMP includes an appendix on TCM, which further de-

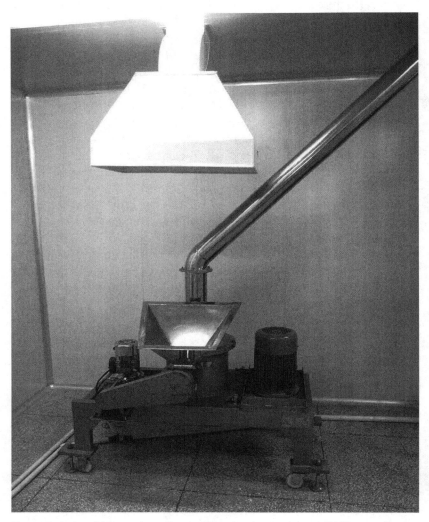

Figure 3.1: An older machine for crushing hard ingredients, GMP compliant ventilation.

fines certain requirements put forward in the main text. Current interpretation by the SFDA seems to be that Tibetan medicine more or less falls within the category of TCM as far as these requirements are concerned. Appendix VII of the Chinese GMP comprises nineteen TCM related articles. Most of them contain simple and reasonable stipulations: the personnel responsible need to possess professional knowledge of TCM, the herbs should not be kept directly on the ground, and so on. In all the discussions I had with Tibetan doctors, factory staff and managers, such requirements were never the subject of complaints. These simple provisions are not considered a goat's head, so to speak, and I do not believe that anybody would see them to be in contradiction with traditional ways of production.

However, a different picture is revealed when looking at the notable exemptions the Drug Administration Law (SFDA 2001) grants TCM, especially in the domain of 'traditional Chinese crude drugs' as the unrefined ingredients of TCM pharmaceuticals are officially called. For example, Chinese crude drugs can be sold at 'town and country fairs' (Article 21) and their production does not have to follow 'national drug standards' (Article 10). The problem is that these exemptions are not applicable to ready-made, refined, multi-component Tibetan formulations, as they do not fall into the category of 'crude drugs'. As a result, the production of Tibetan pharmaceuticals is bound by a set of regulations primarily meant to govern the high-volume production of synthetic biomedical drugs.

Furthermore, drug regulations are also developing rapidly. Since the ushering in of industrial production, new guidelines and decrees have been brought forward frequently (SFDA 2002, 2004, 2005b, 2006a, 2006b, 2007). There are no signs that the jungle of regulations will thin out, that the space of interpretation will diminish, or that Sowa Rigpa will be provided with its own regulations anytime soon.

The Steps of Production

To gain an understanding of the resulting practical conflicts between the current regulations and 'what the Gyüshi says' – including the interpretation of both of them – we need to take a closer look at the actual steps of production of a Tibetan formulation. For a Tibetan pill, the most commonly used form of Tibetan medicine today, the steps of production are roughly the following.

- *Sourcing and storage of raw materials*: Tibetan medicine is based on the notion that everything on this planet has medicinal value. In practice, a couple of thousand ingredients are described in different texts and commentaries and of these a few hundred are frequently used in making Tibetan medicines. Ingredients include minerals, animal parts and, most importantly, medicinal herbs. Most herbs are collected from the wild and dried on the spot. The factories usually buy these dried herbs from intermediary traders. Once the raw materials reach the factory, they need to be stored in a way that they do not lose their properties.
- *Pre-processing*: Before the raw materials can be used in Tibetan medicine, they usually need to be pre-processed. Roots need to be cleaned, flowers and leaves sorted, and certain minerals or plants undergo calcination. Other ingredients, such as mercury, need to be detoxified and their 'coarse potencies' (Dawa 2002: 351–52) removed, which requires more complex procedures.
- *Grinding, mixing and making pills*: Tibetan medicines are multi-component formulations. The ingredients of one formula – involving anywhere between five and more than seventy – are roughly mixed together and then ground into a fine powder. A few special ingredients which are either very precious or difficult to grind with standard equipment are crushed and ground separately. Then, the ground powder is mixed thoroughly to make sure that all the ingredients are well dispersed and the mixture is perfectly homogeneous. Tibetan pills are so-called 'watered pills', made from powder and water. The most commonly used technique is to add, little by little, water and powder into a rotating barrel. The powder starts to clump into small round seed pills, which, by adding more water and powder, are subsequently grown to the required size. Sieving ensures that all the pills have the appropriate size.
- *Drying*: Finally the pills need to be dried. This is traditionally done either in the sun or in the shade, depending on the formula's properties.
- *Packing and labelling*: When the pills are dry they are packed and labelled accordingly.

I will discuss each of these steps of production in turn (except for packaging and labelling, which will be looked at in more detail in

Chapter 6) and show that the problem is not the goat's head but rather the operation of putting it on a sheep's body.

The Sourcing and Storage of Raw Materials

The raw materials used in Tibetan medicine – herbs, minerals and animal parts – are critical for the quality and efficacy of the final compounds. The sourcing of raw materials, however, has seen considerable changes over the last decade, which has had an effect on their quality. This is especially true of medicinal herbs.

Sowa Rigpa's approach to the collection and storage of herbs is described in the Gyüshi. Chapter 12, titled *ngochor* (*sngo sbyor*), of the Gyüshi's Subsequent Tantra, the *chimagyü* (*phyi ma rgyud*), deals with herbal compounds and contains the so-called 'seven essential limbs of medicinal plants' (Dawa 2002: 349–61) or, more briefly: the Seven Limbs or *yänlagdun* (*yan lag bdun*). The Seven Limbs are sometimes called a 'GMP for Tibetan medicine' by Tibetan medicine professionals. Limbs one, two and four contain detailed instructions on how to ensure the highest quality of medicinal plants.

Sowa Rigpa relies, among other things, on a differentiation between hot and cold diseases. Herbs are accordingly categorised as 'hot-curing' and 'cold-curing', or 'cooling' and 'warming' respectively. The first and the fourth of the Seven Limbs describe where to collect and how to process medicinal plants according to their warming or cooling nature. Cooling herbs should be collected on the northern slopes of a mountain and they should be dried in the shade. Direct sunlight should be avoided to maintain their cooling qualities. Plants with warming potencies, by contrast, should be collected from the southern slope of a mountain, exposed to abundant sunshine, and they should be dried in the sun or near a fire. By following these instructions the cooling and warming potencies are best preserved.

The second limb refers to the appropriate harvesting time. It lists eleven categories of herbal ingredients and groups them into four sub-classes – stem, leaves, fruit and bark. For each of these sub-classes of *materia medica* the correct harvesting time is defined. The stem sub-class (which includes root, branches and stems) should be collected in late autumn, the ninth lunar month of the Tibetan calendar; the leaf subclass (leaves, latex and shoots) in late summer; the bark subclass (bark, resin, cortex) in the middle or late phase of spring.

Fruits and flowers, which form the fruit sub-class, are more complex. Some should be harvested when the flowers bloom or the fruits are ripe while for others the best time is the eighth month of the Tibetan calendar (autumn). The second limb ends on the following note: 'The collection of medicinal plants and their parts is considered a very important procedure. On an auspicious time and day, during the waxing phase of the moon of the collecting month, the process of herb collection is done by medical students reciting the mantras of Medicine Buddha and the *rten 'brel snying po* (the essence of interdependence)' (ibid.: 351).

While GMP says nothing about harvesting times, the *Chinese Pharmacopoeia* sometimes does. The monograph on safflower (*Carthamus tinctorius*) or *tsa gurgum* (*rtsa gur gum*), for example, which is among the few Tibetan medicinal plants included in the *Chinese Pharmacopoeia* (SPC 2005: 55), states that 'the drug is collected in summer when its colour turns from yellow to red, and dried in the shade or in the sun'. This is perfectly in line with traditional Tibetan best practice as mentioned in one of the standard Tibetan texts on the sources and identification of medicinal herbs (Gabe Dorji 1995: 101). As safflower has cooling properties, a Tibetan *amchi* may choose to dry it in the shade. The often-voiced complaint that the Seven Limbs are no longer followed and the quality of herbal ingredients is therefore decreasing refers to the growing importance of commercial trade and not to conflicting Chinese regulations.

In terms of storage, the fifth limb states that, unless a decoction is prepared, herbs should be used within one year. GMP's Article 43 (Kuwahara and Li 2007: 105), on the other hand, stipulates a maximum shelf life of three years for all materials, 'unless otherwise defined', meaning that exemptions from the three-year rule would have to be mentioned in the material's monograph in the official *Chinese Pharmacopoeia*. A quick look at the aforementioned monograph on safflower, one of the more sensitive herbs in terms of storage, reveals that there is no specific exemption in terms of shelf life. The official regulations therefore define three years as the plant's maximum shelf life. By contrast, the fifth of the Seven Limbs suggests only one year. Evidently, the traditional guidelines are stricter than GMP in this respect, and the new regulations should therefore not interfere with traditional best practice. In reality, however, many herbal ingredients, especially roots, are stored for more than one year before they are used, regardless of what the Gyüshi, GMP, or the *Pharmacopoeia* say.

For one ingredient, GMP's stipulated three years could nevertheless be a problem: the mineral *biitog* (*bul tog*), a water containing a carbonate known as trona. Tibet Information Network's report on Tibetan medicine mentions that traditionally the best *biitog* was considered to be that which had been stored away in a container for many years. The report cites a pharmacist who complained that GMP's specification of three years of shelf life interfered with this tradition (TIN 2004: 77).

Apart from the question of shelf life, the actual practice of storage has also seen changes. GMP stipulates, for example, that bags of herbs should not be stored directly on the ground but on pallets or shelves (Annex VII, Article 17). Furthermore the bags should be labelled properly and the labels should include information about the origin of the herbs, the date of purchase, and so on (Annex VII, Article 12). In accordance with GMP's general approach to quality control, the storage facilities of the factories I have visited always featured spatially separated channels for the herbs that had already been tested (usually marked with green labels), those rejected, and those not yet tested (marked with red and sometimes yellow labels, respectively). These simple principles of organising storage facilities are usually seen as an improvement in the domain of management.

In summary, my point is that in some cases the traditional approach sets the bar higher than the contemporary drug regulations. In other cases, the Chinese regulations and the Seven Limbs simply have different outlooks. They may contain different notions of quality but they do not necessarily contradict each other. GMP focuses on the actual manufacturing process, and the monographs in the *Chinese Pharmacopoeia* are mainly concerned with biochemical identification tests. Neither gives regard to the selection of individual plants according to their habitat and properties. However, neither precludes the detailed procedures described in the Seven Limbs.

When Tibetan medicine professionals complain about inferior quality of contemporary medicinal herbs when compared to pre-industrial times, the reasons given are more to do with the surge in trade volumes, longer supply chains and the increasing reliance on commercial plant traders than GMP and its associated regulations. These will be discussed in more detail in Chapter 4.

Simple Pre-processing: Washing, Trimming, Sorting

Most raw materials require some amount of pre-processing before they can be used as medicinal ingredients in a compound. Pre-processing includes simple things like cleaning roots or bark, removing unwanted parts of a plant, or sorting out foreign matter and rotten pieces. For some raw materials, pre-processing involves more complex processes, such as calcination or the detoxification of substances such as mercury. I will discuss the simple pre-processing first and then turn to the more complex procedures.

On a textual level, the third of the Seven Limbs deals with pre-processing and emphasises the importance of removing 'coarse potencies'. It says:

> It is extremely essential to remove the coarse potency of the collected medicinal plants or plant parts such as root, stem, branch and leaf as they possess coarse potency. For instance, the bark of a root, pith of a stem, node of a branch, petiole of a leaf, sepal of a flower and endocarp of a fruit possess coarse potency. (Dawa 2002: 351–52)

However, the Seven Limbs are not very detailed in this respect, and other important medical texts and commentaries, such as De'umar Geshe Tenzin Puntsog's eighteenth century *Crystal Rosary* (De'umar Geshe Tenzin Phuntsog 1986), need to be consulted for more specific instructions. In addition, the more complex forms of pre-processing involve much practical knowledge, which is often orally transmitted from teacher to student.

On the side of the PRC's drug regulations, the monographs of raw materials in the *Chinese Pharmacopoeia* usually include simple provisions, for example, that ingredients should be purged of foreign matter, or freed from foreign stones and soil by washing. Besides the instructions in the monographs, the *Pharmacopoeia* also contains two appendices relevant in this context: Appendix II (SPC 2005: A24–25) deals with the sampling, quality control, identification and processing of crude drugs and Appendix IXa (ibid.: A54) describes a straightforward method for the determination of foreign matter. While these regulations are very detailed with respect to how samples from a bag of herbs should be taken, how they should be tested, and how the percentage of foreign matter should be calculated, they do not say anything about the practical side of pre-processing.

Looking at GMP we find that it lists only a few general requirements in relation to the premises and the equipment used. GMP stipulates, for example, that the surfaces of the workbenches for the sorting, trimming, washing and cutting of herbs 'shall be flat and not contribute material to the crude drugs' (Annex VII, Article 6), and that 'Premises for processing, such as steaming, parching, stir-frying and calcining of Chinese crude drugs, shall be suitable for the production capacity, and be equipped with ventilation, de-fuming, dust collection, and cooling facilities' (Annex VII, Article 7).

Compared with other areas of production, pre-processing is not a primary focus of the Chinese drug regulations. The provisions in GMP and *Chinese Pharmacopoeia* are not meant to introduce new techniques but rather to ensure that the existing techniques are carried out in proper circumstances. I have not heard any complaints about the regulations' interference with the ways in which pre-processing was carried out before the introduction of GMP.

The methods employed and the amount of labour dedicated to pre-processing varies greatly between companies. In some factories roots are peeled by hand rather than washed, for example, and safflower is in some cases carefully sorted by hand while some companies forego sorting at all.

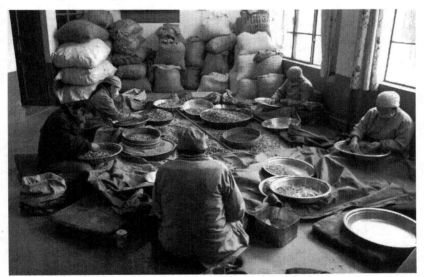

Figure 3.2: Manual pre-processing at the Men-Tsee-Khang in Dharamsala.

In general, there is no evidence that pre-processing has improved under the regime of GMP. On the contrary, one might argue that the orientation towards markets and profit actually encourages less careful approaches to pre-processing, as it remains one of the least mechanised areas of production and is therefore not easily scalable. A case in point is the Men-Tsee-Khang in Dharamsala (India), which is not bound by GMP regulations and allocates a tremendous amount of manual labour to the simple tasks of pre-processing.

The *baru* fruit (*ba ru*, belleric myrobalan, *Terminalia belerica*), for instance, undergoes very careful triage at the Men-Tsee-Khang. The fruit contains a hard seed or stone considered a coarse potency. The seeds are usually removed before the fruits are dried and traded. However, even the best quality *baru* sold on the market still contains a few seeds as well as other foreign matter. At the Men-Tsee-Khang factory in Dharamsala each and every bag of *baru* is sorted manually. By contrast, many factories I have visited in Tibet process *baru* without further sorting. Given that *baru* is one of the most common ingredients in Tibetan medicine and a medium sized factory easily processes five to ten tons per year, the manual sorting of *baru* entails considerable labour.[4] Leaving the Men-Tsee-Khang out of the equation, however, I have no evidence that the larger, more profit-oriented factories in Tibet invest less in careful pre-processing. On the contrary, Arura and the TAR Tibetan Medicine Factory, the two major players in the Qinghai and the TAR respectively, dedicate much more effort to pre-processing than some of the private, *amchi*-run, non-GMP pharmacies I have visited.

As with the sourcing and storage of raw materials, no fundamental incompatibilities between traditional texts and China's current drug regulations can be discerned. The substantial differences in approach to pre-processing observed between factories cannot be explained by a clash of conflicting rationalities. They are rather the result of pragmatic choices in specific situations. My point is that manufacturing Tibetan medicines always requires pragmatic choices and compromises, regardless of what classic texts or new regulations say. Labour invested in one area of production is missing in another, and factory managers regularly have to deal with the allocation of labour resources. In different factories these choices are made according to different priorities.

Complex Pre-processing and Tsothal

Besides simple processes like washing, trimming and sorting, Sowa Rigpa entails more complex procedures to remove the 'coarse potencies' of raw materials. Such procedures often involve practical knowledge deriving from local circumstances and can be extremely sophisticated, as the following account by Pema Gyatso demonstrates:

> Do you know how iron can be used for medicine? Boil it with *aru [Terminalia chebula]* and put it in an air-tight container. Make sure no air gets in or out. Store the container in a place with a temperature between fifteen and twenty degrees Celsius for three years. Now, do you think such a place can be found in Tibet? Yes! Look for a place where sheep are kept, a shelter half-way covered by a roof on the south slope of a mountain. Dig a hole and put the container there, facing south. During day time it absorbs the warmth of the sun and at night the sheep come back and keep it warm with their bodies. After three years, open the container. The medicine has turned from black to blue. It tastes sweet like sugar cane and is greatly reduced in quantity. It is a very effective ingredient in formulas for eye and liver diseases.

Such methods, one would expect, are more prone to be in conflict with the scientific outlook on which GMP, the Drug Administration Law and the *Chinese Pharmacopoeia* are based. While pre-processing may not be a priority in China's drug regulations, patient safety and potential contamination are. The foreword of the *Chinese Pharmacopoeia* states: 'Under the active leadership of the Chairman of the *Chinese Pharmacopoeia* Commission, the issue of pharmaceutical safety is emphasised particularly. In Volume I, atomic absorption spectrophotometry and inductively coupled plasma mass spectrometry are applied to determine the deleterious elements (lead, cadmium, mercury, arsenic and copper) and the limits of these elements have been stipulated' (SPC 2005: xvii).

In spite of these high-tech precautions for fighting the contamination of traditional medicines by heavy metals, a remarkable blind spot in the Chinese regulations and their enforcement exists with regard to one of the most famous ingredients of Tibetan medicine: *tsothal*, which contains traces of mercury.

Tibetan medicine features a special group of remedies called 'precious pills' or *rinchen rilbu* (*rin chen ril bu*). These remedies are considered to be the most potent of Tibetan formulas. They contain from twenty-five up to more than seventy ingredients, including precious substances such as *latsi* (*gla rtsi*, musk), gold and precious stones. Precious pills are shrouded in mystery as many details about their production are considered to be secret knowledge. Probably due to this appealing mixture of mystery and potency they have become the most sought after commodity, and for a good part they are driving the growth of the Tibetan medicine industry. Precious pills have come to symbolise the high art of Tibetan pharmacy, in exile as well as in Tibet. *Tsothal* (*btso thal*), which contains mercury in a purified form, is one of the key ingredients in the most famous precious pills, including Ratna Samphel (*rat na bsam 'phel*), Rinchen Drangjor (*rin chen sbrang sbyor*), Rinchen Mangjor (*rin chen mang sbyor*) and Tsotru Dashel (*btso bkru zla shel*).[5]

A series of incidents relating to the mercury content of Tibetan precious pills has stirred a heated debate about the safety of Tibetan drugs in the West as well as in the exile community in India and, to a lesser extent, in China. In 2001, for instance, a patient in Switzerland showed signs of mercury poisoning after taking Tibetan medicine. This led to an official warning being issued by the Swiss authorities against Tibetan pills (Moser 2001; Neue Zürcher Zeitung 2002; SDA 2002; Winteler 2002). Tibetan doctors and pharmacists are well aware of the potential risks of mercury but insist that when properly purified, as in *tsothal*, there is no danger to the patient.[6] However, if the established procedure of making *tsothal* is not followed with utmost care, there is general agreement among Tibetan doctors and pharmacists that it can be very dangerous.

The practice of making *tsothal* is considered to be the most difficult and complex in Tibetan pharmacy. Apart from mercury it contains eight precious stones and metals, such as gold, silver and copper. The preparation of *tsothal* takes about one month and involves many steps, including the calcination of minerals and metals. One of the pharmacists involved in the production proudly explained to me: 'None of the materials can be skipped when you make *tsothal*, otherwise it cannot be burnt. It is the same with gold. Chinese people don't believe that we are able to burn gold into ashes. But with our wisdom and science, we can do it'.

The making of *tsothal* is a symbol of the refinement of Tibetan pharmacy. As such, it has become a realm for the celebration of the industry's Tibetanness, especially since it includes a strong religious component. The making of *tsothal* relates to Indian alchemy (Samuel 2010) and much of it was and partly still is meant to be transmitted orally from master to student. However, many aspects of this secret knowledge have now been published (Dawa 2004: 412–51).

It is said that Ogyanpa Rinchenpal brought the practice of making *tsothal* to Tibet in the early thirteenth century, where it was passed on to the Third Karmapa and the famous fifteenth-century physician Zurkhar (Gyatso 1991). One of the secret names for mercury is *lhachen mahadeva* (*lha chen ma ha de wa*), a reference to Lord Shiva (in his 'subdued' Tibetan form) and the myth that mercury originates from his semen. The processing of mercury is sometimes referred to as *dülwa* (*'dul ba*). *Dülwa* means 'subjugation' – a very important concept in Tibetan Buddhism, by which the wild and virile is pacified or domesticated. The term is also used to denote monastic discipline (Drungtso and Drungtso 2005: 109, 214).

One might expect that a substance containing mercury, purified using largely secret, religious and alchemical procedures would be a prime target for the PRC's drug regulations. It is difficult to reconcile with the scientific epistemology on which GMP, the Drugs Administration Law and the *Chinese Pharmacopoeia* claim to rely. In a biomedical context, the use of mercury, purified or not, is hardly justifiable, as it is seen as dangerous contaminant. On a production line where medicines containing mercury are produced it is practically impossible to guarantee that there will be no traces of mercury in all the other medicines that do not contain it as an ingredient.

However, the Chinese regulations do not touch on the preparation of *tsothal* at all. Although the *Pharmacopoeia* lists 'atomic absorption spectrophotometry' as the method of choice to determine mercury (SPC 2005: A35, A54–56) in traditional medicinal substances, there is no reference to this method in the monographs of the *rinchen rilbu* in question. *Tsothal* is not even listed as an ingredient in the monographs of Ratna Samphel (*qishiwei zhenzhu* in Chinese), Rinchen Drangjor (*renqing changjue*) and Rinchen Mangjor (*renqing mangjue*). The Ratna Samphel monograph, for example, mentions simply: 'Qishiwei Zhenzhu pills are a prescription used by the Tibetan Nationality, and prepared from Margarita, Lignum Santali Albi , Lignum Dalbergiae Odoriferae, Jiuyanshi, Stigma Croci, Calculus Bovis and Muschus, etc.' (ibid.: 584). As the monographs in the *Pharmacopoeia* usually list all ingredients including their composition, the omission of sixty-three out of seventy raw materials is remarkable. This omission is a result of the inclusion of all three *rinchen rilbu* mentioned above in the list of so-called 'national heritage drugs', meaning that these formulas are considered secret knowledge and only selected companies are legally entitled to produce them.[7]

Tsothal has also remained outside the scope of GMP. From the perspective of GMP *tsothal* is just another ingredient. However, since January 2008 the production of so-called 'prepared slices of Chinese crude drugs' also falls under GMP (*People's Daily* 2008). The term 'prepared slices' refers to cut, cleaned or processed ingredients used as intermediates in TCM. Arguably, *tsothal* is such a prepared slice. However, by the end of my research the rule had had no effect on the production of *tsothal*.

When I asked the director of production at one of the factories about *tsothal* and GMP, he answered: 'It's a secret. The authorities do not know that Ratna Samphel contains *tsothal*'. Contrary to this claim, *tsothal* does have at least some kind of official existence. In 1988 the Lhasa Mentsikhang applied for a patent filed as 'Method for Processing Traditional Tibetan Medicine (Zuotai Powder)' (Gamaqupei 1990). The patent was granted by the State Council of the PRC in 1992. Furthermore, *tsothal* was also included in the first batch of items on the UNESCO inspired, Intangible Cultural Heritage list in 2006. In both cases mercury is explicitly mentioned.

Taken together, these strands reveal a remarkable picture: on the one hand, *tsothal* is officially acknowledged as a part of Tibetan cultural heritage, to which each and every Tibetan should have a right; on the other hand, *tsothal* is covered by one company's patent. Regardless of both, the right to produce *tsothal*-based *rinchen rilbu* is held not by one and not by all but by a limited number of companies. This, in turn, does not hinder the majority of excluded factories from continuing to manufacture the *rinchen rilbu* in question, so that in reality a variety of different brands is readily available in pharmacies throughout Tibet. Meanwhile, *tsothal* is on all counts in conflict with the proposed methods for fighting mercury contamination in traditional medicines, a fact that does not, however, hinder *tsothal*-based formulas driving the industry's success. And for all that, the practice of making *tsothal*, so far untouched by government interference, has become an important marker of the industry's Tibetanness.

In terms of complex pre-processing methods, exemplified by *tsothal*, there is clearly a conflict between the rationalities found in traditional texts and China's drug regulations. When it comes to ritual and alchemy, the Buddhist epistemology on which Sowa Rigpa is based clearly contradicts the scientific epistemology in which the drug regulations are embedded. The clash of rationalities and epistemologies, however, does not translate into a confrontation at the level of practice, and the making of *tsothal* has not (or not yet) been affected.

Grinding, Mixing and Making Pills

Comparing industrial to manual manufacturing, the grinding of raw materials is certainly the step of production that has seen the biggest change. Before mechanical grinders were introduced, ingredients were crushed with a pestle in a stone mortar and then sieved. The remains were crushed and sieved again and the whole procedure was repeated until all ingredients were finely pulverised. The resulting powder was checked with the tongue in order to ensure that no solid pieces remained. 'If it feels like eating mud then it is acceptable for use in medicines', Shongpalhachu's founder Pema Gyatso explained to me.

Everyone who has witnessed the drudgery this procedure involves will agree that mechanical grinding has made the production of Tibetan medicines infinitely easier. In fact, large-scale production of Tibetan medicines could not be imagined without mechanical grinding. However, as noted in the previous chapter, mechanical grinding was introduced long before GMP, and the new regulations therefore cannot be regarded as responsible for mechanisation as such.

The relevant Chinese regulations for grinding are found in Appendix I of the *Chinese Pharmacopoeia*, where it is simply stated that 'watered pills are made of [a] fine powder of crude drugs using water … as [a] binder' (SPC 2005: Annex I, A5). What fine powder means is further elaborated in Appendix XIb, Method 2, where a 'double particle size sieve method' is stipulated rather than the use of the tongue. GMP itself does not say anything specific about grinding at all. The Chinese GMP (Kuwahara and Li 2007: 83–90) lists several general provisions for equipment, stating for example that surfaces of machines should be easy to clean and corrosion resistant, lubricants should not come in contact with the medical materials, and equipment should be easy to operate and maintain. Annex VII of the GMP mentions that dust-collection facilities 'shall be provided where needed' (ibid.: 255). The mills I have seen in non-GMP factories would probably not meet these criteria, especially in terms of dust collection and easy-to-clean surfaces. When the GMP factories were built they were usually equipped with new grinders. The question is, therefore, how these new grinders compare with the ones they replaced.

Palden Dorji, an *amchi* who both runs a private clinic and also works as an employee responsible for grinding in one of the major factories, was quite explicit in his assessment of the new machines: 'Grinding has improved. Before we had this grinding and sieving process [older machines required sieving after grinding]. But sometimes this was not so good, the mixture was less perfect. In addition, [with the old machines] we had to grind one medicine six times. Now all the medicines, except for one, need to be ground only once'. Although Palden Dorji shared the opinion of the majority of Tibetans that GMP had generally not increased the quality of medicines, he insisted that as far as grinding was concerned things had definitely improved.

The difference between grinding in a GMP production line and an older, non-GMP factory is indeed striking. In the Men-Tsee-Khang factory in Dharamsala, two older generations of mills are still in use. The newer one is considered to be better than the older one, but both create an enormous amount of noise and dust, and need to run almost permanently in order to keep up with the production volume. The dust collection facilities, closed designs and much quicker operation of the mills used in GMP factories certainly make for much better working conditions.

Palden Dorji's account ties in with Rinchen Wangdu's observation that the grinder they had been using before GMP did not produce such fine powder. Contrary to Palden Dorji's assessment, however, Rinchen Wangdu (the retired manager with a sharp analytic mind) was of the opinion that this was not necessarily a good thing. The perceived loss in the quality of the medicines produced under GMP might well be associated with this, he reflected. Moreover, the newer machines would grind much faster and the ingredients were getting very hot, which might also be problematic, he added.

Rinchen Wangdu was not alone in his assessment. One of the GMP-certified factories I visited went back to secretly using the old grinding equipment, lacking dust collection and closed designs, because of a perceived advantage over the new GMP-compliant grinder they had purchased. In addition, Cheezheng, the biggest Tibetan medicine company, was working on a new design for a mill that would again grind more slowly and thereby keep the temperature low. But as with all the changes that came with GMP, the effect of faster and finer grinding was never evaluated, never 'validated' in GMP parlance. It is therefore impossible to single out which changes in production had which effect.

Sienna Craig highlights another concern her interlocutors voiced during GMP introduction, namely that GMP stipulates separate grinding of all ingredients as opposed to the traditional way of combining the ingredients of one formula before grinding them to powder (Craig 2006: 206). This concern, however, turned out to be a misconception. GMP does not demand separate grinding. In fact, monographs in the *Tibetan Drug Standards* and the *Chinese Pharmacopoeia* specifically mention that all ingredients should be ground together, with the exception of some precious substances like musk and saffron. These provisions are in line with well-established traditional practices, and all the factories I have visited seem to follow them. Nevertheless, the initial fear that GMP would require separate grinding is an indicator of the general uncertainty about the complex regulations and their interpretation that surrounded their coming into force.

In summary, we can say that GMP brought more gradual than radical changes in terms of grinding, mostly because mechanical mills had been in use long before the factories were rebuilt between 2002 and 2004. The gradual changes that came with new machines are appraised differently by people in the industry.

However, compared to the 'golden age' of manual production, grinding has changed profoundly. Consequently, the criticism voiced with regard to grinding was mostly aimed at mechanised production as such and not the introduction of GMP. Pema Gyatso elucidated what he believed the problems were:

> There is no comparison between the modern machines and using stone grinders to grind and mix. The main thing that affects quality is ... for example, if *rinchen rilbu* get in contact with iron, their efficacy will be lost or damaged. Therefore when we produce *rilkar* [one of the precious pills]

in our factory, we use a special grinder. The lower part of the grinder is
made of stone and the upper part of marble.

In fact, such grinders — modelled after the traditional mortar-
and-pestle system, usually with mortars made of stone and three
mechanised pestles featuring marble heads — can be seen in several
factories. However, these machines are used only for special ingredients, and most herbs are ground in conventional mills made of
stainless steel.

Whether stainless steel is to be considered a form of 'iron' remains
an open question. Generally, the view that stainless steel is not the
same as deprecated iron and therefore not directly in contradiction
with traditional ways seems to prevail among the doctors and factory
personnel I talked to. When I asked a senior pharmacist at the Men-
Tsee-Khang factory in Dharamsala, usually a guide to traditional
ways of production, what his view on the topic was, he answered,
'Probably there is not much difference in terms of quality [between
stone and stainless steel]'. In this sense, the Gyüshi's warning against
iron and the GMP requirement of corrosion-resistant materials can
also be seen as aimed at achieving the same goal.

After grinding, the powder has to be mixed in order to guarantee
complete homogeneity. As with grinding, mixing was mechanised before GMP was introduced, and the differences between old and new
equipment are not especially revolutionary. Depending on the size
of the factory, different styles of mixers are used and they all seem
to work just fine.[8] The ground and mixed powder is finally used to
make pills. Most commonly, an open, rotating barrel made of stainless steel is used to this end. Small amounts of water and powder are
added by turns until the powder clumps and small 'seed' pills start to
form. Slowly, these 'seed' pills grow though adding water and powder
in increasing amounts. When the desired proportion is reached, the
pills are taken out of the barrel and sorted according to size. This is
achieved with two vibrating sieves, an upper and a lower one. The
pills that pass through the upper sieve but not the lower one have
the correct size. The pills that are too small fall through both sieves
and are again put into the barrel to be made bigger. Those too big to
pass through either of the sieves are usually ground again or simply
dissolved in water and rolled once more into pills.

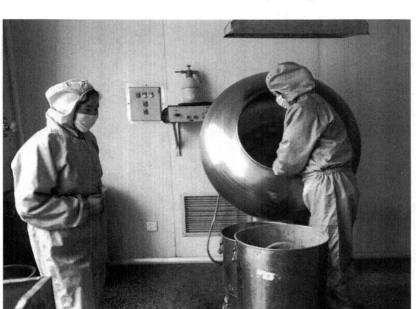

Figure 3.3: Making pills.

This technique is used in GMP and non-GMP factories without notable differences. Nevertheless, certain provisions put forward by GMP and the *Chinese Pharmacopoeia* relate to the process of making pills. Tolerable weight variation, for example, is defined as plus or minus 9 per cent, and the time span between ingestion and complete disintegration in the stomach, the so-called maximal disintegration time, is specified as one hour. However, some of the Tibetan compounds listed in the *Chinese Pharmacopoeia* are exempt from the latter (SPC 2005: A5–6).

Furthermore, the *Pharmacopoeia* monographs define both the weight and size of pills. This is sometimes at odds with traditional ways. Tenpa Wangchuk explained how Shongpalhachu's Chumar 70, their most important product, was affected by these regulations:

> In 1996, our Chumar 70 was about this size [he spread his fingers] and its weight was 1.5 grams … This Chumar 70 was effective, good and famous … But after the introduction of GMP it was stated that the size of Chumar 70 should be one gram only and so it lost its original weight. Still we have

the old Chumar 70. [The] taste and smell of these bigger pills are much stronger and they are much more effective than today's Chumar 70.

The standardisation of pill sizes is more an outcome of a general trend towards standardisation than the result of scientific scrutiny. It cannot be explained by the rationales on which GMP and its associated regulations are based.

In spite of these issues, grinding, mixing and making pills are not seen as the main problems associated with GMP production. While on a conceptual level conflicts such as 'stone' versus 'iron' may exist between traditional texts and new regulations, in practice Tibetan pharmacists and doctors judge them in different ways and seldom see them as critical. As grinding, mixing, and making pills underwent mechanisation before GMP was introduced, the transition to GMP-compliant equipment implied more gradual than radical changes.

Sterilisation

Traditionally, grinding and mixing were directly followed by making pills. All the GMP factories I have visited, however, featured large industrial microwaves guarding the entry points through which the powdered ingredients were brought into the clean area of the factory – allegedly to sterilise them.

This in itself is a remarkable enterprise. The natural ingredients on which Tibetan medicine relies, the herbs endowed with the potencies of a pure, unspoilt, high-altitude environment (as it is frequently referred to in advertising) are suddenly seen as potential sources of contamination. Whereas people have to don special clothes, wear face masks and carefully wash their hands, herbs need to undergo microwave treatment before they qualify for access to the clean production areas.

Most people in the industry see the use of microwaves as potentially harmful to the potency and quality of raw materials. One of the bigger and better equipped factories carried out a validation study on the efficacy of microwave ovens. The study showed that the ovens' ability to kill bacteria and other germs was rather limited. It also showed, however, that micro-organisms were generally not a problem for Tibetan medicine factories on the Tibetan Plateau. By contrast, to the best of my knowledge, no studies have so far been carried out to test the idea that microwave treatment does not harm the potency of the ingredients.

One might suspect that microwave sterilisation is a GMP requirement, but as a matter of fact it is nowhere mentioned. GMP's lapidary comment is simply that 'sterilization of Chinese crude drugs, intermediates, and finished products shall not affect their quality' (Kuwahara and Li 2007: Annex VII, Article 19). The *Pharmacopoeia* (SPC 2005) offers some more guidance. Annex XVI lists methods for removing 'viable micro-organisms'. The proposed methods are steam sterilisation, dry-heat sterilisation, ionising radiation [*sic!*], gas sterilisation and filtration. Remarkably, using microwaves is not listed among the methods and is also not mentioned as an option under dry-heat sterilisation. Despite my repeated attempts to find out what regulation microwave ovens were based on I never found an answer. The most plausible explanation seems to me that they fall within the realm of interpretation by the SFDA.

The microwave ovens I have seen in different factories have much in common: it is usually the same model made by the same company that is used (the JWYM2 by San Li), and all the devices look spotlessly clean and brand new. During a site visit with one of the vice-directors of a smaller company I asked him how the machine was used and what all the knobs and buttons (labelled in Chinese) were for. 'I have no idea', he answered. 'We never use it'. In fact, several managers of different factories told me with astonishing frankness that their microwave ovens were only there to satisfy the inspectors and that is was better not to use them, as they would harm the potency of medicines.

The history of these ovens remains elusive: the regulations which allegedly made them a requirement cannot be found and their function as guardians of the factories' inner realms is simply ignored. As neither the Gyüshi and its commentaries nor the current drug regulations refer to using microwaves, one cannot speak of an incompatibility on the textual, conceptual level. As in reality they are simply ignored, neither does a real conflict exist at the level of practice.

Well-cleaned but otherwise neglected, the microwave ovens are reminders of schemes and plans that were never really thought through – a fate they share with other expensive machinery, ranging from a fully automatic blister packaging machine I saw in one factory to chromatography devices in the laboratory of another. But these unused machines not only stand for failures in planning. They also mark the considerable leeway between regulations and the choices factories make in the absence of permanent control. What some may see as incomplete implementation others may judge as a means of following traditional, more Tibetan, ways.

Drying

Because pills are made with water they need to be dried. Pills, just like herbs, have cooling or warming properties and should be dried accordingly: warming pills in the sun (or near a fire) and cooling pills in the shade. The complaint most often heard in relation to GMP is that all pills, irrespective of their cooling or warming properties, have to be dried indoors with hot air in an electric dryer. These electric dryers, which look like industrial pizza ovens, are said to be responsible for a considerable part of the perceived loss of quality associated with GMP production. This is especially true for the cooling medicines, which should not be exposed to heat.

Basic regulations about the drying of watered pills can be found in Annex I of the *Chinese Pharmacopoeia* (SPC 2005: A5-6). Here, the maximum moisture content of watered pills is defined as 9 per cent. In addition, maximum drying temperatures of 80°C and 60°C for normal watered pills and pills with 'high amounts of volatile constituents' are stipulated respectively. An exception is made for 'thermolabile pills', which should be dried 'with other proper methods'. However, Tibetan pills are apparently not considered to be 'thermolabile', despite Tibetan claims to the contrary, and therefore the standard drying procedures apply.

There is no article in the GMP that directly opposes the traditional distinction between drying in the sun and drying in the shade. On the contrary, one could argue that a guiding principle of GMP is that no step of production should in any way affect the quality or potency of the product. But indirectly there are several GMP requirements that make outdoor drying impossible. Article 23, for instance, stipulates that the air used for drying 'shall be filtered to comply with the requirements for production', and the rules for factory design would make it difficult to justify pills being taken out of a factory's clean area in order to be dried. The ban on outdoor drying is therefore a side-effect of GMP – a side-effect that is arguably in contradiction with fundamental principles of GMP itself.

Now, drying indoors or outdoors is not the same as drying in the sun or in the shade. For the drying of hot medicines one could argue that

an electrical dryer is a close enough equivalent to the method of drying 'near a fire' proposed in the Seven Limbs. As a matter of fact, most
people I talked to see fewer problems with the drying of hot medicines
in electrical dryers. But still, depending on the model of dryer and the
mode of operation, it is considered to be less than ideal.

A possible solution would be to build an indoor sun-drying facility
with a glass roof. I have seen one factory that features such a facility;
but rather than for pills, it is used for the drying of ingredients after
they have been washed and cleaned. As the climate inside this facility was fairly damp and hot, I can fully understand that it is not an
adequate substitute for the Tibetan Plateau's intense sun and dry air.

The drying of pills with cooling properties, on the other hand,
raises different questions. The appropriate traditional method of drying them in the shade is mostly done indoors anyway. There seems
to be no obstacle to building GMP-compliant indoor drying facilities
where pills are dried slowly with cool, filtered air, fully in line with
the traditional ways outlined in the Gyüshi. Indeed, a few companies
have constructed such facilities and successfully certified them. But
the vast majority of factories lack such indoor drying facilities and
therefore all pills are dried with hot air in electric driers.

Drying is also mentioned in the official *Pharmacopoeia*. We learn
that 'drying in the shade' is actually an official requirement for several of the sixteen Tibetan formulas listed. Of course, what 'shade'
means is again subject to interpretation by the SFDA; but arguably, the absence of direct sunlight in an electric drier is not enough
to meet the condition. Nevertheless, I have not heard of any case
where an SFDA inspector found fault with the absence of a cold
drying room. All the factories without such a facility passed GMP
certification successfully, regardless of whether they produced one
of the formulas that officially require 'drying in the shade'.

Remarkably, the single most common complaint about the harm
GMP does to Tibetan medicine could as well be interpreted as a vio-
lation of current regulations. Obviously, there is room for interpretation and some regulations seem to be considered more important
than others. But the question still remains: why do most factories
not use indoor drying rooms? The answer, I argue, is simple: because they were not part of the design for GMP plants. The quick
and forced introduction of GMP did not leave the companies time
to gain experience and carefully evaluate the new equipment. The

new factories had to be certified quickly, and once the production lines were built, architectural changes were practically impossible to realise. The lack of indoor drying facilities is therefore a side effect of the rapid way GMP was introduced rather than a result of GMP rationality being in conflict with traditional Sowa Rigpa.

In the light of these major concerns about electric drying I was surprised to learn that the Men-Tsee-Khang in Dharamsala, known for its adherence to traditional ways, has recently bought such a dryer, more precisely a 'solar dryer'. The machine is based on the same principle as conventional electrical dryers: heat and ventilation. But given that the sun is shining, the heat is produced by a solar thermal collector on the roof. If there is no sun, it operates as a conventional electric dryer. The Men-Tsee-Khang's purchase of a dryer and other measures such as the construction of cold storage rooms have to be seen in relation to Dharamsala's climatic conditions. Being located on the south side of the Himalayas, Dharamsala gets heavy and long monsoon rains and is generally much more humid than the arid Tibetan Plateau. Dharamsala's weather rather than imposed government regulations being the main motivation behind the purchase, the dryer was never seen as a threat to the quality of medicines – quite the opposite, as the Men-Tsee-Khang's newsletter proudly announced: 'With this system in use Men-Tsee-Khang envisions the safer production of medicinal pills especially during the long rainy season in Dharamsala. This system will speed up the drying process and eventually leave no chance for fungal and moisture growths in the medicines' (Men-Tsee-Khang 2006).

One might suspect that by installing a 'solar dryer' instead of a conventional electric one it was easier to present the introduction of new technology as perfectly in line with traditional methods of production. But the reasons for relying on solar energy as much as possible is more pragmatic. The Men-Tsee-Khang simply cannot draw enough power from the local grid to operate the dryer's two chambers at once. Above that, the operating costs of a solar dryer were lower. The local shortage of power also triggered an unexpected innovation. Early tests with the new machine showed mixed results, especially with pills containing sticky substances, such as pomegranate seeds (*Punica granatum*), known in Tibetan as *setru* (*se 'bru*). Mixed results and a chronic power shortage prompted the idea of running the machine's ventilation system without the heating element so that the pills were dried 'cold'.

This cold drying mode yielded very good results and became standard practice for some of the formulas. Besides, the Men-Tsee-Khang generally used lower drying temperatures compared to the factories I visited in Tibet; a maximum of about 45 degrees Celsius was used, compared to 60 to 70 degrees in Tibet.

This being said, there is also considerable variation among the factories in Tibet in terms of drying procedures. Some factories claim to use the same temperature for all pills. As the different formulas contain different ingredients and some dry faster than others, different drying times are used to meet the 9 per cent moisture limit. Other factories claim to use different temperatures depending on the pills. At least one factory, I was told, faced the problem that the pills on the upper shelves in the drying chamber dried much quicker than those on the lower shelves, and as a consequence they had to raise the temperature. The director of another factory explained to me that they tried to reproduce natural climatic patterns, alternating hot with cold phases and adding more or less 'wind' at different times. Yet another factory relied on heating the dryer for thirty minutes and letting it slowly cool down again, which they did three times in all. All this variation is in accordance with the current regulations, which only stipulate a 9 per cent moisture limit but no detailed procedures, intervals or temperatures (except for the maximums given above).

All in all, the practice of drying pills underwent a tremendous change with the introduction of GMP. Before, pills were mainly dried outside in the sun or in well aired indoor drying rooms. Now, the majority of pills are dried in electric dryers. But as was the case with the production steps discussed above, the regulations themselves can hardly be blamed. It is not GMP and its associated regulations as such but the tight schedule, the actual process of implementation, and the socio-political circumstances in which it took place that are responsible for the current discontent. The GMP manufacturing plants were quickly constructed between 2002 and 2004. The architectural decisions taken then, such as the absence of cold drying rooms, now make it difficult to follow both established traditional best practices and current regulations at the same time.

Remarkably, the same equipment facing so much criticism in Tibet is seen as a blessing in Dharamsala, partly because it is operated at lower temperatures, and partly because the reasoning and circumstances that led to its purchase were completely different.

Rationales, Practicalities

Is the sheep with a goat's head, the chimera evoked at the outset, just an illusion or is it reality? Is Sowa Rigpa as a system of knowledge really being superseded by GMP and its associated regulations? And does GMP really interfere with the traditional practices of producing Tibetan medicines?

The steps of production discussed above allow for a simple typology, which may serve as a first step towards an answer to these questions: a conflict may or may not exist either at the level of rationales or at the level of practices. Accordingly, four dispositions can be distinguished: (1) no conflict at all; (2) a conflict in practice but not between rationales; (3) a conflict between rationales but not at the level of practice; and (4) a conflict at both levels.

The sourcing and storage of raw materials as well as simple forms of pre-processing (washing, trimming, sorting, and so on) belong, by and large, to the first disposition: neither on a practical nor on a theoretical level is there a substantial conflict. The Gyüshi's Seven Limbs and the current drug regulations simply entail different vantage points. Neither do they contradict each other, nor do they cause friction at a practical level.

The drying of pills, the most heatedly discussed area of production, exemplifies the second disposition. Considering that GMP entails the philosophy that no step in production should in any way negatively affect the quality of the drugs, and that some official monographs even explicitly call for 'drying in the shade', there is no fundamental incompatibility at the level of concepts. However, there is a conflict at the level of practice. Most factories find themselves forced to operate according to procedures they consider to be wrong. Here, the side effects of GMP introduction are most evident.

The third disposition, a clash of rationales but no conflict at the practical level, is exemplified by the making and usage of *tsothal*. There is clearly antagonism between Sowa Rigpa and scientific epistemology with regard to the use of mercury, purified with alchemic procedures embedded in Buddhist ritual. Yet, there is no actual relevance to this antagonism in reality, as the practice of making *tsothal* has so far not been subjected to any kind of government control.

The microwave devices meant to sterilise ground ingredients may also be classified here. Whereas using microwaves mirrors the drug regulations' general concern for contamination, the microwave devices are largely ignored in practice and simply relegated to the role of pleasing the SFDA inspectors. The microwave devices, on the other hand, are also reminiscent of the first disposition, as using microwaves is absent in both traditional texts and current drug regulations. The use of microwaves is an outcome of the aura of scientific epistemology in which drug regulations are enshrouded, but not of the regulations themselves.

Remarkably, no step of production falls into the fourth disposition, which would entail both a conflict in practice and a conflict of underlying rationales. Conflicts on the level of rationales either do not extend to the realm of practice (*tsothal*) or else they are solved pragmatically (microwave ovens). The conflicts in practice, on the other hand, do not stem from conflicting rationales or epistemologies but rather from the side effects of the actual implementation of GMP.

This ties in with James Scott's hypothesis about well-intended modernist schemes that rely on *techne* rather than *mētis* (Scott 1998). His argument is that such schemes tend to fail because the thin simplifications of *techne* are just not good enough to capture complex realities. Scott describes *mētis* as contextual, practical knowledge while *techne* is universal:

> The universality of *techne* arises from the fact that it is organized analytically into small, explicit, logical steps and is both decomposable and verifiable … The rules of *techne* provide for theoretical knowledge that may or may not have practical applications. Finally, *techne* is characterized by impersonal, often quantitative precision and a concern with explanation and verification, whereas *mētis* is concerned with personal skill, or 'touch', and practical results. (ibid.: 320)

In principle, both GMP and Sowa Rigpa encompass at once abstract, universal knowledge in the sense of *techne* as well as the practical, localised knowledge of the *mētis* type. Just as Tibetan doctors will agree that the Gyüshi is organised analytically in small and logical steps, GMP specialists involved in large-scale production of synthetic drugs will confirm that GMP entails much practical knowledge and personal skill. However, the *mētis* of GMP production gained in the factory halls of 'Big Pharma' is not easily transferable to the context of Tibetan medicine. As a consequence, GMP arrived in Tibet almost purely as *techne*, as a global form to be recontextualised. Therefore, Scott's *mētis* and *techne* suggest themselves as descriptive labels for the different forms of knowledge encountered above.[9] Practices such as burying iron and *aru* for three years at a sheep shelter on the south slope of a mountain exemplifies the *mētis* type of knowledge; defining cleanliness classes by reference to the maximum permitted numbers of particles and micro-organisms per cubic metre of air clearly resonates with *techne*.

There are, however, also crucial differences between the present case and the failed schemes Scott describes, such as Soviet collectivisation, forced 'villigisation' in Tanzania, scientific forestry and agriculture and high-modernist cities. While the scope and speed of GMP introduction in Tibet indeed bears the marks of high-modernist planning fervour with little regard for any *mētis*, the style and content of GMP relies on corporate responsibility and continuous assessment. As argued in the Introduction, GMP implementation in Tibet is the child of two different visions of modernisation, two layers of modernity. The results are particularly apparent in two important principles of GMP's approach to quality control: validation and self-inspection.

Validation

The concept of validation (*yanzheng*) basically means that all planned changes in production require proactive testing in order to demonstrate that the changes have no negative effect on quality. Articles 57 to 60 of the Chinese GMP deal with validation (Kuwahara and Li 2007: 123, 127, 131). They stipulate that any modification to premises, equipment or operation requires a scientific validation study, which has to follow a written protocol defined in advance. The analytical results and the data of this study have to be documented, and a validation report needs to be produced and approved. Furthermore, revalidation is necessary whenever primary raw materials or production processes are altered.

The problem is that validation was simply ignored during the creation of the industry. To the best of my knowledge, no validation studies have ever been performed to justify the changes in production processes or equipment that accompanied GMP introduction and the construction of new factories. Neither electrical drying nor adjusting pill sizes, adopting microwave sterilisation or using newer and faster grinders were ever validated. The age of validation only started when the new factories had been built and successfully passed GMP certification. Once GMP was introduced and the factories were built, the new status quo became the base line from which any future change would require validation.

On a conceptual level GMP's validation requirement ties in with Tibetan medicine's traditionally cautious and at times downright conservative approach to change. Both take into account that even small changes in production can have unforeseen effects on the quality and efficacy of medicines. At the level of practice however, the two have not played well together. First, the traditional cautiousness had to be left behind during the transition to GMP while GMP's validation requirement was not yet in force. The changes resulting from this rapid transition were therefore moderated by neither Sowa Rigpa nor GMP. The speed and scope of GMP introduction precluded the regulations from being implemented according to their own content and spirit as well as Sowa Rigpa practitioner's traditional cautiousness. Second, the validation requirement ignores the way innovation used to take place in Sowa Rigpa. It thereby endangers one of Sowa Rigpa's major strengths, namely, its capacity for adaptation. Being practised from Mongolia to Nepal and from the Kalmyk Republic in Russia to Yunnan province in south-west China, Sowa Rigpa has proved to be capable of adapting itself to a variety of climatic and ecological conditions. In Buryatia, for example, the Russian borderlands north of Mongolia, over the course of two centuries more than 80 per cent of the original *materia medica* has been replaced with locally available herbs (Dashiyev 1999). This far-reaching but slow, step-by-step transformation was enabled by Sowa Rigpa's abstract and structured approach to pharmacy. In addition to being categorised as warming or cooling, an ingredient is also classified as possessing one of six tastes (*ro*) and one of eight potencies (*nus pa*).[10] This system of classification enables a Tibetan pharmacist to search for a suitable substitute possessing the same combination of taste and potency if a specific ingredient is not available (see Aumeeruddy-Thomas and Lama 2008: 172–75).

Faced with the looming scarcity of several medicinal plants, such substitution may well become important for Sowa Rigpa's survival in the future. Yet the validation requirement, together with the standardised formulas defined in the monographs and the centralised drug registration regime, now legally prohibit such adaptations. In this sense, it is fair to say that the introduction of GMP, which has been heralded as boosting the innovation of Sowa Rigpa, may become a major obstacle for innovation and adaptation to changing circumstances. This, however, depends on whether the validation requirement is strictly enforced. For the time being, it is not. Validation shares this fate with many other rules and regulations, looming and waiting to be applied one day.

This leads to the second crucial difference between the present case and Scott's high-modernist schemes, namely the party-state's flirtation with neoliberal governance and its effects in Tibet.

Self-inspection

The introduction of GMP and a national system of drug registration have to be seen against the background of a shift in government policy that went along with privatisation and the launching of a 'socialist market economy'. Gary Sigley argues that the party-state was fully aware that the new economic freedom it introduced would also require adaptations in the style of government, a process officially referred to as *zhengfu zhineng zhuanbian*, 'the changing function of government'. In this context a different kind of vocabulary emerged, emphasising 'management' (*guanli*), 'governance' (*zhili*) and 'autonomy' (*zizhi*) instead of 'planning' (*jihua*) and 'administration' (*xingzheng*) as the state's primary tasks (Sigley 2006: 496). This shift in vocabulary and outlook mirrors a similar tendency in the discourse of the World Bank, the WHO and other international organisations starting in the late 1980s, subsumed under the idiom of 'good governance'. As the party-state chose to rely on private initiative and entrepreneurship as the motor behind China's economic success it opted for less direct techniques of government in order to manage these dynamics.

With privatisation and the 'socialist market economy' the state has, in some respects, retreated from domains formerly managed and controlled directly. Yet, despite the emphasis on governance the party-state has not become weaker, Sigley maintains (2006); its power has simply transformed. Both Sigley (2006) and Lisa Hoffman (2006) argue that Foucault's notion of governmentality is worth revisiting against this background.[11] The term governmentality (*gou-*

vern-mentalité) captures Foucault's working hypothesis about the reciprocal link between power and knowledge. Power techniques, forms of governing, have to be understood in relation to the rationalities on which they are based, the mentalities or modes of knowledge (Lemke 2001: 191). Foucault introduced the concept in his 1978 lectures at the Collège de France to analyse the gradual transformation of the 'state of justice of the Middle Ages' to a modern 'administrative state', where the central focus of government turned towards managing populations, economies and territories (Foucault 1991: 102).

Both Sigley and Hoffman are well aware of the pitfalls that lie in an attempt to transpose a Foucauldian framework derived from the analysis of European history to contemporary events in the PRC – an endeavour that easily results in an 'artifice of history' (Chakrabarty 1992) where Europe remains at the conceptual heart of the analysis. Sigley cites Deng Xiaoping to make clear that an analysis of governance and governmentality in contemporary China is more than an academic artefact: the Chinese Communist Party elite has actively and consciously sought to 'learn from other countries, including the developed capitalist countries, all advanced methods of operation and techniques of management that reflect the laws governing modern socialized production' (Deng 1994, cited in Sigley 2006: 48).

In his 1979 lectures, Foucault used the concept of governmentality to scrutinise the rise of neoliberal rationality after the Second World War. He focused on the formation of neoliberal discourse (Lemke 2001: 192–200) and related it to a specific, complex and subtle form of power in a society where its members play an active role in their own self-government.

Foucauldian neoliberal governmentality clearly resonates with GMP. Articles 83 and 84 (Kuwahara and Li 2007: 211–12) of the Chinese GMP, for instance, stipulate that self-inspection should be regularly conducted and documented; Articles 80 to 82 (ibid.: 207–11) mandate the establishment of procedures for handling customer complaints and adverse reaction reports. Like most contemporary quality management systems, GMP does not rely on permanent external supervision but on an internalised, comprehensive philosophy of quality control. Whereas the existence of self-inspection reports and a system for handling complaints can be verified by SFDA inspectors, their content lies fully within the responsibility of companies. Therefore, GMP is not meant to prevent active attempts to circumvent it. The point is, however, that Tibetan scepticism against GMP (which will receive fuller treatment in Chapter 4) precludes a philosophy of quality control considered as foreign and unsuitable from being fully accepted and internalised. For the majority of the people I talked to, the ethically right thing to do is to circumvent GMP whenever necessary and feasible in order to make it comply with the traditional best practices of Sowa Rigpa.

In addition, it is important to mention that the shift in governmental style to forms of governance that emphasise management and autonomy instead of planning and control remains a partial one in the context of Tibet. Robert Barnett argues that public space may have become less susceptible to close supervision in inland China, especially in metropolitan areas such as Beijing, but not in Tibet (Barnett 2006a: 36). The shift from planning and control to management and governance has been less pronounced in the TAR than in inland China. On the one hand, there is a strong notion that Tibet is lagging behind, development needs to be accelerated and the recipes that proved to be successful in inland China should also be applied to Tibet. On the other hand, the security question often takes priority. A widespread mistrust of Tibetans – all Tibetans, including cadres and business people (Barnett 2001a) – has led to a situation in which policies related to the 'changing function of government' are not or not fully implemented once they arrive in Tibet.

In this context, GMP and its associated regulations have given rise to a legally grey area, a space of uncertainty but also one of leeway and opportunity, in which the loopholes are as important as the rules and regulations themselves. As we will see in the next chapter, this also applies to the sourcing of and trade in medicinal plants.

Notes

1. The following is an expanded version of an argument presented at the workshop of the Research Group on Body, Health, and Religion (BAHAR) in Cardiff in January 2011 and published in *Medical Anthropology* (Saxer 2012).
2. Immel (2000) argues that Upton Sinclair's famous novel *The Jungle* (Sinclair 1906) lies at the origins of GMP. Sinclair depicted the reality of early industrial meat production in the USA in such horrible detail that it caused

a public outcry. This outcry led to the Pure Food and Drug Act of 1906. The law can be seen as a direct predecessor to GMP.

3. When discussing *pharmacopoeia* monographs in this chapter I will concentrate on those included in the 2005 edition of the *Chinese Pharmacopoeia*. The highly criticised *Tibetan Drug Standards* published in 1995 follow an older, less detailed format. They also lack links to the various appendices of the *Chinese Pharmacopoeia*, which are binding law for Tibetan medicine as well.

4. At the time of my research, even the Men-Tsee-Khang in Dharamsala was looking into mechanised means of pre-processing in order to reduce employees' workloads and to free up capacity for other tasks. In December 2008, tests were being carried out on the prototype of a new machine that was supposed to filter out sand and little stones using strong vibrations and several different-sized sieves. It remains to be seen whether or not the Mentsikhang in Lhasa considers this prototype to be suitable for their own purposes.

5. *Tsothal* is not the only source of mercury in Tibetan medicines. Several formulas contain cinnabar *(mtshal)*, which is mercury sulphide in chemical terms. Mercury sulphide is considered to be relatively harmless. For a more detailed discussion about the different forms of mercury in precious pills, see Aschoff and Tashigang (1997).

6. This view is supported by a clinical study carried out at the Men-Tsee-Khang hospital in Dharamsala in cooperation with universities in Israel and the UK. It shows that the consumption of Tibetan medicines containing mercury does not lead to an accumulation of mercury in the human body. No signs of mercury poisoning were found among the patients who participated in the clinical trial (Sallon et al. 2007).

7. The list of 'national heritage drugs' also has noteworthy implications for the debate about intellectual property rights, which will be discussed in Chapter 5.

8. By contrast, the manual mixing of ground ingredients was attributed great importance in some Sowa Rigpa traditions. In Buryatia (Russia), for example, mixing is traditionally embedded in a Buddhist ritual that lasts several days and is considered to enhance the potency of the compound (Saxer 2005: 23). Against this background, mechanical mixing indeed implies a radical departure. During my research in Tibet, however, I never heard complaints about mechanical mixing.

9. Scott's usage of the terms *mētis* and *techne* follows Marta Nussbaum's (2001) and is markedly different from that of other authors. Stephen Marglin, for example, employs the term *techne* in much the same way as Scott uses *mētis*. Marglin contrasts *techne* with *episteme*, which is very similar to Scott's *techne* (Marglin 1990: 231–37). Marglin's usage is also closer to Foucault's, defining *techne* as practical rationality in relation to episteme, which denotes the (unconscious) structures underlying the production of knowledge (see Foucault 2005).

10. The six tastes are sweet *(mngar)*, sour *(skyur)*, salty *(lan tshwa)*, pungent/acrid *(tsha ba)*, bitter *(kha ba)* and astringent *(bska ba)*; the eight potencies

include heavy *(lci)*, light *(yang)*, oily *(snum)*, coarse *(rtsub)*, cool *(sil)*, hot *(tsha)*, blunt *(rtul)* and sharp *(rno ba)*. Furthermore, three post-digestive tastes and seventeen secondary properties are distinguished in Tibetan pharmacy. Taste and potency, however, are the most important when looking for a substitute.

11. That the party-state's power has not weakened can be seen in the light of Vivienne Shue's (1995) observation that in terms of size and complexity, the state apparatus (and especially local bureaucracy) was initially growing during the 1990s. Greater economic freedom coincided with a more active role in monitoring and regulating the burgeoning sector of private business. Shue speaks of 'state sprawl' and concludes that private trade 'has not been developed at the expense of local state power or authority – the two have been rising together' (ibid.: 101). However, with the more recent emphasis on a leaner and more efficient state, efforts are being made to downsize local government administration (Barnett 2006a: 53), as can be seen in the re-transferring of power from local authorities to the central SFDA.

✤ Chapter 4
Raw Materials, Refined

The sourcing of raw materials has become a major challenge for the Tibetan medicine industry. As the industry is still largely based on wild herbs, concerns over the sustainable use of medicinal plants are growing. Besides the issue of drying pills, ensuring steady supplies of raw materials in good and consistent qualities was often mentioned as increasingly difficult by doctors and factory staff.

With soaring output, the factories have come to rely more and more on commercial harvesters and traders to secure their supplies. The more commercial traders and middlemen are involved and the longer supply chains get, the less control factories have over the origin, time of harvesting and overall quality of herbs. In order to ensure the orderly transition from a product of nature to a medical raw material, as required for the production of standard, quality-controlled formulas according to China's drug regulations, the unruliness of the wild is being tackled in new ways. However, at the intersection of ecological concerns and commercial trade, Sowa Rigpa's relation to nature is being reconfigured.

In this chapter I look at factories' strategies for dealing with the problem of sourcing, namely, their efforts at cultivating medicinal herbs and at establishing direct relations with village-based plant collectors. Both strategies have their limits, as we will see. Moreover, many raw materials used in Tibetan medicine are not native to Tibet, and herbs imported from India and Nepal constitute a considerable part of Sowa Rigpa's *materia medica*. Therefore, cross-border trade is essential for the industry. Based on a journey I undertook with a commercial trader to buy herbs in Nepal, the second part of this chapter provides a discussion of recent changes in import regulations, the dilemmas they created and the pragmatic ways in which a trader deals with them.

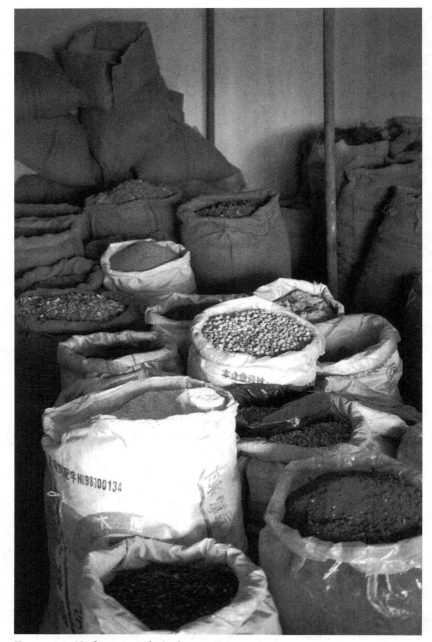

Figure 4.1: Herbs in a trader's shop in Xining.

Domestic Sourcing Strategies

We saw in the last chapter that *amchi* and factory managers generally regard commercially traded herbs as inferior to those collected in the traditional way following the procedures described in the Gyüshi's Seven Limbs. Before GMP was introduced and the industry's output started soaring, most of the producers of Tibetan medicines tried to follow the second limb's suggestion: they relied, at least to some extent, on summer expeditions of their own staff or students to collect herbs in the nearby mountains. These expeditions were usually guided by an experienced *amchi*.

A second popular way to get good quality herbs, especially for the larger producers, was to trade medicinal plants for ready-made pills with Tibetan doctors coming from rural areas (cf. Hofer 2009a: 190). Nowadays, however, most factories buy from commercial traders. The consequences of this are well summarised in the following quote by a senior Tibetan doctor: 'If you buy from traders you don't know whether [the herbs] have been collected at the right time or not. When they are not collected at the right time, then the quality is affected. Nowadays, whenever something is found, it is picked'. In addition, commercial harvesting is made responsible for over-exploitation. Several herbs have already become difficult to find, prices are generally increasing, and most people I talked to expressed deep worries about the situation. The availability and quality of medicinal herbs is a major concern for the Tibetan medicine industry. Again, Rinchen Wangdu's view stands for that of many others: 'Recently, we started to introduce Tibetan medicine to the Chinese market and the whole world. That means we have all these additional factories and we have to produce a lot to meet the demands from domestic and international markets ... If we continue like this ... [then] in less than ten years we will be running out of herbs'.

Several well-known herbs used in Tibetan medicine feature prominently on lists of endangered species. *Üpal ngönpo* ('*ut pal sngon po*, a *Meconopsis* species known as blue Himalayan poppy) is among them, as well as *bongkar* (*bong dkar, Aconitum heterophyllum*), *solomarpo* (*sro lo dmar po, Rhodiola crenulata*), *gangachung* (*gang ga chung, Gentiana urnula*), *sumchu tigta* (*sum chu tig ta, Saxifraga* sp.) and *pangpö* (*spang spos, Nardostachys grandiflora/jatamansi*, Spikenard). Nevertheless, it is extremely difficult to assess the extent to which these plants are really facing extinction due to the industry's rocketing demand.

A case in point is *üpal ngönpo*, the blue Himalayan poppy, usually the first example mentioned by my interlocutors when I asked which plant they considered to be the most endangered. Despite this, 2009 was apparently a very good year for *üpal ngönpo*, at least in some areas in Central Tibet. In one of the factories in the TAR I witnessed a considerable quantity of newly harvested Himalayan poppy, which had just been purchased from traders and had originated from the area around Tingri. As the plants had been bought fresh, the company resorted to drying them on the floor of an unused part of the factory – an unusual sight in the clean area of a GMP-certified manufacturing plant. The herbs were worth 200,000 yuan ($29,000), I was told proudly.

At a general level, there is ample evidence from several studies carried out in other parts of the Himalayas that commercial trade has an influence on harvesting patterns (see Olsen and Larsen 2003; Larsen and Smith 2004; Ghimire, McKey and Aumeeruddy-Thomas 2005a, 2005b). Ghimire, McKey and Aumeeruddy-Thomas (2005a) have shown, for example, that *amchi* possess more knowledge about plants than commercial collectors, and that their knowledge expands in a certain way into the communities in which they live. The authors argue that this knowledge translates to harvesting patterns, whereby *amchi* follow a much more selective approach than commercial collectors. The authors' claims are based on a field study in Shey Phoksundo National Park and in its buffer zone in Dolpo, north-west Nepal. One of the herbs investigated is *pangpö* (*Nardostachys grandiflora*). The plant is listed in Appendix II of the Convention on International Trade in Endangered Species of Wild Fauna and Flora (CITES), which both Nepal and China have signed (Dutta and Jain 2000: 52–54).

Nevertheless, the species is actively traded and contributes substantially to household incomes. Whereas in Shey Phoksundo National Park only the *amchi* collect, commercial collection is also taking place in the bordering buffer zone. The researchers found that harvesting levels were different in the national park from those in the buffer zone, and that harvesting patterns also varied considerably. *Amchi* harvest in September and October at the end of the growing period and they only take the rhizomes from mature plants, which are considered to be medically more potent. Commercial collectors work around the year and collect rhizomes from any specimen they can find.

This difference in harvesting patterns is significant because germination rates of perennial plants at high altitudes tend to be very low. The maturation and survival of adult plants is therefore crucial for maintaining population levels. As indiscriminate commercial harvesting techniques are more likely to target these plants at vulnerable stages of their life cycle, such techniques decrease their population density much more than the traditional harvesting patterns employed by *amchi* (Ghimire, McKey and Aumeeruddy-Thomas 2005a). When a certain species becomes harder to find a vicious circle starts, as Rinchen Wangdu explains: 'Today, since the scarcity of these herbs has become evident, people have to rush to get ... even low quality herbs. They have to fight to get them. This society and all the people, they are never thinking about future generations, just about profit and benefit. They don't have any kind of longer perspective'.

Ghimire, McKey and Aumeeruddy-Thomas's argument and Rinchen Wandu's remarks tie in with a complaint I frequently encountered about commercial harvesting techniques of *bongkar* (*bong dkar*), an aconite most commonly identified with *Aconitum heterophyllum*. *Bongkar* is also a perennial high-altitude plant. It features two tubers and traditionally only one of them is harvested. This ensures the plant's survival. Commercial harvesters, however, are said to collect both tubers. This was repeatedly given as the reason for the sharp decrease in *bongkar* populations to the extent that the herb has become difficult to find in areas where it was abundant a mere decade ago. Its decreasing population density has inevitably also led to an increase in price. In 2007, 1 kilogram of *bongkar* cost around 1,000 Nepalese rupees in Kathmandu ($14). By March 2008, the price had doubled to 2,000 rupees, although it went down again to about 1,700 rupees in November 2008 after the new harvest came in. A Tibetan trader from Kathmandu told me that the *bongkar* he was getting was inferior to the one he used to see a couple of years ago. Now, he often received the whole plants, including stems and both tubers.

Harvesting patterns even have the potency to alter the phenotype of plants themselves. Ethnobotanist Jan Salick and her team carried out a research project on Himalayan snow lotus or *gangla metog* (*gangs lha me tog, Saussurea laniceps*) in the Khawa Karpo area of Yunnan. Comparing the current size of plants with herbarium specimens collected in the region since 1872, they found a significant decline in size over time. As plant collectors prefer bigger specimens, the smaller plants have a higher chance of survival and the population of snow lotus has adapted to continuous harvesting pressure. In the vicinities of Khawa Karpo, which are considered sacred and where traditionally no commercial collection took place, no such 'human-induced dwarfing' was found (Law and Salick 2005: 10219).

Long-term Relations with Village Collectors

As mentioned above, the producers of Tibetan medicine have ambivalent relationships with commercial traders. The factories rely on them but they are fully aware that their control over collection, drying, storage and transportation is limited. As a result, factories are looking for more direct access to herbs whenever possible. One approach to this is to foster direct and long-term relations with private herb gatherers, village cooperatives and small village traders. With such arrangements, defined quantities of specific herbs can be ordered, collection is carried out on demand, and big commercial traders are largely circumvented.

Ties to family and hometown are often used to establish and maintain such arrangements. If an employee responsible for buying raw materials or an *amchi* working at a factory is from a region with abundant medicinal herbs, their first choice is to rely on their own social network. The closer and better the contacts are, the more reliable the quality of the herbs will be. In addition, the prices paid in such arrangements are comparatively low because there is little or no intermediate trade involved.[1] Collecting herbs has remained a low-income occupation in Tibet, despite soaring demand and generally increasing prices. A manager responsible for purchasing herbs in one of the smaller factories complained that people in her home town had become reluctant to engage in medicinal plant collection; rising standards of living rendered the drudgery of climbing mountains and gathering herbs increasingly unattractive.

Indeed, in places where other sources of cash income are available, medicinal herbs are usually left untouched. A friend of mine, who had been my research assistant for a while and knew about medicinal herbs because his grandfather had been an *amchi*, kept repeating that many of the herbs frequently mentioned as almost extinct or increasingly difficult to find in Central Tibet were still abundant in his village. Nobody would pick them, nobody was interested, because the area was known for *yartsagunbu* (*dbyar rtswa dgun 'bu*, *Ophiocordyceps sinensis*), the caterpillar fungus famous as a general tonic and said to possess a virility-boosting effect. Picking *yartsagunbu* is also hard work but it is much more profitable than collecting other medicinal herbs. In a good season, which lasts for only six weeks in April and May, my friend would make up to 70,000 yuan ($10,000) harvesting *yartsagunbu*.

Daniel Winkler estimated that around fifty tons of *yartsagunbu* were collected in the TAR in 2004, amounting to a staggering 1.8 billion yuan ($263 million) or 8.5 per cent of the TAR's total GDP – more than mining and industry together. The role of *yartsagunbu* can hardly be overestimated. It is often by far the most important source of rural cash income today. In prime production areas the fungus accounts for 70 to 90 per cent of local income. Between 1997 and mid 2008 the value of *yartsagunbu* increased nine fold; in 2004 the best quality was sold in Shanghai for up to $32,000 per kilogram (Winkler 2008a, 2008b: 291, 2010). Where *yartsagunbu* is found the collection of other medicinal herbs is simply not worth the effort by comparison. It is probably not far off the mark to claim that the *yartsagunbu* boom has basically excluded large areas of the Tibetan Plateau as potential collection sites for other medicinal herbs.

Competition from other sources of income can also be observed in the Solu Khumbu region in Nepal. According to an *amchi* running a clinic in Namche Bazaar the region was blessed with abundant medicinal herbs of excellent quality. People in Solu Khumbu took no notice of the herbs, he said, as they were only interested in tourists. One would rather sell Coca-Cola to a thirsty trekker on his way up to the Everest base camp than climb up the mountains to look for medicinal plants.

On the other hand, regions with no other sources of cash income heavily rely on the collection of medicinal plants. A friend of mine from the farming region around Gyantse (TAR) told me that the 2,000 to 3,000 yuan per year made from the collection of medicinal herbs were crucial for the livelihood of his family. For comparison: when his father offered his services as a day labourer, he was paid just 7 yuan per day.

In summary, we can see that the collection of medicinal plants for Tibetan medicine is not only a question of availability. Collection is directly linked to local economies and livelihoods. If there are other, more profitable options, people tend to opt out.

In the absence of comprehensive and reliable data on medicinal plant populations on the Tibetan Plateau – an impossible task in view of the sheer size of the area – it is difficult to say whether complaints about the scarcity of a specific plant are really an indication that it is actually endangered. It might well be that the balance between the drudgery of collection (which quickly increases when a species gets rarer) and the expected revenue has changed. Areas blessed with quick money from tourism or *yartsagunbu* might still feature vast populations of otherwise rare medicinal plants. While tourism and *yartsagunbu* collection are often blamed as a threat to the fragile ecology of the Tibetan Plateau, they might also turn out to be a boon to the survival of certain medicinal plant species.

Competition from other sectors of income is a problem for both the factories and commercial herb traders. The latter also get their supplies from villages, sometimes directly and sometimes through one or several intermediate traders. Moreover, the model of direct relations between villages and factories only works for raw materials found inside Tibet and in areas where one has established relations of trust. The imported herbs pose a different set of problems, as we will see later.

Cultivation

The second obvious strategy to regain better control over the quality of medicinal plants is to cultivate them instead of relying on wild-grown supplies. Cultivation features prominently in most factory brochures and has been high on the state's agenda (SFDA 2001: Article 3). Companies starting cultivation projects can count on financial incentives from the authorities, and the Chinese press frequently enthuses about the success of such projects (CTIC 2006b, 2006c, 2007a, 2007b). The reality, however, is different. Although most companies had high hopes for cultivation at one time, many have since given up on their initial efforts. The plantations I have seen personally seldom gave the impression that they were meant to contribute substantially to a factory's supplies. Moreover, where cultivation is actually done it focuses almost exclusively on a few medicinal plants which are easy to grow and not particularly rare, such as *manu* (*ma nu*, *Inula racemosa*), *ruta* (*ru rta*, *Saussurea lappa*), and *chumtsa* (*lcum rtsa*, *Rheum palmatum*).

The reasons why the factories' initial ardour has somewhat cooled are manifold. There are basically two approaches to cultivation: either to try growing a plant in its natural habitat (*in situ*) or in a dedicated herbal garden (*ex situ*). *In situ* cultivation clearly has advantages, as many high-altitude plants require a specific habitat. But the procedure is much less convenient and requires considerably more effort, given the difficulty of reaching the cultivation site. To the best of my knowledge, *in situ* or 'wild' cultivation has hardly been tried in Tibet on a large scale. Furthermore, *in situ* cultivation offers no guarantee of success. In Jan Salick's research project on snow lotus mentioned above, the team observed the *in situ* germination of *Saussurea laniceps* and *Saussurea medusa* for two consecutive years. While the seeds of *Saussurea laniceps* germinated in one year but not the other, the seeds of *Saussurea medusa* failed to germinate in both years. The team concluded that germination in these species was highly variable from year to year (Law, Salick and Knight n.d.).

In view of these difficulties, growing high-altitude plants away from their natural habitat appears even more precarious. Even if the seeds germinate and the plants finally grow, it is not sure whether the cultivated herb matches the properties and quality of the wild one. Rinchen Wangdu had his experiences with cultivation himself and presented the difficulties as follows:

> We are thinking about cultivating these [rare] herbs, but there are so many problems: climate, altitude, etc. Even if you find a solution to cultivate some of the herbs, it takes three years until you can harvest the first samples [of a root medicine]. When you assess the quality of such a sample, you [often] find that it is totally different from the wild one, so you cannot use it.

What to do then? Start all over again? But which parameters have to be changed if one does not know what exactly went wrong?

Establishing plant gardens in the vicinity of a usually urban-based factory can be a challenge for other reasons as well, such as the availability of suitable land and motivated, skilled labour. I accompanied a Tibetan doctor working for a government-sponsored research institute on a visit to their plant cultivation sites in the outskirts of Lhasa, amidst the greenhouses of Chinese vegetable growers. While we were working in the field, watering the crops, a young Chinese couple approached us. They were immigrant farmers looking for land to breed pigs. Arable land close to cities is costly and in high demand. When I came back a year later, the research institute had relocated their cultivation project to a smaller site further away from Lhasa. The benefit of cheaper tenure, however, came at the expense of a greater distance to the site.

In addition, factories often rely on hired labour, which brings into play another type of incentive problem. A lesson learned from collectivisation schemes in China and elsewhere is that output tends to be poor when agriculture is based on the labour of people not directly affected by its success or failure (Crook 1973; Lin 1990; Kung and Putterman 1997; Bramall 2000). One could argue that community-based approaches in which smallholders profit directly from the yields and quality produced may have a better chance of success.

In this regard, it may not come as a surprise that the most successful attempt at growing large quantities of a medicinal plants used in Tibetan medicine focused from the very beginning on rural income generation and environmental protection rather than being initiated by a company looking to secure its supply. The project was started by The Mountain Institute (TMI), an international NGO with an office in Kathmandu, and aims at the cultivation of *gyatig* (*rgya tig*, *Swertia chirayita*) in the Taplejung and Kanchenjunga areas of far eastern Nepal. *Gyatig* belongs to the category *tigta* (*tig ta*), a group of medicinal plants known for their bitterness ([*kha*] *tig* means 'bitter' in Tibetan). The first syllable of the name, *rgya*, refers to *rgya gar* – that is, India – and denotes the herb's origin. However, most *gyatig* actually comes from Nepal. *Chirayita*, as it is called in Nepal and India, is also widely used in Ayurvedic medicine and is therefore in high demand. It grows in parts of Tibet as well, but the variety considered to be the most potent is usually from Nepal. Initially, TMI's project was aimed at providing a local monastery with stable revenue. Soon, the initiative expanded to include local farmers who used to collect *gyatig* in and around the Kanchenjunga National Park. According to the NGO, the percentage of wildcrafted *gyatig* decreased from around 70 per cent to 30 per cent within half a decade.

Gyatig proved to be an ideal cash crop for the region. It is planted along the walls of terraced fields or in narrow strips of otherwise unused land close to people's houses; yields are very high and the crop requires relatively little additional work. The quality of cultivated *gyatig*, contrary to the case of many other species, seems to be in no way inferior to the collected one. None of the Tibetan doctors and traders I asked found a difference between wild and cultivated supplies. Most of the *gyatig* I saw in herb stores in Nepal and Tibet was said to come from the region covered by the project.

TMI has paid much attention to maintaining sufficient genetic variety. Seeds are collected in different locations in the wild. In 2008, more than 5,000 farmers were involved in the project and *gyatig* contributed substantially to their household incomes. The project was managed by TMI's Karma Bhutia, a man from the region who had gained the farmers' trust. In addition, farmers who joined the project early on were now teaching others about their experiences.

Although there are many lessons that could be learned from this project for similar ventures in Tibet, it cannot be taken as a model that guarantees success. TMI was invited to share its experiences with the Himalayan Amchi Association (HAA) and to help with setting up a similar project in Nepal's Upper Mustang. Unlike the Kanchenjunga area, which gets abundant monsoon rains, Mustang, like the Tibetan Plateau, lies in the rain shadow of the High Himalayas. On the high, arid and windswept plains of Mustang, the cultivation methods developed in eastern Nepal yielded mixed results (HAA 2009).

The success of the *gyatig* project in eastern Nepal rests on the combination of favourable parameters: good growth in a nearby *in situ* environment, a focus on income generation, good quality, and a growing demand that has, at least until now, outpaced the increase in supply provided by the participating farmers. The latter is not always the case, even with otherwise successful cultivation projects. In Bhutan, for example, the Department of Agriculture initiated a project for the cultivation of *ruta* (*ru rta, Saussurea lappa*). The factory, part of Bhutan's National Institute for Traditional Medicine (NITM), agreed to buy the herbs for a guaranteed price which was far higher than the market price in India or Nepal – a premium they were willing to pay for better quality, locally grown *ruta*. Many farmers had high hopes and yields were good – too good. The NITM soon had great difficulty absorbing the quantities produced and the farmers now increasingly face a sales problem.[2]

In general terms, cultivation only plays a minor role in today's Tibetan medicine industry. In the companies I visited most herbs were still sourced from the wild. Ecological, agricultural as well as socio-economic factors make large-scale cultivation a difficult task. Given the urgency of the problem, it is astonishing how little energy actually goes into serious, long-term programmes to overcome the difficulties. At the Lhasa Mentsikhang's research centre, for example, only two or three out of twenty-six researchers, one of them an intern, were working on cultivation issues in 2009. Most of the research centre's energy is dedicated to pharmacological or clinical studies of herbs and compounds and the publishing of old medical texts. Moreover, there is reason to believe that the official agenda to encourage cultivation has not always yielded the intended outcome. When I visited one company's sizeable cultivation project in Kongpo, the manager in charge complained that somebody had stolen the sign that had marked the turn-off from the main road to the dirt track leading to the fields. Reading the puzzled expression on my face – Why would somebody steal a sign and why was it an issue for a highly profitable company like this? – my host explained that the signs were very important. Most of the plant gardens in the region actually consisted of not much more than a sign on the road, he complained. Once a project had received government funds, the money was often used for other purposes. Of course, their own cultivation site was an exception, he added with a smile.

Commercial Traders[3]

Whenever cultivation or direct ties to village collectors are not feasible, factories rely on commercial traders. Sometimes they work together with one trusted trader, sometimes they rely on several. During fieldwork I came in contact with about a dozen herb traders and developed closer relations with four of these. One of them was Penba. I met him in Lhasa where he ran a herb business together with his father.

The family's business had been started by Penba's father, a man from a poor rural family in Golog, Qinghai province. He made a living by touring the area, buying sheep and yak skins, and selling them in the province's capital, Xining. He also started trading clothes, which he would buy in the city and bring back to Golog. Later, he ventured into the booming business of selling cheap Chinese textiles via Lhasa across the border in Nepal. Once he had acquired enough knowledge of the cross-border trade and built up a network of business partners and friends at the border, he recognised the prospects offered by the herb trade. In 2002, the family moved to Lhasa and started a small herb shop. In 2005, Penba's father established a second branch back in his hometown, and since then Penba has been in charge of the shop in Lhasa.

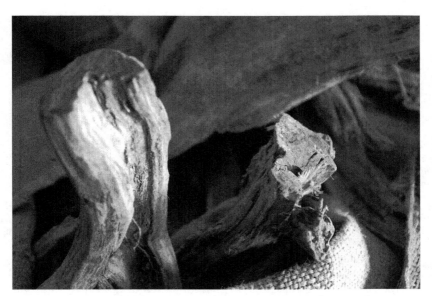

Figure 4.2: Agar, the resinous, mould-infected heartwood of an *Aquilaria* tree.

Penba and his father are newcomers in the medicinal herb trade. Nobody in the family was an *amchi* or had a specific interest in Tibetan medicine. But being familiar with cross-border trade, Penba's father was quick to understand the opportunities the burgeoning industrialisation of Tibetan medicine was creating. In this sense, the Norling Herb Store, as I will call it, is a typical by-product of the industry's creation.

The Norling Herb Store traded in 132 different kinds of medicinal raw materials, mainly herbs but also some of the most common minerals and a few animal ingredients. Bags of herbs were piled up along the walls of the store. In the middle of the room, providing a display of the range and quality of the store's products, samples of each material were displayed in open bags. Near the windowed door facing the courtyard, the brightest spot in the otherwise dim storeroom, there was an old balance used to weigh the goods.

Penba, the eldest son of the family, was in his early thirties, married, and had a young son. Adjacent to the storeroom, there was a small office with a desk, two chairs and a couch, providing comfort for the customers to chat, smoke and drink tea. There was a laptop computer on the desk and Penba usually kept it running. Every few minutes a blip signalled that one of his instant messenger friends had come online or had left. Sometimes his son would take a nap on the couch or play in the office. The little boy owned a rabbit that once in a while escaped from the office into the storeroom and enjoyed itself, hopping from open bag to open bag, making a big mess to everybody's amusement.

There is a sharp contrast between the world of the herb trade and the factories in terms of cleanliness. While protective clothes have to be worn and hands washed and disinfected before entering the clean area of a factory, in herb stores people would smoke with one hand and rummage in a bag of herbs with the other. This is not to say that the traders I have come to know are negligent about the quality of their goods – they are very careful, just in a different way. The clean room atmosphere of GMP production plants seems somehow illusory when compared to the reality of how herbs are collected, transported, traded and stored. The Norling Herb Store was one of the cleanest and neatest I have seen. But for Penba, as for any other herb trader I came to know, the medicinal plants were first and foremost a form of merchandise, a commodity.

Remarkably, the domestic herb trade has so far largely remained outside the scope of Chinese regulations, despite the emphasis on patient safety and the general trend towards tighter control of the pharmaceutical industry. Many of the existing rules and standards do not, or do not yet, apply to Tibetan medicine. A case in point is China's 'good agricultural practices' (GAP), which have not yet been declared a binding standard (SFDA 2002; WHO 2003: 33–41). The GAP guidelines were developed in the spirit of the WHO's recommendations for 'good agricultural and collection practices' (GACP). Remarkably, the 'C' standing for 'collection' in the WHO's document has been omitted in the Chinese approach. As the Tibetan medicine industry relies mainly on wild-grown ingredients and China's GAP is not yet binding, the standards hardly affect the Tibetan medicine industry at present.

More important, however, is the status TCM is being granted within China's drug regulations. Although the 2001 Drug Administration Law defines the term 'drug' in a broad way that encompasses TCM raw materials, the so-called Chinese crude drugs (SFDA 2001: Article 102), it also stipulates far-reaching exemptions for the latter. Chinese crude drugs, under which Tibetan medicinal plants, minerals and animal ingredients[4] fall by default, are neither required to obtain drug registration nor do retailers need special licences to trade in them (ibid.: Article 31, 21). Due to these special provisions for TCM and its crude drugs, the sourcing of ingredients for Tibetan medicine within China has not been brought into the domain of state control so far.

Of the 132 types of medicinal materials Penba traded in 2008, 80 per cent originated from within the territory of the People's Republic of China and about 20 per cent were imported from India and Nepal. In terms of volume, however, the herbs imported from Nepal and India accounted for around 50 per cent, largely due to the big trade volumes of *aru* (*a ru*, *Terminalia chebula*), *baru* (*ba ru*, *Terminalia belerica*) and *kyuru* (*syku ru*, *Phyllanthus emblica* or *Emblica officinalis*). The 'three fruits' – *dräbusum* (*'bras bu gsum*) – as *aru*, *baru* and *kyuru* are collectively called, are an indispensable part of Tibetan pharmacy,[5] and can be found in the majority of Tibetan formulas. *Aru*, the myrobalan fruit, is also the most widely used symbol for Tibetan medicine. The Medicine Buddha is usually depicted holding a myrobalan plant and many company logos feature it as well. In addition to *aru*, *baru* and *kyuru*, many of the most highly valued ingredients are imported from abroad. Examples include the so-called *zangpodrug* (*bzang po drug*) – the six superior medical substances[6] – as well as black eaglewood (*ar nag*, *Aquilaria agallocha*), sandalwood (*tsan dan*, *Santalum*) and ocean crabs (*sdig srin*).

The problem is that the exemptions and special provisions granted to Chinese crude drugs do not apply for these imported raw materials. This brings us to the issue of transnational trade.

Transnational Trade and Border Regimes

Transnational trade, I argue, is conditioned by several border regimes. The term 'border regime' is meant to describe administrative efforts at regulating the transition of herbs and traders across borders. Spatial borders thereby very often coincide with conceptual boundaries. Border regimes keep separate spatial and conceptual spheres – the foreign product of nature from the domestic crude drug, the illegal migrant from the official trader, or officially declared merchandise from smuggled protected species. Simultaneously, the task of border regimes is to enable controlled and orderly flows between these spheres.

The notion of 'border regime' contains a paradox. On the one hand, 'regime' connotes state power. The 'border', on the other hand, is a liminal space where state power is potentially rendered vulnerable. Border regimes are intended to tackle this vulnerability with administrative, architectural and spatial measures. A border regime is entangled but not equal to the state's larger apparatuses. Border regimes are more flexible, manipulable and prone to rapid change than the related apparatuses and legal frameworks on which they are based. They only exist while they are being actively enacted, and as long as they are enacted they provide a glimpse of the malleability and unruliness of state power and its instruments.[7] I argue that the contemporary trans-Himalayan trade in medicinal plants is shaped by a set of three such border regimes and the traders' tactical manoeuvres to deal with them.

Import Licences

The first and most important of these border regimes stems from the fact that the exemptions granted for domestic Chinese crude drugs do not apply to imported raw materials. For imported drugs, the Drug Administration Law makes no difference between an antibiotic and a medicinal herb. Imported drugs need to be sampled, tested and cleared by the respective drug testing offices (SFDA 2001: Article 40).

At the outset these rules failed to have an impact on the cross-border trade in Tibetan medicinal plants. They were simply not enforced. But in 2005 the SFDA issued more specific provisions on the import of crude drugs, which came into effect in February 2006 (SFDA 2005a, 2006b). These provisions reiterated the line adopted by the 2001 Drug Administration Law. They called for traders to obtain a licence from the SFDA in Beijing and they repeated that drugs had to be imported via authorised ports and tested by a local drug-testing office. Although it was announced that the provisions would come into force from July 2006, there was no immediate effect on the cross-border trade of medicinal plants between Nepal and Tibet. In 2007 and early 2008 I met several traders who did not have such licences but were not especially worried about it. However, with generally tighter border controls coming into effect after the riots of 14 March 2008, the provisions began to be strictly enforced during the following summer and a new border regime was set up. Cross-border trade has since become much more difficult.

The new system works as follows: Each herb requires a separate licence, which is valid for two years and entitles the holder to an indefinite number of imports. The licence document is basically an official certification of a long-term business contract between an importer and a specific supplier, for example a wholesaler in Kathmandu. These provisions tie in with the general direction the SFDA has set in the recently published 'Guidelines on the Protection of Traditional Chinese Medicines' (SFDA 2009). These guidelines state that raw materials should come from a designated source with stable supplies and a traceable origin in order to make quality controllable (C-Med 2009).

None of the people I talked to raised objections to the idea of traceable origin and stable supplies. But unfortunately, the new system, which entails tying an importer to a trade partner abroad for the purchase of a specific herb, is not very practical. How, in the end, would one know if the trade partner named on an import licence had a specific herb in stock? And who would guarantee that it was of good and consistent quality? What if the trade partner started abusing the fixed terms of the system and suddenly demanded higher prices? What, if they went out of business? In short, the provisions completely fail to capture the realities of the plant trade.

In addition to the licence entitling the owner to import a specific herb over the period of two years, each instance of an import necessitates an import permit, which has to be obtained beforehand. The import permit is issued by the local authorities and specifies the volume of the planned import. The permit is required for customs clearance at the authorised port of entry. In the case of cross-border trade between Nepal and China, the only authorised entry port is Dram (or Zhangmu) on the Friendship Highway between Kathmandu and Tibet. The testing of imported drugs is done in Shigatse or Lhasa.

For the Tibetan plant traders based in Kathmandu, the new requirements were almost impossible to meet. The rules were designed for large enterprises in China importing crude drugs from abroad but they were not meant for Nepal-based traders who used to travel to China and sell their goods there. I came to know a well-established plant trader, a Nepali citizen of Tibetan origin based in Kathmandu. He was a trusted supplier of many factories in Tibet and claimed to ship up to fifty truckloads[8] per year of *aru, baru* and *kyuru* from Nepal to Tibet, as well as many other medicinal herbs.

In addition to exporting herbs from Nepal to Tibet he was also importing herbs from Tibet to Nepal and India. He would spend about four months a year in Lhasa. During this time he would live in his storeroom on the Barkor and go to villages to buy herbs. Under the new border regime, the import–export business permit under which he had been operating was no longer considered to be sufficient and in summer 2008 he was put out of business.

Furthermore, the new border regime penalised the smaller cross-border traders. The importing enterprise on the Chinese side has to be in possession of an SFDA issued Drug Manufacturing Certificate or a Drug Supply Certificate, which is simply out of reach for many of the smaller traders. Moreover, each imported batch of herbs has to be tested and approved by the drug-testing offices in Shigatse or Lhasa, and each test costs about 1,800 yuan ($260), regardless of quantity. Thus, the bigger the batch, the smaller the additional cost per kilogram.

Apparently, the rules even apply to the import of samples of herbs. A factory in Nyalam near the Nepal border, for example, used to order herb samples from Nepal. Only if the quality of these samples was satisfactory would they order larger quantities. Sampling before bulk ordering is a standard practice in the domestic trade. Being close to the border, the factory also followed the practice for their imported herbs. Under the new border regime this is becoming increasingly complicated. According to the director of the factory:

> The central government suggested that we may want to get samples from Qingdao or Shanghai instead. But then the price would just go up and the factory could not cope with that. So right now we still use our old relations with the customs in Dram and try to get samples across. And we also petitioned the SFDA for permission to import the samples.

When I returned to Nyalam in 2009, they had found no solution to the problem and had indeed started to import herbs via inland China. The herbs now travel all the way from Nepal to India, by sea to Shanghai or Hong Kong and then overland back to Nyalam, an hour and a half from the border with Nepal. Despite official claims by China and Nepal that they are fostering trade along the Friendship Highway, recent developments on the Chinese side have made cross-border trade of medicinal plants considerably more difficult.

Another immediate consequence of the new border regime was that it affected trade using border crossings other than the Friendship Highway. Over the last decade, many new roads have been constructed within the TAR, extending China's road network south to the Nepal border. As a result, many of Nepal's northern border areas are now closer to the road network in China than the roadheads in Nepal's Terai. From the high mountain valleys in Nepal's north it is often only a day's walk to the Chinese border and the Tibetan roadhead, whereas transport to the roads in Nepal's south takes several days.

The new roads in Tibet are used to trade Chinese goods with remote northern areas in Nepal. Rice, flour, noodles, soap, candles, shoes, clothes, blankets, beer, liquor, batteries, solar panels, television sets, kitchen utensils, entire stoves and blue metal roofing are carried across the Himalayas from China to Nepal. These remote border crossings, known from the pre-1959 salt trade (Hagen and Thapa 1998: 189), have become welcome alternatives to the road between Kathmandu and Lhasa.

The Mountain Institute, the NGO running the successful *gyatig* cultivation project, carried out an unpublished study on 'taxes' (that is, bribes) collected on the way from north-eastern Nepal to the Indian border. They found that a trader had to pay twenty-seven bribes along the way. When the Maoists seized power in the region, they took their share of these taxes, but the total number and sum of the bribes did not change substantially. These enormous transaction costs induced a re-orientation of the herb trade towards Tibet and across remote border posts. Under the new import regime, however, a truckload of *pangpö* was seized by the Chinese border authorities at one of the remote crossings in 2008. The requirement that medicinal herbs must be imported via an authorised entry port affected the informal trade of medicinal plants between Nepal's northern regions and Tibet.

The current situation remains unclear. In addition to the entry ports authorised for drug import (Dram being the only one between Nepal and Tibet), the 2006 provisions on the import of crude drugs provide for special 'frontier ports' through which crude drugs produced near the border may be traded (SFDA 2005a). This might be applicable to some of the remote border crossings. Indeed, by August 2009 the cross-border trade of medicinal herbs was allegedly possible again, at least at one of these crossings in far eastern Nepal – whether informally or officially I do not know.[9]

Trader Tactics

The Norling Herb Store was in the lucky position of having good relations with one of the major Tibetan medicine companies in the TAR. The factory applied for import licences on Norling's behalf and the licences enabled Penba and his father to continue and even expand their business during the troubled year of 2008. Several times a year, a member of the family travelled to Nepal to buy herbs.

In autumn 2008, I had the opportunity to join Penba on such a business trip. The plan was to buy around 20 metric tons of herbs, which represents a considerable investment. For some time our departure had been delayed because the family was still trying to secure the necessary cash for the purchase. For Penba it was his first journey to Nepal as a businessman. His father considered himself to be too old for the hardships of the road. Penba felt the burden of responsibility on his shoulders. 'My wife says that I have such a good life, travelling to Nepal and all. But actually, it is a big responsibility and not really fun', he told me before we left.

Our journey started in Lhasa, where I met Penba at his house. He had organised sharing a taxi to Shigatse, about 300 kilometres from Lhasa on the way to the Nepalese border. We left early in order to reach Shigatse in time to get the necessary paperwork done and to collect the required import permits. On the road from Lhasa to Shigatse there are several checkpoints where the time of passage is carefully noted and checked. As a reaction to frequent accidents on this section of road and as a measure to reduce the speed of the traffic, a minimum travel time between checkpoints has to be honoured, increasing the total driving time to almost double. Our driver, a jolly middle-aged Chinese woman from Sichuan, convinced the first checkpoint that she had a passenger on board who was suffering from altitude sickness (me) and needed to get to Shigatse as quickly as possible. To everybody's delight, the stamped and certified slip of paper took us through all the subsequent checkpoints without any waiting time. Shigatse is in fact higher than Lhasa and the story of the passenger with altitude sickness made no sense at all. This anecdote, as trivial as it may sound, has allegorical value. Throughout Penba's journey, the 'truth' stamped on a piece of paper was often more relevant than the reality to which it purportedly referred.

We arrived in Shigatse early and had plenty of time before the relevant offices closed. Penba decided to buy some presents for the officials he was about to meet. 'I don't want to come empty-handed', he said. We went to a nearby supermarket and for more than half an hour we wandered up and down the aisles, looking for a convenient gift. A bottle of alcohol? Maybe too expensive. And what if the official was a woman? Just fruit? Probably not enough. Something more special, chocolates maybe? But which ones?

Although the task that lay ahead was not a particularly difficult one – Penba had the import licences, so obtaining the import permits was a mere formality – the risk that something could go wrong, that a necessary paper was missing or not perfectly in order, always loomed. More detailed and strictly enforced regulations did not mean greater certainty about the exact requirements. On the contrary: the new import regime meant new offices with officials yet to be befriended and it was therefore better to create a good impression from the outset.

Finally, Penba settled on fresh fruit and some assorted sweets and set off for the office. Two hours later he came back, smiling and obviously relieved. 'Everything OK!' he said. And the presents? 'Oh, I gave them to the wrong person. She was not even in charge! But no problem'.

Penba had shown me a list of the two dozen herbs he intended to buy in Nepal. But when I asked him if I could see the licences and import permits, he only had two. 'This is enough', he explained. 'Last time we had five, but that was too much, a waste of money'. The current situation was apparently that, without licences and import permits, cross-border trade was simply impossible; however, it was not necessary to have a different license for each herb.

The experiences the Norling Herb Store had gained under the new import regime, especially with the drug-testing office responsible for clearing imported herbs, were ambiguous at best. Penba told me that the testing took several months. As long as the herbs were not cleared they could not be sold. Testing was carried out in a laboratory by laboratory staff. But the testing as such was not to be trusted, and the officials involved were largely ignorant when it came to Tibetan medicine: 'The people in this drug-testing office, they know nothing about Tibetan medicine. You bring them a sample of *aru* and they ask, what is this? – *Aru*. – How do you spell it? They have no idea! They just put everything in their machine and wait for the results'.

Penba told me the story of a sample one trader brought in for testing. It failed the test. But when another trader went with a second sample from the same bag, it passed. 'It's like a gambling machine. If you are lucky, you win, otherwise you lose', he said. Indeed, the family had lost almost 50,000 yuan ($7,300) when two batches of herbs Penba and his father imported in summer 2008 were rejected and confiscated.

I related this story to a Tibetan doctor who was responsible for buying herbs for a major factory, and he mentioned that they had encountered similar problems with *zati* (*dza ti, Myristica fragnans*) – nutmeg. The variety of *zati* from Nepal was not the same as the variety used in China. *Zati* from Nepal is oilier and therefore considered to be of better quality than the Chinese variety. The official test for *zati*, however, was based on the Chinese variety, he explained, and consequently *zati* from Nepal was prone to fail the import test.

I was unable to confirm these accounts and I do not know the exact reasons why Penba's herbs were rejected and confiscated. Neither was I able to witness how the tests are actually carried out. Most likely, testing is based on microscopy and chromatographic fingerprinting as specified by the identification tests listed in the *Chinese Pharmacopoeia*. But as only a few medicinal plants used in Tibetan medicine are mentioned, the standard according to which all the other herbs are tested remains unclear. The *Tibetan Drug Standards* includes more species but lack the detailed laboratory procedures included in the *Chinese Pharmacopoeia*.

Taxonomy and Legibility

Regardless of these uncertainties, the anecdotal evidence surrounding the import tests points to potential problems with taxonomy and translation. Licences and import permits, as well as the *Chinese Pharmacopoeia*, feature botanical (Latin) and Chinese names; Tibetan names are not included. However, it is often the case that a single Tibetan name may cover several botanical names, while the Tibetan nomenclature may recognise several varieties of a species designated by one botanical name (cf. Clark 2000). The licences, permits and import tests meant to increase patient safety and control by rendering cross-border trade more legible fail to identify the very objects they target. Omitting Tibetan names is yet another 'thin simplification' characteristic of *techne*, to use Scott's terms once more (Scott 1998: 309).

An example is necessary to illustrate the scope of these difficulties. Kletter and Kriechbaum, for instance, list seven different species that have been mentioned in the literature as botanical equivalents of *bongkar* (*bong dkar*): *Aconitum fischeri* Reichb., *Aconitum grandiflorum*, *Aconitum heterophyllum* Wall., *Aconitum naviculare* Stapf., *Aconitum tanguticum* (maxim.) Stapf., *Geum strictum* Ait. *and Nepeta sibirica* L. (Kletter and Kriechbaum 2001: 32). This variation can be explained in part by the fact that there are probably hundreds of aconite species in the Himalayas, and Tibetan doctors have come to rely on the locally available ones. The distinguishing criterion in Tibetan pharmacy is the colour of the interior of the tubers. The second syllable of *bongkar* – *kar* (*dkar*) – means 'white' in Tibetan. Other aconites used in Tibetan medicine include *bongmar* (*bong dmar*) and *bongnag* (*bong nag*) that respectively feature red and black tubers.

On the other hand, the biological classification system based on Linnaean taxonomy also has its history. By adding the name of the botanist who first described a species as a suffix (Stapf., Reichb., Royle and so forth) it pays tribute to the fact that classification is carried out by humans. The distinction between species found in different locations is often fluid, and many plants have been 'discovered' more than once and now have different botanical names. With regard to *bongkar*, Kletter and Kriechbaum mention that. 'in the Flora of Pakistan *A[conitum] cordatum* is listed as a synonym of *A[conitum] heterophyllum* var. *heterophyllum*, although the original description of *Aconitum cordatum* Royle apparently matches that of *A[conitum] heterophyllum* var. *bracteatum*' (ibid.: 34).

The problem gets still more complex when adding variants of the Tibetan name to the mix. Kletter and Kriechbaum (ibid.: 32) give several Tibetan synonyms for *bongkar*: *shingtudugme* (*shin tu dug med*), *sosordugme* (*so sor dug med*) and *gangkizhungchung* (*gangs kyi zhun chung*). Dr Dawa, a former director of the Men-Tsee-Khang in Dharamsala, goes even further in distinguishing two varieties of *bongkar*: variety one (*rigs dang po*) he identifies as *Aconitum heterophyllum* Wall. *ex* Royle; variety two (*rigs gnyis pa*) he simply classifies as *Aconitum* sp. – an undefined aconite species (Dawa 2002: 44, 46).

117

To make matters more complex still, *Aconitum heterophyllum* is also widely used in Ayurveda, where it is commonly known as *atis* (Kletter and Kriechbaum 2001: 36). However, a plant trader from Humla (Nepal) I came to know in Kathmandu insisted that the *atis* used in Ayurveda and the *bongkar* of Tibetan medicine were not the same type of aconite. He traded with both Ayurvedic doctors and Tibetan *amchi*.

Despite these complexities, taxonomy has not constituted a major problem in the day-to-day interactions of plant traders, Tibetan doctors and factory pharmacists. People know what they are talking about and neither Chinese nor botanical names are used in this milieu. With import tests, however, this situation may well change radically. Under these circumstances the safest option for a cross-border trader was simply to avoid the official procedure as far as possible. In order to accomplish this, the licence was a precondition, even if its ambit was not necessarily relevant. A licence was more like an entry ticket; in much the same way as our Chinese taxi driver had been able to rush us to Shigatse, the mere existence of a licence enabled the officials involved to present coherent documentation to their superiors, regardless of whether a truck was actually passing the border with a couple of dozen herbs instead of two. Once this basic 'document truth' was established, the officials involved were still able to reap the benefits of turning a blind eye to the details of a specific import. The traders, for their part, managed to maintain sufficient leeway to do business and escape the quirks of a utopian licensing and testing system.

Penba was not overly concerned with all these things. He considered dealing with officials and with ever-changing rules as an integral part of doing business in China. He was confident that there would always be loopholes that provided pragmatic solutions. The 'fees' paid to this end were usually reasonable. 'When the drug testing people come, sometimes two, sometimes three, we usually give them about 500 yuan each', he said.

Penba was more nervous about dealing with the Nepali wholesalers in Kathmandu. While he was telling me these stories, sharing a freezing-cold hotel room in Shigatse, Penba was jokingly practising his English for these envisioned encounters. He owned a fancy Chinese mobile phone with a built-in language trainer that stuttered sentences like 'He is attracted to fast cars' and 'I could really use a drink right now'.

Business Cultures

A Land Cruiser evacuating an altitude-sick tourist (this time a genuine case) agreed to take us to the border. The Friendship Highway runs across the arid Tibetan Plateau until the peaks of the High Himalayas finally appear in the distance. From the southern rim of the Tibetan Plateau, the road leads down into the steep canyons towered over by snow-capped mountains. The vegetation changes from the high, arid plateau, which lies in the rain shadow of the Himalayas, to the lush and humid valleys of Nepal. It is in these steep valleys, carved into the Himalayan range, that many of the herbs used in Tibetan medicine grow. As in Eastern Tibet, enormous differences in altitude make for a large variety of different habitats.

The border town of Dram lies on the steep slope of one such valley. A narrow road winds down to the town and finally to the Nepalese border post of Kodari. The hundreds of trucks trying to pass one another on the narrow road cause a permanent traffic jam and attest to the importance of the Friendship Highway as a trade route.

We spent a day and a night in Dram, where Penba had to withdraw sufficient cash from the bank and change it into Nepalese rupees. Negotiating the exchange rate and counting the hundreds and hundreds of bills four times, twice by Penba and twice by the money changer, took hours. Equipped with a bag of cash we finally headed for the Friendship Bridge, which marks the actual border between Nepal and China.

The little bridge straddles the boundary between two very different worlds. Coming from China, the far side of the bridge marks the immediate and sudden beginning of the Indian subcontinent. Smells, aesthetics, behaviour, etiquette, humour, ways of doing business and dealing with authorities, truck drivers and their habits – all are completely different from Tibet. The new and fancy border checkpoint on the Chinese side, an index of correctness and control where everybody wears a uniform, stands in stark contrast to the casual and somewhat disorganised atmosphere in Nepal's immigration office. Crossing the border, Penba and I caught sight of a Nepalese truck on which slightly imperfect Olympic rings were drawn. Beneath the rings an inscription proclaimed: Nepal Olympics 3057 – an ironic comment on the state of affairs in Nepal, something that would never have been tolerated in China, given the symbolic sensibilities surrounding everything related to the Beijing Olympics.[10]

This contrast between the two worlds – one might call it a difference in habitus (Bourdieu 1979) or social aesthetics (MacDougall 1999) – is crucial for an understanding of the subtle quirks of
the cross-border trade. Doing business in China and doing business
in Nepal require different sets of skills, different approaches and
tactics. Creating trustful relationships across these worlds can be a
challenge, especially as contemporary cross-border trade along the
Friendship Highway lacks the stability of traditional trading connections between Tibet and the Indian subcontinent, which were
encouraged by long-established friendship ties, etiquette and ceremony (Fürer-Haimendorf 1975: 295–97; Ross 1982: 44; Fisher
1986; Rizvi 2001: 20).

Tibetans often complain about Chinese business culture, considering it unethical, solely oriented towards money making, and so
on. Remarkably, I have heard Nepali herb traders using almost the
same words for their Tibetan customers: difficult to deal with, always smart, bargaining incredibly hard and invariably looking to turn
things to their own advantage. Yet again, a big Indian wholesaler
based in Delhi and Kathmandu complained to me about how difficult it was to do business in Nepal, as everybody just tried to cheat
and extort as much money as possible from the situation. Cross-
border trade inherently makes all parties outsiders in some contexts
and insiders in others.

When we arrived in Kathmandu, Penba started calling friends of
his father's to help him with his mission. The people he contacted
were not just other Tibetans but almost exclusively people from
Amdo or even from his hometown. Penba felt ill at ease among the
exile Tibetans. He spent the first night in a hotel in Boudha, the part
of Kathmandu around the famous stupa where many exile Tibetans
have settled, but soon moved to a Chinese business hotel in the tourist area of Thamel where he felt much more at home. We usually had
dinner in an Amdo restaurant hidden in a dark courtyard, where the
menu was in Chinese and the noodles almost as good as back home
in Amdo. In Dram we had spent the night in an Amdo hotel, and the
money changer he had chosen was a woman from Amdo. Even the
little Kathmandu hippie-style bag that Penba used to carry his cash
in had been bought in a shop run by an Amdo woman. Throughout
our trip we kept meeting people from Amdo and they were always
ready to help us.

The obvious approach to tackle the problem of being an outsider in Kathmandu was to rely on these ties of shared place,[11] especially as relations between the different groups of exile Tibetans are not always easy. While the first wave of Tibetans that emigrated in the late 1950s and 1960s was mainly from Central Tibet, the 'new arrivals', as they are called, predominantly come from Amdo and Kham. The well-established exile Tibetans often regard the new arrivals as overly Sinicised (Moynihan 2003: 318; Yeh 2007).

One of Penba's Amdo friends accompanied us on a tour of Kathmandu's wholesalers. In the past, Penba's father had bought herbs from a Marwari[12] trader family in Kathmandu. We went to their shop, located in a tiny alley tucked away between New Road and Durbar Square, known as one of the best places to buy medicinal herbs. The Deoras, as they were called, ran a modest little shop amidst many similar ones. Nothing betrayed the fact that they were actually among the biggest wholesalers in Kathmandu. Their retail outlet in the alleyway primarily served as a contact point; their offices and storerooms were located in other parts of the city.

The shopkeeper had one of his servants bring us to the family's house by taxi. Stuck in one of Kathmandu's traffic jam, Penba listed what he thought to be Nepal's biggest problems. 'First, the roads are bad', he complained, 'and second, there are always power cuts, no electricity. Third, the *bandhs*; there is always a *bandh* somewhere.[13] And fourth, the traffic, oh the traffic ...'.

We were received by Arjun and Raksha, two brothers of the family, and were offered tea and Indian sweets. As they had never met Penba before, the brothers treated him with a degree of scepticism. When Penba asked a question about this or that detail of transportation or the tax levied by the Nepalese Forest Department, Arjun and Raksha lectured him in a slightly arrogant way, making it clear that he could either risk organising everything by himself or take the precaution of enlisting their aid.

But the Deoras were also dependent on Penba. Arjun had previously ventured into the Chinese market, shipping a large consignment of medicinal herbs via Mumbai and Hong Kong. Being unfamiliar with Chinese business culture, he had been tricked and cheated, and had lost a large amount of money. Finally, he had called Penba's father and asked him if he could store his herbs until they found a buyer. Penba had taken care of the matter and rented storage space in Xining. He had organised transport for Arjun's goods and the herbs were still waiting to be sold. Although transportation by sea had been cheap, all the additional fees for opportunistic intermediaries had added considerably to the cost of the merchandise. The Deoras counted on Penba to buy the herbs from them and to find a buyer himself. Now it was Penba's turn to show the two brothers how naive they had been. 'For this quality at this price I cannot sell them', he made clear.

Penba explained that while shipping herbs out of Mumbai by sea to Hong Kong or Shanghai may be relatively cheap, transport within China was still comparatively expensive. On the other hand, transport from the border to Lhasa and further to Xining benefited from the fact that most trucks were going in the other direction, carrying goods from China to Nepal, and were usually empty on the return journey.[14] As long as one was familiar with the situation, shipping herbs from Nepal to Tibet via the Friendship Highway was a relatively inexpensive matter. A truck from Dram to Lhasa currently cost around 4,500 yuan ($660) and from Lhasa to Xining around 7,000 yuan ($1,000). As a Chinese truck could carry about 20 metric tons, the added cost per kilogram of transported goods was therefore only 0.225 yuan to Lhasa (about 900 km) and 0.575 yuan to Xining (1,900 km). On the Nepal side, transport from Kathmandu to the border, a mere 111 km, was 1.5 Nepalese rupees per kilogram (or about 0.15 yuan in November 2008). Per ton and kilometre, transport from Kathmandu to the border amounted to 1.35 yuan, compared to 0.25 yuan between Dram and Lhasa and 0.3 yuan between Lhasa and Xining. All in all, Penba calculated 2 yuan per kilogram for transport to Xining, including taxes, customs, testing and other costs.

Although frustrated at times about the business cultures of the respective others, Penba as well as the Deoras were well aware that this type of insider knowledge combined with the right connections were crucial for a cross-border trader's success.

CITES and the Nepalese Authorities

In addition to transport, customs and testing expenses, an export tax of 3 Nepalese rupees per kilogram had to be paid to the Nepalese Forest Department. This tax was strictly enforced. Penba was under the impression that only a trader in Kathmandu equipped with the requisite export license was allowed to handle the payment of this tax. The Deoras explained that anybody could do so, but that the Nepalese border authorities were known to be difficult to deal with.

Here, the second border regime comes into play. Its underpinning rules stem, at least in part, from the Convention on International Trade in Endangered Species of Wild Fauna and Flora (CITES). Several commonly used ingredients in Tibetan medicines are listed in CITES Appendix II, which means that they are potentially endangered and, unless special permission is granted, trade across international borders is prohibited. As Nepal is a CITES member state it is required to control the export of restricted species. The species in question include *pangpö* (*spang pos*, *Nardostachys grandiflora*, Spikenard), *tsandan marpo* (*tsan dan dmar po*, *Pterocarpus santalinus*, red sanders or red sandalwood), and *agar* (*a gar*), the resinous heartwood of *Aquilaria* trees infected with a specific type of mould.[15]

The border regime in relation to CITES was a cause of great uncertainty because the extent to which the export restrictions were actually being enforced by the Nepalese authorities appeared to be arbitrary. Despite being a listed species, trade in *tsandan marpo* was booming, and prices rose tenfold between 2003 and 2008. The CITES listing was amended in 2007 as to include powdered and extracted forms of *tsandan marpo* (the original listing from 1995 had only included logs and wood chips). When I was in Kathmandu in March 2008, several traders I interviewed claimed that it was still permissible to export *tsandan marpo* in ground form (as a medical ingredient for Tibetan medicine); only solid wood was banned. In November 2008, none of the Kathmandu traders I was in contact with was taking the risk any longer. The technically illegal but tolerated informal trade of red sandalwood across the Friendship Bridge had come to an end. *Tsandan marpo* was now smuggled secretly across the border. In August 2009 I witnessed several dealers offering the wood for sale on the Chinese side of the border in the streets of Dram.

Later, when we got to know the Deora brothers a little better, Raksha told us that his younger brother had served six months in prison because of an alleged attempt to smuggle sandalwood. 'All the paperwork was OK', he said, 'but there is no rule in Nepal'. Because of this incident the family had decided to focus their business more on India and to explore other avenues of trade with China.[16] Although Penba had no plans to import any of the listed species this time, the stories about the unruliness of the Nepalese border regime worried him. He decided that it would be safer to hire a middleman through the Deoras who would take responsibility for his goods on the Nepalese side of the border.

After this exchange of information on the problems associated with transport and crossing the border, Penba and the two brothers agreed to discuss the future of the Deoras' herbs in Xining at a later stage, and to concentrate instead on the herbs Penba intended to buy. Slowly, the atmosphere warmed up. Penba had a list of about two dozen herbs, and a discussion about the available qualities and their prices ensued.

The question of herbs and prices requires closer attention. As mentioned before, the general agreement among traders and people in the Tibetan medicine industry was that herb prices were increasing year by year. With Penba's help I compiled a list of the 2005, 2007 and 2008 prices of all the 132 materials he sold in his shop. Based on this data, the average annual increase in price over the previous three years was 13.6 per cent (9.7 per cent inflation-adjusted),[17] while the average increase between October 2007 and October 2008 was 22.6 per cent (15.7 per cent adjusted). For the 28 species imported from India and Nepal, the three-year-average rise was also 13.6 per cent (9.7 per cent adjusted); between October 2007 and October 2008, however, the average increase in price was 25.8 per cent (18.9 per cent adjusted). From these numbers we can see that the increase in prices has accelerated, and that this acceleration has been even more pronounced in the case of imported herbs. The latter difference would have been even bigger in Nepalese rupees. However, as the Nepalese rupee has seen a steep devaluation against the Chinese yuan, the price increase of imported herbs has been cushioned on the Chinese side.

These numbers corroborate the general observation that herbs have become more expensive. Their robustness, however, is limited. First, the numbers are based on the prices of only one herb trader. Second, the variation from one herb to another is considerable. While one herb, Qinghai *tigta* (*mtsho sngon tig ta*), has seen a 40 per cent decrease in price within one year, the prices of other herbs have doubled within the same period. And third, herb prices tend to fluctuate seasonally. The prices of a particular herb are usually much lower right after the harvesting season.

Penba and I compiled the inventory in October 2008, before our trip to Nepal. The prices Arjun and Raksha were now presenting to us were again considerably higher. Penba had a list of the prices his family had paid the Deoras five months previously and he was quite shocked to hear the brothers' current charges. He decided to compare these offers with the prices proposed by other wholesalers and insisted that he had to see the herbs before he could make up his mind.

One of his Amdo friends was acquainted with another Indian trader known for his competitive prices, and I was also eager to introduce Penba to a couple of traders in Kathmandu. The next days were hectic. We met several wholesalers, went through the same procedure of asking prices and insisting on actually seeing the herbs. Some of the storerooms we were brought to were in questionable condition – humid, with crumbling walls, and infested with rats. Penba started to tell everybody that high quality was imperative, as the herbs would otherwise fail the import test. Furthermore, it turned out that most wholesalers actually did not stock the quantities Penba needed, and would have to import them from India first, or buy them from other wholesalers.

While discussing each and every herb in detail would go beyond the scope of this chapter, a closer look at two examples will provide an insight into the dilemmas Penba was faced with and the pragmatic decisions he had to take. In the following, I briefly discuss *baru* and *gyatig*.

Baru

Aru, baru and *kyuru* are the three basic ingredients imported in large quantities to Tibet. Penba planned to buy five metric tons of each. All three fruits are harvested in autumn. While *aru* was available in large quantities and of good quality, *baru* and *kyuru* were more of a problem. It was already early December but the *baru* we were shown was from the previous year. The new harvest was just about to come in, we were told. We would only have to wait for another two weeks or so. This put Penba in a difficult position, because the import permit he had obtained in Shigatse was only valid for one month and he was increasingly afraid that he might miss this deadline if he agreed to wait and see whether the new harvest or the promised better quality product brought from Nepalgunj or even from Delhi would materialise or not. Although the quality we were shown was mediocre, he felt that it was too risky to wait. Who could be sure that the herbs would arrive in time? And what if the quality was still not satisfactory?

Most of the *baru* sold in Nepal comes from the lower hills in the western part of the country and Nepalgunj has become an important trading hub. I learned from a well-established trader that wholesalers were increasingly reluctant to ship large quantities to Kathmandu. 'Before, Kathmandu was the main centre of trade. But now, Nepalgunj has become more important because you have to pay so many bribes on the way to Kathmandu', he said. As most of the *aru*, *baru* and *kyuru* was sold to India anyway, Nepalgunj was an ideally located trading hub. As a consequence of this shift, and in combination with the time constraint Penba faced due to the limited duration of his import permit, he finally settled on buying the previous year's lower-quality *baru*. Although he was not happy with it he felt that this was the best course of action under the given circumstances.

It should be noted that the Chinese system of licences and import permits, aiming at ensuring steady supplies and stable quality, was in this case the immediate cause of Penba's purchase of inferior *baru* for the production of Tibetan medicines.

Gyatig

As mentioned in the section on cultivation at the beginning of this chapter, *gyatig* belongs to the family of *tigta*. A substantial part of it is now cultivated in Nepal's Kanchenjunga area. This type of *tigta*, usually identified as *Swertia chirayita*, is regarded as the best.

The herb is also widely used in Ayurveda. The market for *gyatig* has seen a veritable boom over the last few years and prices have been increasing steadily, albeit with considerable seasonal fluctuation. In March 2008, the price was around 350 Nepalese rupees per kilogram in Kathmandu. A trader working for a factory in Lhasa, who was also one of Deora's customers, had paid 390 Nepalese rupees in summer 2009 as an advance for the new harvest that was scheduled to arrive in the autumn (although, by the time I left Nepal he had not managed to get the necessary licences and permits and had not been able to collect his goods). The price the Deoras wanted now in early December was higher still: 470 rupees per kilo. Penba wanted

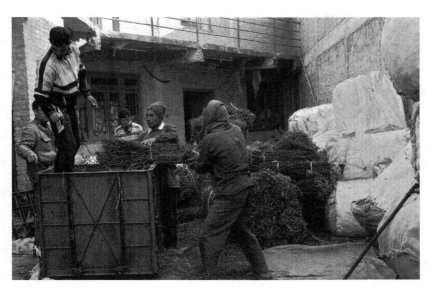

Figure 4.3: Pressing *gyatig* into bales.

to buy two metric tons of *gyatig* and Deora turned out to be the only wholesaler we could find who had this quantity in stock.

With *gyatig*, the whole plant is used in Tibetan medicine, and as the dried plants are relatively light but bulky they are usually strapped into compressed bales for transport. Deora had a machine to make such bales, and so it was agreed that he would hire his usual labourers to do the job. It took a full two days to package the two tons of *gyatig*. Penba was nervous and wanted to be present while the bales were made. Anxiously, he told me, 'You don't know what they put into the bales. You find grass, dirt and many other things if you don't check carefully'.

When we arrived at the packing site, work had already started and Penba did not like what he saw. The *gyatig* was still humid and parts of it had turned black. Turning to Raksha for an explanation, he received the reply that this was the condition in which the herbs had been bought from intermediary traders. The monsoon had been long and Dasain, a major Hindu festival celebrated throughout Nepal, had fallen early this year. As people in the villages needed cash for the festival, they had harvested a couple of weeks earlier than usual, while the late monsoon was still going on, and the plants had not yet completely dried. But the quality, Raksha insisted, was still excellent.

In fact, Penba was not too concerned that some of the herbs had turned black. 'I can still sell them', he said; 'it does not affect the quality too much'. What bothered him, however, was the potential loss of money. Once in Tibet, the herbs would dry fully and thereby lose weight, making the price paid to the Deoras seem even greater. Penba tried to find a solution and to negotiate a discount of 10 per cent in order to compensate for the moisture content. But Raksha argued that he would lose money if he agreed. Being aware that Penba had limited time and that the Deoras were the only whole-saler who had enough *gyatig* in stock at the moment, Raksha knew that Penba had hardly any room for bargaining.

While we were overseeing the making of the bales, a middle-aged man with a thick moustache dressed in simple clothes entered the courtyard and approached Raksha. Judging from his behaviour I guessed that he was either a tenant or a distant cousin of the Deora family, coming to ask for money or a favour. But the man turned out to be a policeman coming to ask for a 'donation'. The policeman complained that Raksha's father had only given them 2,000 rupees for Dasain, but the goat they had bought had cost 4,000 rupees! Deora turned him away, saying that he was busy now, and that he should come back tomorrow. After the policeman had left, Raksha complained, 'Protection! What kind of protection can they give us? Nepalis are just lazy; they only want money but don't offer anything in return'. He mentioned that the Maobadi[18] were much more de-manding than the police in this respect. The family paid them be-tween 40,000 and 50,000 rupees per year.

Penba and I were surprised. We found the plainclothes police-man's appearance as a humble suppliant remarkably different to the much more self-confident demeanour of their Chinese counterparts. Although this incident can hardly be taken as representative, it illus-trates how different dealing with officials in Kathmandu can be from dealing with officials in Tibet.

In the end, Penba bought the *gyatig* at Raksha's price. He had to accept the Deoras' terms because he had no other option. Raksha agreed to instruct the workers to leave the wettest and the most rot-ten bits and pieces aside but Penba was still very unhappy about the course events had taken.

Again, the quality of the herbs, which would finally be used in the production of Tibetan pharmaceuticals, was not directly dependent on the trader's knowledge and careful selection. A long monsoon and an early Dasain, combined with the local need for cash for the festival, defined the context of this purchase. The example also highlights the peculiarities of the wholesale trade. Buying two tons of *gyatig* is not the same as buying a few hundred kilograms. For smaller quantities, Penba would have had several options. Most traders in Kathmandu had some *gyatig* in store. But the Deoras were the only wholesaler able to deliver the required quantity within Penba's time frame.

Back to Tibet

After a week of herb shopping, Penba and I parted. While he was busy with the last details of his purchase and sorting out transport, I travelled on to India. Eight months later, in August 2009, I met Penba again in Lhasa and he told me what had happened on his way back to Tibet.

All his plants except the *aru*, for which he had a licence, had been confiscated at the border. The deputy customs officer at Dram, a Tibetan, informed him that importing herbs without a permit was no longer tolerated. Penba went to see the chief customs officer, a Chinese. He explained that this was the first time he was importing herbs under the new regime and that he had not been clear about the exact requirements. The Chinese officer almost agreed to turn a blind eye to the affair, but finally called in his deputy, who was very upset that Penba had tried to bypass him. The Chinese officer reversed his stance and Penba's herbs were seized.

However, Penba was granted a reprieve of three months to secure the necessary permits for the other herbs. Meanwhile, his goods were kept in a storeroom at the border. Of course, three months were much too short a period within which to apply for and obtain all the permits. After six months Penba had at least managed to get a permit for the *gyatig*. He went back to the border and for two weeks he kept going to the customs office every day, trying to find a solution. He started to befriend everybody in the office and, in the end, he managed to retrieve all his goods, not just the *gyatig*, and transport them to Lhasa. The *gyatig*, for which he now had a permit, needed to undergo testing, and the results were still pending when I last saw him. The herbs, however, were already in Lhasa, where Penba had them stored in a newly built second-storey addition to his storeroom, which had been built especially. I asked whether he was able to sell the herbs before the results arrived. He said, 'Yes, no problem. If it doesn't pass the test I can always give them another *gyatig*'.

What did Penba do in order to get his herbs back? How much did he pay? 'Some cigarettes and the bill in a restaurant were enough', he said proudly. No bribes were necessary. Later, the two customs officials came to Lhasa and he managed to invite one of them to his house. A subsequent business trip to the Nepalese border passed without further incident. Now that he knew all the officials they were less meticulous about checking his truck; they merely opened a few bags near the rear of the truck, those containing the herbs for which he had a licence. They asked him if he had any other goods in the truck and, when he responded negatively, allowed him to pass.

However, a new problem had emerged in the meantime – the tightening of yet another, a third border regime, not one to regulate the flow of herbs for the purpose of quality assurance or biodiversity protection, but one to control the flow of people: Penba's passport was about to expire, and with less than six months' left on it he had not been able to obtain a visa to go to Nepal in July 2009. Renewing passports has become very difficult for Tibetans over the past few years. Penba was told that he needed an invitation letter from his business partner in Nepal, a copy of his partner's identity card, and a letter from the Nepal Forest Department, all this in addition to the import licences and the necessary papers in China. Penba managed to get the invitation letter but not the copy of his business partner's identity card. His business partner – not the Deoras but the official one mentioned on his licences – had initially agreed, but subsequently reneged on the grounds that providing Penba with his identity card might raise problems for his own future business plans in China. In the end, Penba asked a driver in Nepal to give him a copy of his identity card. 'Any Nepalese ID will do', Penba said with a smile. The driver agreed reluctantly and the only thing Penba was lacking when I last saw him was a letter from the Forest Department. 'But maybe I can manage without', he said. 'Let's see'.

Tactics and Strategies

A booming industry confronted by a potential ecological crisis, the state's relative non-interference in domestic plant sourcing and trade, three border regimes governing the transnational flow of people and herbs, and the ways factories and traders deal with this situation – these are the elements of the industrial assemblage discussed in this chapter. All the actors involved – the factories, the traders, and the authorities – deal with the same problem: efforts at cultivation, maintaining contracts with village-based collectors, developing legislation and setting up border regimes, and bypassing distrusted import tests are all attempts at coming to terms with the unruliness of nature.

Let me, in summary, revisit each of these threads. In a government White Paper published in 2003 on Tibet's environment and ecology, the issue of medicinal plants was not even mentioned (IOSC 2003). Since then, awareness of the issue has certainly grown but official China's approach to the problem has not seen nearly as much fervour as projects like GMP. Despite frequent claims by companies as well as the authorities that cultivation is crucial for a sustainable industry, most people in the industry agree that what has so far been accomplished is not enough. On the part of the companies, the difficulties associated with cultivation, especially of rare high-altitude species, have led to a certain degree of disillusionment. Apart from a few easily cultivated species, the industry still relies mostly on wild-crafted herbs. On the part of the government, the incentives meant to boost cultivation have not yielded the envisioned results. Furthermore, the collection of and trade in wild medicinal plants within China has remained outside the state's regulations up to now, due to the exemptions granted to TCM and its crude drugs.

China's relative non-interference in terms of cultivation, collection and domestic trade stands in sharp contrast to the situation regarding cross-border trade, where three border regimes, two in the People's Republic of China (PRC) and one in Nepal, aim at regulating the flow of people and goods across the border between the two countries. These border regimes illustrate what James Scott has described as 'the utopian, immanent, and continually frustrated goal of the modern state … to reduce the chaotic, disorderly, constantly changing social reality beneath it to something more closely resembling the administrative grid of its observations' (Scott 1998: 82).

I suggested the term 'border regime' to describe the conditions in which herbs and traders move both across international borders and conceptual divides. The three border regimes encountered above can thereby be seen as answers to certain problems.

The first border regime responds to the problem of patient safety, which is related to surging trade volumes and industrial production. Increasing legibility (licences, import permits, authorised entry ports) and control (quality assessment of imports) are the means of choice in this attempt at 'cultivating the wilds'.[19] The second border regime, enforcing Nepal's CITES obligations more strictly, can be seen as a reaction to dwindling resources and the general concern over ecological balance; and the third border regime, constraining the number of Tibetans who can legally visit Nepal and India, is the way in which the PRC's security apparatus responds to the fragile political situation.

The corresponding spatial and conceptual divides are the following. The first border regime separates the imported, untested, raw product of nature from the approved, 'civilised' medicinal raw material, thereby reinforcing the divide between the sphere of nature on one side and culture, society and technology on the other. The second border regime stemming from Nepal's CITES obligations emphasises the same divide, although for other reasons and with opposite signs. Here, it is not humans who have to be protected from the potential dangers of the wild nature and its raw products but nature itself, which needs protection against transnational capitalism as a form of encroachment. And third, by making a simple passport renewal a most difficult procedure for Tibetans (but not for Chinese), the party-state's security apparatus aims at maintaining a distance between the Tibetans in the PRC and those in exile, who are blamed for conspiring against the party-state. Again, the spatial divide between China and exile is also a conceptual one: the Communist Party's truth against the exiles' lies.[20]

There is very little reason to believe that a stricter import regime leads to better quality imported herbs. On the contrary, Penba's dilemmas and decisions suggest that the unintended side effects of such regulations can affect the quality of medicinal ingredients negatively. However, as the border regimes' quest for legibility and control is never fully realised, there is room for a certain flexibility in the ways they are enacted. This flexibility cushions the negative effects to some extent.

Here, the distinction between tactics and strategies is useful. In de Certeau's (1988) sense border regimes are strategies: they are linked with institutions and based on political, economic and scientific rationality. Tactics, on the other hand, are the 'ways of operating' within the spaces defined by strategies. They include 'clever tricks' and 'knowing how to get away with things'. Whereas strategy defines space, tactics depends on time. The distinction brings us back to the notion of *mētis*: the systems of tactics 'is always on the watch for opportunities that must be seized "on the wing". Whatever it wins, it does not keep. It must constantly manipulate events in order to turn them into "opportunities" [...] The Greeks called these "ways of operating" *mētis*' (ibid.: xix).

Tactics, cleverness and 'knowing how to get away with things' are apt descriptions for the skills of a successful trader. However, traders are not the only ones who rely on them. The officials in charge of a border regime are not only responsible for legibility and control; they also have to make the border regime work on the ground, or at least they must make it appear to work. Whereas import licences are issued in Beijing, drug testing and import permits fall in the domain of local authorities, and the actual enforcement of new regulations is left to the customs authorities in Dram. With ever-changing policies and regulations that are often impossible to meet, local authorities are in a difficult situation. On the one hand, they have to implement policies forged in Beijing; on the other hand, making them work, or at least appear to work, often requires bending rules and turning a blind eye towards technically illegal but well-established practices.

Bending rules is, then, much more than mere corruption; it is a structural feature of a constellation that is neither particular to the herb trade nor the case of Tibet. The local officials' reluctance to report problems with targets and policies from above is widely known and acknowledged (Brown 2002; Tsai 2008). Cai (2000), for example, argues in his article on local cadres and statistical reporting in rural China that the manipulation of statistical data by local officials is rooted in the institutional arrangement of the administrative system itself. Since lower-level officials are dependent on the goodwill of their higher-level counterparts in terms of their career prospects, they are held more accountable to their superiors than to the public. Reporting problems with the implementation of a specific policy is not expedient in this context and local officials enjoy considerable autonomy in the absence of permanent supervision (ibid.: 784).

In the case of the TAR, however, it is important to mention yet another aspect: as a majority of government officials – especially in the lower ranks – are Tibetan (Conner and Barnett 1997: 40, 214; *People's Daily* 2001), the need to ensure their compliance is considered to be especially important (Barnett 2006a: 47–50). In this sense, frequent, quick and far-reaching changes in policy – be it on purpose or not – also combine two 'benefits' in terms of control: first, pressure is maintained on all actors involved to move in the direction defined by Beijing. And second, in a situation in which officials and business people are constantly violating one rule or another, they are all, inevitably, permanently vulnerable and need to keep good and friendly relations with the office above or the superiors in charge.

In short, while the border regimes in the present case are designed to regulate and render legible the transits of traders and herbs, their justification derives not only from their capacity to exercise control but also, even more importantly, from facilitating successful trade. Ironically, the survival of a border regime rests to some extent on both officials and traders breaking its rules in order to make it work.

Nevertheless, as constituent parts of doing cross-border trade, the border regimes push a particular outlook on nature and medicinal plants. The emphasis on careful selection and harvesting according to the procedures described in the Gyüshi's Seven Limbs, for example, is hardly relevant when the focus lies on tactical navigation across unruly borders and conceptual spheres. Despite the latitude the border regimes entail, they reconfigure Tibetan medicine's relations with nature. In this sense, the companies' concerns about commercial trade are certainly justified.

Notes

1. However, a 2004 report by the Tibet Information Network suggests that the prices the factories pay are still higher than what local *amchi* are able to offer. The commercialisation of raw materials is therefore having a paradoxical effect on rural *amchi* practice. Whereas commercial trade made it easier for rural *amchi* to obtain certain raw materials from far away, the increasing competition by the factories rendered local ingredients more expensive and therefore less accessible, the report argues (TIN 2004: 80).

2. Personal communication with Ugyen Dorji, Project Director of the Medical Plants Phase II Project of the Bhutanese Department of Agriculture, September 2009.

3. A version of the following section of this chapter was presented at the 7th International Conference on Traditional Asian Medicines (ICTAM VII) in Bhutan in 2009, and published in a special issue of *Asian Medicine* (Saxer 2011).

4. Sowa Rigpa classifies medicinal ingredients into eight categories (*sman rgyu'i dbye ba brgyad*): *rinpoche (rin po che)* – gems and precious metals; *sa (sa)* – soils; *do (rdo)* – stones; *shing (shing)* – wooden plants; *tsi (rtsi)* – aromatic; *thang (thang)* – shrubs; *ngo (sngo)* – herbs; and *sochag (srog chags)* – animal products (Dawa 2002: 27).

5. The full Tibetan names are *arura (a ru ra), barura (ba ru ra), and kyurura (skyu ru ra)*. Generally, the two-syllable terms are used. Instead of the expression *dräbusum ('bras bu gsum)* – which can also refer to three other fruits (*a 'bras, sra 'bras and 'jam 'bras*) – the concatenation *a-ba-kyu-sum (a ba skyu gsum)* is sometimes used.

6. Nutmeg – *zati (dza ti)*; clove – *lishi (li shi)*; great black cardamom – *kakola (ka ko la)*; green cardamom – *sugmel (sug mel)*; saffron – *kache gurgum (kha che gur gum)*; and bamboo concretion – *chugang (cu gang)*. Chugang, however, also refers to a mineral found in the Kailash region.

7. Sociologist Gesa Lindemann (2002; 2009) also uses the term 'border regime', although in a different context. She speaks of socio-biological border regimes guarding the conceptual divide between life and death in the emergency rooms of hospitals.

8. This number refers to trucks in Nepal. A truck in Nepal usually loads up to ten tons, the Chinese trucks on the Tibetan Plateau about twenty metric tons. The fifty truckloads therefore equal five hundred metric tons, which seems very high. I have not been able to confirm this claim.

9. Personal communication from Karma Bhutia of The Mountain Institute in Kathmandu, August 2009.

10. The year 3057 in the Nepali calendar equals the year 3000AD.

11. See Samten Karmay (1994; 1996) for a discussion of the political significance of place for Tibetan identity.

12. The Marwaris, an ethnic group originally from Rajasthan (India), are well known for their extensive trade and business networks throughout the Indian subcontinent.

13. *Bandh* literally means 'closed' and denotes a common form of strike in Nepal. Businesses and markets are forced to close and road traffic comes to a standstill. These strikes have become so frequent that a website, www.nepalbandh.com, offers a regularly updated calendar with all announced *bandhs*.

14. Tina Harris (2009) argues that the phasing out of exports from the Indian subcontinent to China is a relatively recent development, which has been further accelerated since the railway link to Lhasa was opened in 2006.

15. Several species of the *Aquilaria* tree can be the source of *agar*. Whereas originally only one species, namely *Aquilaria malaccensis*, was listed in Appendix II, all species were finally included in 2004. However, several member states have raised objections against this inclusion, which have not yet been resolved. The situation therefore remains unclear. See www.cites.org, documents > appendices; and documents > reservations, respectively.

16. Harvesting rare herbs, poaching endangered animals and smuggling the goods across the border to China, often with the help of officials in charge, is a topic frequently discussed in Nepal's newspapers. See, for example, Shahi 2010; Neupane 2010; Himalayan News Service 2010.

17. Inflation adjustment was calculated on the basis of the consumer price index in China, published by TradingEconomics (www.tradingeconomics.com).

18. The term 'Maobadi' refers to the members of the CPNM (Communist Party of Nepal [Maoist]) – since January 2009 officially the Unified Communist Party of Nepal – commonly known as the Maoists. Between 1996 and 2006 the Maoists led the 'People's War' in Nepal. Although the Comprehensive Peace Accord, signed in November 2006, officially put an end to the Maoist practice of extorting money from the population in support of their People's War, the practice seems to continue in some areas.

19. I take the expression 'cultivating the wilds' from a panel at the 2009 International Congress on Traditional Asian Medicine in Thimphu, Bhutan, organised by Sienna Craig and Denise Glover.

20. These divides are reminiscent of Bruno Latour's (1993) analysis of the 'modern' project. He argues that the notion of modernity, in whichever incarnation, implies the idea of such 'great divides': the ancient from the modern, nature from culture, humans from non-humans. A constant effort is necessary to keep these spheres apart, a continuous 'work of purification' in Latour's terms. However, as phenomena in the real world regularly criss-cross these great divides, Latour emphasises that in reality the 'work of translation' remains a permanent necessity. This is an apt description of the purpose of all three border regimes of the present case.

Chapter 5
Knowledge, Property

With the advent of industrial production, the issue of to whom Sowa Rigpa belongs has gained considerable relevance. As knowledge of Sowa Rigpa acquires potential market value, new questions arise: Who is entitled to use the formulas and who is eligible to reap the benefits from producing them? In the preceding chapters knowledge has been discussed in relation to the strategic *techne* and tactical *mētis* of production and trade; in this chapter knowledge will be examined as part of the industrial assemblage in yet another form, namely, as intellectual property.

In the context of Sowa Rigpa and the industrial production of Tibetan medicines, the notion of intellectual property rights is as much a political and moral issue as it is an economic and legal one. In an editorial in *Tibet's Environment and Development Digest*, an exile publication, Tashi Tsering cited a Tibetan doctor from Amdo who had expressed his concerns that *amchi* would soon be barred from producing certain medicines as Chinese companies were gaining patents. Tashi Tsering writes:

> Surely, the ultimate subversion of the Tibetan medical tradition would be if the Tibetan people themselves were forced to purchase medicine invented by their own culture and made from their own land, at a higher cost, and from a Chinese company because of a contrived patent system set up to benefit large industries to the exclusion of local practitioners. (Tashi Tsering 2005)

In a reply to Tashi Tsering's editorial, Tsultrim Tsering Gyaltsen (2005) went a step further and suggested that companies not owned by Tibetans should pay royalty fees for using plants from the Tibetan environment. He argues that companies substituting Tibetan plants with foreign medicinal herbs should not be allowed to call their products 'Tibetan'. A committee consisting of people with an 'intimate understanding of Sowa Rigpa' should be entitled to issue certificates for authentic Tibetan medicine. 'This is the only way to insure the continued efficacy of the medicines and to prevent the bastardization of the Tibetan medical tradition for profit' (ibid.).

These provocative statements lead right to the centre of the issue. First, linking authenticity to the origins of the *materia medica* used in Tibetan medicine is, despite being meant to protect Tibetan interests, a delicate proposition. As mentioned in Chapter 3, it has been common practice throughout the history of Sowa Rigpa to substitute ingredients that are difficult to obtain. Substitution and variation were and are responsible for the remarkable adaptability of Sowa Rigpa, which has allowed it to be successfully practised from Buryatia to India and from Bhutan to the Kalmyk Republic. Gyaltsen's proposition denies one of the major strengths of Tibetan pharmaceutical knowledge, namely, its openness and adaptability. Moreover, what would such a suggestion mean in terms of the raw materials not native to the Tibetan plateau? Much of this *materia medica* imported from India and Nepal, for example, is also used by other medical systems, including Ayurveda and Unani. The idea of denying companies using plants of non-Tibetan origin the right to call their medicines 'Tibetan' would necessitate a complete reinvention of Sowa Rigpa. If Gyaltsen's propositions were followed, none of the producers, neither in Tibet nor in exile, could claim to be making authentic Tibetan drugs.

Second, the idea of royalty fees for the use of Tibetan genetic resources and knowledge also raises the question of whether Tibetan medicine producers in turn would have to pay royalty fees for the imported ingredients they use. This would neither benefit companies nor private *amchi* in Tibet.

And third: when is a company Tibetan? Tibetan ownership is not easily definable, as we have seen in Chapter 2. How to assess a company whose stock is held by a variety of Tibetan and non-Tibetan investors? And would a company owned by a local government of the Tibetan Autonomous Region (TAR) be considered Tibetan-owned? From the exile perspective, the Chinese government equals encroachment and occupation. It therefore has no moral right to any form of stewardship nor ownership. From the perspective of the People's Republic of China (PRC), the state is naturally predestined to be responsible for the protection of Tibetan medicine against possible encroachments from outside. Who else could take this role?

My aim in this chapter is not to find an answer to these questions but to examine what happens to Sowa Rigpa as a system of knowledge when it is conceived of as intellectual property. The concept of intellectual property rights itself is, again, a global form. I intend to show that its recontextualisation within the industrial assemblage affects the Tibetan knowledge of healing in a particular way.

Owners and Pirates

The polemical propositions from exile outlined above have to be understood against the backdrop of ongoing global debates about genetic resources, rights of access, biopiracy, sharing benefits in the form of royalty fees, and the patentability of traditional knowledge. As we will see, these debates are of only limited applicability to Sowa Rigpa, as well as to any scholarly Asian medicine, for that matter. Nevertheless, they have gained a great deal of influence in shaping the modes in which knowledge becomes conceived of as a question of intellectual property rights.

The trigger for the biopiracy debate was a series of cases in which Western, mostly North American, companies filed patent applications for plants in foreign countries. One of the most famous of these cases involved a patent over the extraction of azadirachtin, a pesticide, from the Indian neem tree. A patent was granted to New York-based W.R. Grace and Co. in 1992 (Wolfgang 1995). The neem tree (*Azadirichta indica*) is known as the 'blessed tree' or the 'curer of all ailments' in India and has been used for centuries in medicine and agriculture. The patent could have meant that Indian farmers would have to pay royalties to an American corporation. Jeremy Rifkin, an activist and outspoken critic of patenting traditional knowledge, initiated a successful campaign against this ruthless act of biopiracy. The patent was legally challenged and finally revoked.[1]

China has also had experiences with global biopiracy. Monsanto, for example, applied for a patent over a variety of wild soya. The application was filed simultaneously in over 100 countries – an illustration of the vast financial and organisational powers of a major transnational corporation. After enormous pressure from China and several NGOs, including Greenpeace, Monsanto finally withdrew the application. Other problematic cases include the granting of a patent over the extraction of an anti-malarial substance from *Artemisia annua* by Rhone-Poulenc and GlaxoSmithKline, respectively French and British pharmaceutical giants (Qin 2009: 226), and a patent over 'ginseng royal jelly', which was granted to a US company (Jia 2005: 64). These and many other cases mobilised NGOs and governments around the globe. Bioprospecting, the systematic screening of large numbers of plants for potential medicinal value by transnational biotech companies, came under attack because it was seen as a prelude to biopiracy (see Cox and Balick 1994; Balick and Cox 1996).

Despite the fact that large-scale bioprospecting is based on advanced biotechnology, the relevance of indigenous knowledge should not be underestimated. Biotech companies often take indigenous knowledge as a lead in their bioprospecting activities. Farnsworth (1988: 95) showed that 74 per cent of the plant-derived drugs in his sample were employed in the same or a related manner as they had been traditionally. Undeniably, traditional knowledge guided the 'discovery' of these drugs, and it is therefore a valuable asset in bioprospecting.

An important discursive strategy in campaigns against the exploitation of traditional knowledge has been to couple bioprospecting and biopiracy with the loss of biodiversity, which became a matter of increasing concern during the 1980s. NGO campaigns argued that indigenous knowledge was a vital aspect of any strategy for the preservation of biodiversity, and that bioprospecting activities (and the possible subsequent exploitation of knowledge and plants) were a threat to local, sustainable harvesting patterns. Indigenous knowledge, biodiversity, large-scale bioprospecting, and biopiracy thus became linked in the discourse of NGOs, scientists and social movements. Their campaigns gained considerable momentum (see Escobar 1998).

The most significant outcome of these campaigning efforts can be seen in the United Nations' Convention on Biological Diversity (hereafter: Biodiversity Convention), signed at the Earth Summit in Rio de Janeiro in 1992. China was among the first countries to ratify the Convention the following year. Apart from the conservation of biodiversity and the sustainable use of its components, the convention also touches on the question of traditional knowledge. Article

8(j) requires all parties to 'respect, preserve and maintain knowledge, innovations and practices of indigenous and local communities' and to 'encourage the equitable sharing of the benefits arising from the utilization of such knowledge, innovations and practices' (United Nations 1993: 149). The article has sparked an ongoing debate about terminology. Is it traditional, local or indigenous knowledge that needs to be protected?

Graham Dutfield compiled a catalogue of characteristic criteria for the definition of traditional knowledge. He contends that traditional knowledge is, generally, recorded and transmitted orally, gained through experience, enhanced, checked and revised on the basis of day-to-day observations, and based on an intuitive mode of thinking. It is mainly qualitative and rooted in a holistic world-view, which emphasises the social and spiritual relations of all life forms (Dutfield 2001: 241).

However, that knowledge is enhanced, checked and revised on the basis of day-to-day practice is probably true of any medical practice, including biomedicine. And, while an orally transmitted, 'intuitive mode of thinking' may be adequate to describe certain modes of knowledge transmission in medical systems, it is hardly suitable to describe the highly structured approach of the Gyüshi. In short, Sowa Rigpa (as well as any scholarly Asian medicine) is not really 'traditional' in the sense of this definition. Moreover, Sowa Rigpa is neither local nor by any standards indigenous knowledge.[2]

Above all, Sowa Rigpa has not been a major target of biopiracy activities so far. Transnational biotech firms are mostly interested in single plants from which an active ingredient can be extracted to treat a specific condition. Tibetan multi-component formulas largely elude bioprospecting as their biochemical mechanisms are too complex – and therefore too expensive – to investigate (cf. Adams 2002: 675).

But even as international corporations have so far not shown much inclination to appropriate Tibetan medicine, and the entire debate seems not particularly germane to Sowa Rigpa, it has reverberated in the field. The idea of biopiracy provides a discursive space for local actors to voice their concerns and justify their claims. There is a heightened awareness about bioprospecting and rights of access to Himalayan medicinal plants.

A case in point is Laurent Pordié's analysis of how the discourses linking biopiracy and intellectual property rights are used to various ends in Ladakh (Pordié 2008). The fear of biopiracy has led to significant scepticism about outsiders working on medicinal plants, regardless of their motivations. Pordié describes the case of the Plant Foundation, an NGO dedicated to the conservation of medicinal herbs, to make his point. The organisation is run by a retired Dutchwoman who started working in Ladakh in the late 1990s. She came under suspicion of 'stealing' plant knowledge for an imaginary pharmaceutical company and was finally expelled from Ladakh – despite the fact that she had been recommended by a well-known Tibetan Rinpoche who guaranteed her good intentions (ibid.: 137).

In this context, Ladakhi *amchi* who are willing to cooperate with foreigners run the risk of being incriminated by their colleagues. On the other hand, those *amchi* at the forefront of defending Ladakhi resources and intellectual property ascend to powerful positions, Pordié argues. The expulsion of the Dutchwoman who came with the blessing of an eminent Buddhist master was also an expression of local power struggles, namely between Ladakhi *amchi* and the Tibetan exile community. Pordié recalls that her expulsion was locally seen as 'refusing subservience to the will of the Tibetans'. The topic was hotly debated among leading Ladakhi *amchi*. Finally the biopiracy allegation won the upper hand, going against the will of an important lama (ibid.: 149). Pordié notes that, 'intellectual property rights are retranscribed as a reason for power; their plasticity permits the assertion of power for the benefit or the disadvantage of a single person, while systematically encapsulating the presumed community interests' (ibid.: 137).

This is not devoid of a certain irony. We saw above how concerns of Tibetans in exile about Chinese encroachments on Tibetan knowledge and resources are couched in terms of biopiracy allegations. Now, the exile Tibetans are increasingly facing resistance by local groups, in Ladakh and elsewhere in the Indian Himalayas, who rely on the very same discursive strategies to voice their claims. The branch clinics set up by the Dharamsala Men-Tsee-Khang throughout the Indian Himalayas, for example, came under suspicion for serving as a disguise of the Men-Tsee-Khang's attempt to gain access to local plant resources.

These examples from the Indian Himalayas clearly show that biopiracy discourse has the capacity to reconfigure local power relations, regardless of whether biopiracy is actually happening or not.

This is also true for the Tibetan medicine industry in the PRC, as I will argue shortly.

The Problem of Patents

A matter of much debate is whether or not intellectual property rights are the right framework for the protection of traditional knowledge (Society for Critical Exchange 1993; Brush and Stabinsky 1996; Patel 1996; Posey and Dutfield 1996: 75–92; Coombe 2005: 120; Mgbeoji 2006; Oguamanam 2006). Intellectual property rights, and especially patent regimes, are seen by many critics as predatory mechanisms of appropriation (Shiva 1997, 2001; Mgbeoji 2006: 121).

One argument is that their individualistic construction is at odds with the often communal nature of traditional knowledge held by families, clans or lineages (Dutfield 2001: 254; Oguamanam 2006: 158). This, however, has also been called into question. Patents in capitalist societies are similarly owned by vast and fluid communities, such as the shareholders of a corporation (Oguamanam 2006: 160), and clan or family knowledge, on the other hand, is in some societies a perfectly marketable commodity (Dutfield 2001: 246–47; Geismar 2005).

A second argument is that patents are meant to protect new inventions. Mainstream patent regimes require novelty, an inventive step, and a patent cannot be granted if it is based on 'prior art'. There is good reason to consider traditional knowledge as a prime example of prior art and therefore no patents should be granted. The problem is that mainstream patent regimes tend to give consideration to prior art only if documented and published in a written form – a condition that does not always apply to traditional knowledge. According to US patent law, for example, undocumented knowledge held in a foreign country does not count as prior art and is therefore not excluded from being patented (Dutfield 2001: 247).[3]

A third line of argument emphasises the question of patents on products of nature. In theory, products of nature are excluded from patenting. But as the life-science industry booms, the distinction between a 'field of technology' and a 'product of nature' is becoming increasingly blurred. Mgbeoji (2006) argues that the exclusion of products of nature from patentability has de facto been abandoned.

Courts tend to set the bar low when it comes to assessing human intervention as innovation. The isolation of an active ingredient from a plant may be enough to make it patentable (Oguamanam 2006: 171).

Contrary to these critical objections to the suitability of patents for the protection of traditional knowledge, some experts argue that claiming patents can also serve as a preventive or defensive measure against possible encroachment. Preventive patents, however, are not without problems: patents only guarantee protection for a limited period of time (usually twenty-five years) and many indigenous groups may not have the means either to file expensive patent applications nor to fight possible infringements later on (Dutfield 2001: 251; Oguamanam 2006: 162).

The Biodiversity Convention does not explicitly state that traditional knowledge should be treated as intellectual property; it simply says that traditional knowledge, innovations and practices should be respected, preserved and maintained, and possible benefits should be shared. Member states are free to establish systems of *sui generis* rights beyond the concept of intellectual property. But since intellectual property is the primary means for the allocation of rights over knowledge in the West, it is often taken as a logical starting point in the search for a mechanism that would guarantee an equitable sharing of benefits (Oguamanam 2006: 155).

This also has to be seen in relation to the fact that many of the Biodiversity Convention's signatory states are also members of the WTO and therefore bound by its Agreement on Trade-related Aspects of Intellectual Property Rights, the so-called TRIPS agreement. While giving no regard to traditional knowledge, the TRIPS agreement defines patentability in very broad terms. Article 27 states that patents shall be available for any invention in all fields of technology, regardless of whether they are products or processes, given that they involve an inventive step and are capable of industrial application (WTO 1994: 331). Contrary to the Biodiversity Convention, which leaves the signature states much room in terms of implementation, the TRIPS agreement is meant to harmonise intellectual property regimes across the globe – in other words: to enforce dominant intellectual property regimes globally.

Precious Pills, Precious Properties

How do these global debates resonate in the PRC and how are the international legal frameworks adapted to the context of traditional medicine in China? And how are they relevant to the Tibetan medicine industry?

In 2006 *Legal Daily* published an article arguing that China's government was in 'a passive and disadvantageous position' while 'our own TCM is frequently [the subject of patent applications] by other countries, which reminds us of the serious situation that Chinese traditional medic[al] knowledge is encountering' (*Legal Daily* 2006).[4]

Current legislation in China limits the scope of possible patents. As a socialist country, China defines public property over almost all natural resources in its constitution (Qin 2009: 227). Animal and plant varieties as well as methods for the diagnosis of disease are exempt from patenting (SIPO 2009). In accordance with most patent regimes, China's patent law requires novelty for a patent application, which basically forbids the patenting of traditional formulas. As a consequence, only very few newly designed Tibetan medicines have been patented so far, and almost no new formulas have come to the market since changes in the system of drug registration in 2002. Most patents in the industry refer to production processes and not to formulas.[5] The few examples for patented Tibetan formulas include Cheezheng's pain relief plaster and Jigme Phuntsog's hepatitis drug.

Due to its relatively restrictive patent regime and the limited possibilities of patenting traditional formulas, China has established a set of other measures to protect traditional knowledge. The most relevant for the present case are the Regulations on [the] Protection of Traditional Chinese Medicines (Government of China 1993). Here, novelty is not a requirement. Protection can be granted to Chinese medicines produced within the territory of the PRC and listed as standardised medicines at the state level (Zhang 2007). Companies can apply for a protection certificate for one of these medicines, and during the protection period only those enterprises holding such a certificate have a right to produce the respective formula.

The provisions distinguish between Grade I and Grade II protection. Medicines in the first category are entitled to a protection period of up to thirty years, those in the second category are granted protection for seven years, extendable again for another seven years.

A total of 1668 traditional Chinese medicines had obtained protection by 2005, twelve of them falling under the first category (Jia 2005: 65). However, this number appears to have decreased, most probably due to the expiry of protection periods. In February 2009 only 1,257 medicines were under protection (C-Med 2009).

This form of administrative protection and the exclusive rights that come with it triggered a recent quarrel in the Tibetan medicine industry over the right to produce some of the high value 'precious pills' (*rinchen rilbu*). Most companies used to produce Ratna Samphel, Rinchen Mangjor and Rinchen Drangjor, the three most famous precious pills, but have since lost their entitlement to do so. Currently, only the TAR Tibetan Medicine Factory in Lhasa and Arura in Xining are officially authorised to manufacture these formulas. These exclusive rights led to a legal dispute between Jigme Phuntsog's company Jiumei Tibetan Medicine Co. Ltd. and the Arura Group in Xining. Arura took the chance and applied for a protection certificate for Ratna Samphel and Rinchen Mangjor in 1998. Both medicines were granted Grade II protection in September 1998 and January 1999, respectively. The protection periods were renewed in December 2005 and February 2006. The protection certificates, proudly exhibited in Arura's showroom, gave the company exclusive rights to produce these formulas until September 2011 – seven years from the date of the second application.

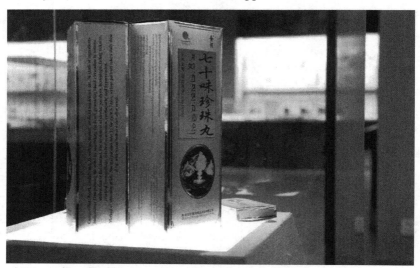

Figure 5.1: Arura's Ratna Samphel.

Jigme Phuntsog, however, challenged Arura's exclusive right on moral grounds: why should he as a Tibetan *amchi* trained in a monastery be banned from manufacturing some of the most potent and well known Tibetan formulas? Tibetan medicine belonged to the Tibetans, he argued. It cannot be appropriated by a single company with good relations with the state. As Jigme ignored Arura's certificates and continued producing the *rinchen rilbu* in question, Arura sued him and Jigme lost the case. Adding insult to injury, the regulations stipulate that any unauthorised production of a medicine under protection 'is to be regarded as the preparation of counterfeit medicine and to be dealt with according to law by the health administrative departments at county level and above' (Government of China 1993: Article 23). Jigme's well-known and highly appreciated *rinchen rilbu* were now officially counterfeit products. But Jigme had no intention to succumbing to what he conceived of as an administrative form of piracy and continued manufacturing the precious pills. He was sued again, fined and banned from continuing. But during visits to pharmacies in Xining I still encountered the lavish boxes of Jigme's now banned *rinchen rilbu*. Whether old stock was still in circulation or the court order had provided a genuine counterfeiter with an opportunity, we will never know.

As mentioned in Chapter 3, Ratna Samphel and Rinchen Mangjor have the status of national secrets, a special form of trade secret. Disregarding the fact that the formulas were widely produced and known throughout the Tibetan world, Arura was granted the protection certificates on the condition that it would not disclose the formulas to anybody. Under the pretext of safeguarding a national trade secret, the state transferred stewardship over traditional knowledge to a single semi-private corporation. In this case, the administrative mechanism to protect traditional knowledge clearly served as a means to strip most traditional knowledge holders of their rights. When I asked a senior manager at Arura why their company alone was granted the certificate, his simple answer was, 'We were first'.

Further adding to the complexity of the matter is the fact that the TAR Tibetan Medicine Factory is also producing both the precious pills in question. According to one of Arura's senior managers, they would technically not be entitled to do so. But Arura appears to be wise enough not to take action against the TAR's most famous, government-run Tibetan medicine company. Moreover, both Ratna

Samphel and Richen Mangjor contain *tsothal,* for which the TAR Tibetan Medicine Factory holds a patent. Therefore, the TAR Tibetan Medicine Factory could argue that Arura does not have a right to produce the *rinchen rilbu* in question. In this situation, Arura's certificate and the TAR Tibetan Medicine Factory's patent can both be seen as insurance against unlikely but possible claims from the other company.

In principle, the protection of varieties of Chinese medicines is not necessarily exclusive. Other *rinchen rilbu* – such as Yunying 25 (*gyu rnying 25*), Mutig 25 (*mu tig 25*), Chumar 25 (*byu dmar 25*), or Tsotru Dashel (*btso bkru zla shel*) – are also considered to have national-heritage status as protected drugs, but this has not led a company claiming exclusive manufacturing rights over them, and they continue to be legally produced by several companies. Zhang Qingkui, head of SIPO's Pharmacy and Biotech Examination Department in Beijing, pointed out that if a medicine granted protection was produced by other companies before its approval, those companies were entitled to reapply for a certificate. Such an application must be submitted within six months from the date of publication of the original certificate (ibid.: Article 23).

In theory, Jigme Phuntsog as well as all the other companies who lost their right to produce these highly valued *rinchen rilbu* would have been free to apply for protection as well. For whatever reason, they did not. In any case, the outcome of such an application would have been highly uncertain. Obtaining a certificate of protection requires not only familiarity with the rules and regulations, but also with the ways they are currently handled. Direct and good relations with all levels of the government are certainly an advantage.

However, the authorities are well aware of the problems with the current protection system for traditional Chinese medicines. Zhang Qingkui, himself a senior bureaucrat at the SIPO, wrote:

> Firstly, it is not always intellectual property that is under protection, as 'novelty' is not required for protection for varieties of traditional Chinese medicines ... It will undoubtedly harm the public interests to authorize certain enterprises to monopolize such existing technologies.
>
> Secondly, the same type of medicine produced by several manufacturers may also receive this protection. As a result, one or more producers of the medicine will be forced to apply for protection and face extra costs. (Zhang 2007)

Furthermore, some experts and doctors feared that the quality and reputation of Chinese medicines would suffer if companies resorted to producing similar products with different names in order to circumvent protected formulas. Sinopharm (2009), for example, complains that a veritable 'imitation craze' was set in motion around 2005 because the strategy to change the dosage or add an ingredient or two to a well-established formula and apply for protection for this new product often proved to be successful. This could result in an even greater strain on the supplies of certain raw materials, critics say (Jia 2005: 70).

In view of these problems, the authorities have recently raised the bar for new applications and tightened control over the extension of protection periods. In February 2009 the SFDA issued new guidelines to this end (SFDA 2009). The guidelines stipulate that the efficacy of Grade II protected formulas has to be clinically demonstrated, new dosage forms henceforth need to be accompanied by scientific studies demonstrating that they are innovative and reasonable, and modified drugs must have a proven advantage over the original (C-Med 2009).

In September 2011 Arura's second protection periods for Ratna Samphel and Rinchen Mangjor ended. Protection cannot be extended for a third period. It remains to be seen how the situation develops but the opportunity for other factories to resume the legal production of these *rinchen rilbu* may be better than a few years ago.

It is important to mention that Tibetan medicine companies, including those that were banned from manufacturing certain *rinchen rilbu*, are not necessarily against the protection of intellectual property rights. Jigme Phuntsog's patented liver drug Chinnä Künchom (*mchin nad kun 'joms*), for example, is vital for his company's economic success. Similarly, Shongpalhachu generates about half of its revenue with its proprietary Chumar 70, and the popularity of Cheezheng's patented pain-relief plaster is the basis of its highly profitable business. The Tibetan medicine industry, like any other industry, naturally has an interest in the protection of intellectual property rights.

Evidently, protecting Sowa Rigpa as traditional knowledge is a balancing act. On the one hand, the global biopiracy threat has necessitated placing the development of protection schemes for traditional knowledge at the top of the PRC's agenda. On the other hand, China's membership of the WTO and its resulting TRIPS obligations has meant placing an emphasis on intellectual property as an internationally tradable commodity. As the Chinese constitution limits possibilities for defensive patents, the provision of administrative protection for traditional medicine has gained in importance. However, as the *rinchen rilbu* case shows, these provisions can lead to a situation where customary knowledge holders are denied the right to continue using that knowledge, now protected under the stewardship of another company.

Filtering Knowledge

There is almost universal agreement among experts in China that traditional knowledge has to be codified and documented in order to protect it. Su Gangqiang of the State Administration of Traditional Chinese Medicine (SATCM), for example, proposes a dual strategy:

> We are well aware of the fact that as a WTO member, China must abide by the WTO agreements and TRIPS Agreement, but we also understand the significance and importance of the traditional IP protection in the context of economic globalization. On the one hand, we hope that the patent law can be implemented in a way that favors the protection of TCM. On the other hand, we are studying hard how TCM can adapt and conform to the requirements for patent protection. (Su 2003)

Su goes on to suggest that new scientific and technological contents should be added to traditional knowledge in order to make it susceptible to the requirements of modern patent systems. Along similar lines, Tsering Drolma advocates 'creative strategies on science and technology' in order to protect 'our intellectual property' (Tsering Drolma 2007). And Jia Qian's proposition reads: 'It is the first step to collect and document TCM knowledge including the minority medicines like medicine of [the] Zang [Tibetan] ethnic minority group' (Jia 2005: 73).

Given the fear of biopiracy and the emphasis on science and technology in China's development strategies, this comes as no surprise. In this process, however, the first question – whether the concept of intellectual property is malleable to traditional knowledge – is superseded by the second: How to conform traditional knowledge to the needs of existing intellectual property regimes. Both the commodification of traditional knowledge and protective measures against its commodification require a new degree of legibility and scientific confirmation.

In this respect, patent regimes and administrative modes of intellectual property protection are closely linked. Both demand that a drug pass the requirements of drug registration, as under the current law only registered, officially sanctioned knowledge is subject to protection. Here, the state's attempts at protecting traditional knowledge intersect with the powerful apparatus of drug administration. However, there is nothing innocent about rendering the invisible visible, as Marilyn Strathern (2000: 309) notes. Making traditional knowledge legible means making it conform to the language and epistemological narratives of science. In this 'filtration of traditional knowledge' (Oguamanam 2006: 145–90) certain aspects are singled out, particularised, validated and documented while other facets, often the cultural, social and spiritual ones, are sidelined.

For Sowa Rigpa this is the most critical fallout of global debates around intellectual property and biopiracy: in order to become eligible for protection, Tibetan medical knowledge first has to be officially verified. Paradoxically, this means that it has to be rendered scientific in order to be recognised as traditional. This paradox, however, is a logical consequence of the scientific episteme's claim to superiority.[6]

The filtration of knowledge at the intersection of intellectual property regimes and drug administration implies a strong preference for certain types of knowledge, namely, knowledge that promises (1) to be translatable to the epistemological narratives of science, and (2) to be worth the effort and money such translation entails. In this context, I argue, both the locus of knowledge production as well as the power relations of knowledge producers and holders are fundamentally altered.

This is best explained by means of an ethnographic example. Early on in my research I heard about an ongoing project aimed at bringing an old but as yet undocumented medicine to the market. The formula in question originated from a well-known *amchi* lineage in Nagchu. The current lineage holders' great-grandfather was the *lamenpa* (*bla sman pa*) – the personal physician – of Reting Rinpoche, who was the regent during the interregnum between the previous and present Dalai Lamas. The family had become especially famous for a formula called Langchenata (*slang chen a rda*). Langchenata is known as an effective treatment for a 'hard liver' – *chimpa tregyur* (*mchin pa mkhregs gyur*). In both Tibetan and biomedical conceptions the condition is frequently linked to the over-consumption of alcohol.

A government-run research institute in the TAR heard of the medicine and approached the family with the idea of commercially developing the formula and having it registered. Langchenata's straightforward indication, which translates well between the different epistemologies and systems of diagnosis, combined with the fact that the formula is a remedy for a rather common condition, made it an ideal choice for such a project. The family was promised a tempting 60 per cent of the potential revenues once the formula was on the market, and one member of the lineage, a young *amchi* by the name of Ngawang Dawa, was offered a position at the research institute.

I got to know Ngawang Dawa in 2008. We met in the apartment of a friend of mine in Lhasa. Nothing in his appearance suggested that he was the holder of a respected *amchi* lineage, nor that he came from a remote, rural part of Nagchu. He was in his early thirties, a handsome young man in fashionable clothes wearing dark sunglasses. Had I met him on the street I would have taken him for a local rock musician or a tour guide. His elder brother, who accompanied him, was clothed in a dark blue jacket in the style of Chinese businessmen. The family owned a Land Cruiser and a house in Lhasa and was certainly not poor. In fact, the brothers were trading in *yartsagunbu*. My friend, himself from a *yartsagunbu* area, recognised them instantly.

The conversation meandered for a while around the subject of that year's *yartsagunbu* season, until my friend's wife served us butter tea and everybody went silent for a moment to perform the little ritual of dipping the tip of the right ring finger into the bowl and sprinkling a little liquid in the air. Ngawang Dawa began to tell his story:

> In the past, there was an old man from Lhundup county suffering from *chimpa tregyur* ['hard liver']. He went to many different hospitals in China and also spent six months at the Mentsikhang clinic [in Lhasa]. But no treatment was effective. He was about to die. Then he was treated by our grandfather and he totally recovered. Thereafter, many doctors started asking him which medicines he had been prescribed, which treatments, etc. Later, some doctors personally came to my grandfather's home.

The knowledge of making this medicine was traditionally only transmitted from father to son. Our ancestors warned that if it was revealed to
anybody else the medicine would lose its effectiveness. It is a secret. But
[when the research institute approached us] our grandfather told us: 'If
this secret is revealed for the benefit of all sentient beings then it is fine.
Do what you think is right'.

Balancing the ancestors' instructions to keep the lineage's formula
secret against the moral obligation to help as many people as possible, the family finally consented to the research institute's proposition. This, they thought, was both economically and morally the
right thing to do.

'Old' and 'New' Knowledge

Despite the fact that the formula had been known and used within
the lineage for generations, Langchenata does not fall under the category of 'traditional knowledge'. For the purpose of drug registration,
all undocumented knowledge is by definition 'new'. As mentioned
in Chapter 2, only the formulas officially documented and locally
registered before 1997 were grandfathered into the current system
as 'old' knowledge. Being a secret lineage formula, Langchenata has
neither been listed in the *Tibetan Drug Standards* nor in the *Chinese
Pharmacopoeia*. This means that the same conditions apply to it as
they do for any other new drug: the formula's efficacy and safety
have to be proven in an comprehensive scientific study.

Remarkably, the PRC's regulatory requirements for a formula
like Langchenata go beyond the requirements in India, and even in
the EU and the USA. India differentiates between two categories of
traditional formulas: the 'classical formulas' and the so-called 'patent and proprietary medicines', marketed as 'Ayurvedic Proprietary
Medicine' or 'Unani Proprietary Medicine'. The classical formulas
are defined as those described in their integrity in one of more than
fifty classical texts. They remain excluded from patenting and every
manufacturer can produce them. Patent and proprietary medicines,
on the other hand, are derived from but not identical to the classical formulas. In order to register a formula under this category it
is enough that its ingredients are mentioned in the body of one or
several of the classical texts. Patent and proprietary medicines are
the property of the registering company and can be sold under its

trademarked brand name. As the ingredients of a proprietary formula are by definition 'classical' and therefore tested by centuries of widespread usage, obtaining drug registration for such a formula is much easier than for a new synthetic drug (Bode 2004: 26; Patwardhan et al. 2005: 468). In India, Langchenata could most probably be registered as patent and proprietary medicine and, for better or worse, no expensive clinical trials would be necessary.

The Indian system is not without problems, however. Critics complain that the way registration of patent and proprietary medicines is handled leaves the door wide open to the abusive use of the term Ayurveda, and many questionable products labelled as such have come to the market. Examples include Swat, a digestive made of 97 per cent sugar, and Proctor and Gamble's Vick's Vapo-Rub, which were both granted registration as 'Ayurvedic Proprietary Medicines' (Cohen 1995: 336; Bode 2004: 27).

Regardless of these problematic cases, comparison of the different approaches in India and China suggests that the linkage between scientific verification and access to protection is an earmark of the PRC's system but not an unavoidable outcome of intellectual property regimes as such. Even in the USA and in the EU, traditional herbal medicines are granted a set of exemptions from the standard process of drug registration. In the US, herbal medicines fall in many cases under the category of dietary supplements and their efficacy and safety does not have to be validated in clinical trials (FDA 1994; Adams 2002: 675). In the EU a remedy is considered traditional and exempt from extensive scientific research if it has been used successfully for at least thirty years in the territory of the European Union (Silano et al. 2004). These rules, of course, benefit European herbal products while basically excluding Ayurvedic, Tibetan or Chinese medicines from being easily registered and marketed in Europe. Nevertheless, if the same rules applied in China, Tibetan formulas would be considered 'traditional' regardless of whether they were included in an official pharmacopoeia at a given point.[7]

The Indian, European and US systems have their own problems, and my intention here is not to suggest that China should adopt any of them. It is noteworthy, however, that the PRC, often lauded for being a particularly fertile ground for traditional medicine, is in certain respects moving towards decisively restrictive policies. That said, it is important to mention that China's regulatory efforts target the industrial production of ready-made formulas and not the archetypal TCM practice, which relies on individualised prescriptions, pharmacists who compound these prescriptions form large stocks of herbal ingredients, and patients who prepare their decoctions from these compounded powders. As argued in Chapter 2, this conceptual, symbolic core of TCM knowledge and practice largely remains outside the requirements of drug registration.

Had Sowa Rigpa been subjected to the same kind of continuous standardisation and documentation efforts as TCM, would Langchenata have surfaced on the radar of the Chinese health authorities and have gained some form of official existence by now? Of course, the question is purely hypothetical. The fact is, however, that only a couple of years lay between the publication of the *Tibetan Drug Standards* in 1995 and the closure of the window for grandfathering in 'old drugs'. Consequently, the chances of a lineage formula like Langchenata becoming officially recognised as 'traditional knowledge', entitled to administrative protection and exempt from the need to prove its safety and efficacy in scientific studies, were indeed very slim. The relatively narrow definition of 'traditional' Sowa Rigpa formulas is clearly linked to Tibetan medicine's late arrival on the national stage.

In summary, we can see that in reality a distinction is not made between 'traditional' and 'new' knowledge but between already documented, filtered and approved knowledge and knowledge yet to undergo this process. The next question is what this process entails and what consequences it has in relation to the present case.

Randomised Controlled Trials

Scientific studies to establish a drug's efficacy and safety typically include pre-clinical experiments to assess the drug's toxicity and properties, followed by a fully fledged clinical trial. In general, clinical trials follow more or less the same three phases in China as in the West. In Phase I, the medicine's safety is tested on a small group of volunteers. Phase II involves a larger group of patients in order to assess the medicine's efficacy. Phase III usually consists of a randomised controlled trial (RCT) involving several hundred patients (SFDA 2007: Article 31).[8]

The scientific research necessary to obtain registration for a 'new' Tibetan formula costs anywhere between 2 and 10 million yuan ($300,000 to $1.4 million), according to various estimates of people working in the industry. When I asked Ngawang Dawa who paid for the Langchenata study he told me that the research institute had applied for funds from the central government. The application had been successful and the institute had been granted 350,000 yuan ($51,000) per annum for this purpose. Over the course of several years about 1.8 million yuan ($260,000) had been spent on the study, he said.

However, the research institute neither had the experience nor the technical means for such a study. 'We got the money, but we could not do it', Ngawang Dawa said. A partner from Jiangsu province was accordingly contracted. 'They research everything', Ngawang Dawa continued. 'Once the research is done, they will return everything to me. Then we will produce it'. In other words, the research funds from the central government, meant to develop Tibetan medicine in Tibet, were directly flowing back to the inland-based research partner.

When I met Ngawang Dawa again a year later in August 2009, the pre-clinical study had shown encouraging results and the clinical trial had just begun. I tried to find out more about the ways these clinical trials were carried out, but Ngawang Dawa had little to tell me, apart from the fact that *amchi* were not involved. The clinical trial was taking place in inland China. 'There are not enough people, not enough patients here in Lhasa', Ngawang Dawa explained. The requirements for statistical robustness precluded the RCT from being carried out in the hospitals of Lhasa.

When I asked Ngawang Dawa whether he had been to Jiangsu province to help with the study, he answered: 'No. All is done by that hospital. Basically, it is decided by the laboratory in Jiangsu province. The Jiangsu lab works for us, we pay them. But they decide all the steps in Jiangsu. Now, they are testing the medicine'. In short, the locus of knowledge production had shifted away from Tibet to the hospitals and laboratories of coastal China. Ngawang Dawa's role had changed as well. His skill and expertise as an *amchi* were of no use in this context. Now, his duty was merely to supply the laboratory in Jiangsu with the powdered ingredients.

RCTs are regarded as the 'gold standard' of evidence-based medicine (Kaptchuk 1998: 431; Phillips et al. 1998; Timmermans and

Berg 2003: 27). During an RCT a medicine is normally tested against a placebo and/or an existing drug for the same condition. Preferably, both patients and administering doctors are 'blinded', meaning that neither of them knows who is getting what. The idea is to isolate the biological efficacy of a drug from the social context of the clinical encounter. The suitability of RCTs for research on traditional medicine, however, is the subject of extensive debate. RCT methodology is criticised for only evaluating therapeutic efficacy but not the overall therapeutic success, the practitioners' appraisal of therapeutic results and patients' valuation of therapeutic quality (Hsu 1996: 38). In other words, the more a study setting is decontextualised and 'clinical noise' in the form of cultural and individual expressions of illness and disease are tuned out, the more internal validity it gains (Waldram 2000: 608). This focus on internal validity comes at the price of reduced generalisability of external validity (Walach et al. 2006).

In addition, important concepts of RCT methodology – such as blinding, informed consent and placebos – are often difficult to translate into other languages, cultural settings and medical traditions (Adams et al. 2005; Miller et al. 2007; Craig 2010). In biomedical terminology, 'placebo' denotes a black box of unspecific properties of a treatment, mostly attributed to a diffuse psychological effect (Harrington 1997; Moerman 2002). What biomedicine acknowledges as the placebo effect may in other medical systems be an integral part of the treatment. A Tibetan doctor, for example, may provide a patient with a specific mantra and instructions to recite it in addition to a stock of pills (Craig and Adams 2009: 3).

Moreover, RCTs rest on the assumption of universal disease categories. When this is not the case – when, for example, a disease in one system is seen as a mere symptom in another – fundamental methodological problems are raised (Adams 2002: 670). Similarly, the validity of the standard RCT methodology is also challenged when a drug considered to have a wide spectrum of effects is tested for a specific disease defined in biomedical terms. The other properties of the drug are then seen as side effects. However, drugs can be specifically used for these 'side effects' and often it is not clear which is the intended main effect (see Etkin 1992). This is true for many herbal medications with a wide spectrum of effectiveness but also for a variety of synthetic drugs like antihistamines and aspirin.

And finally, blinding requires that the tested medicine is not recognisable. In Tibetan medicine, capsules are usually used instead of pills, a procedure that alters the mode of action of a formula according to Sowa Rigpa. In the case of Langchenata, however, the original formula was a powder anyway, to which the capsule is, as some *amchi* argue, a relatively close approximation.

Regardless of these pleas against RCTs as the unquestionable method for securing scientific truth, many *amchi* in Tibet and elsewhere have high hopes that clinical trials will help prove their medicine's efficacy. Ngawang Dawa was no exception. Although for him the entire research process was a black box over which he had no control, he still saw it as a necessary intermediate step to gain recognition. Ngawang Dawa had no doubt about the outcome of the clinical trial, as the medicine had been used for generations and its efficacy had been proven in many cases.

Vincanne Adams argues in this respect that the RCT is both seductive and problematic. It is seductive because the desire for scientific confirmation of Sowa Rigpa obscures how 'uneven the epistemological playing field really is' (Adams 2002: 670); and it is problematic because the outcome of clinical trials is uncertain and renders Tibetan practitioners vulnerable in two ways: 'First … they are potentially criminalized by transporting into the market both their drugs and their magical thinking. Second, entering the research field exposes them to the theft of their intellectual property' (ibid.: 670). Both can be seen in the present case. First, asking Ngawang Dawa whether his family was still producing Langchenata in their hometown, he stated that this was no longer possible. Only with a registration number could it be sold. Now that the formula was being tested in an expensive clinical trial it had finally surfaced on the radar of the health authorities. But of course, Ngawang Dawa added, the family's *amchi* were still using it sometimes for their own patients. And second, for the purpose of the clinical trial, the formula for Langchenata was altered. Out of the original twenty-one ingredients, only fifteen were selected. Furthermore, the formula traditionally distinguished between three different versions: one for the morning, one for the afternoon, and one for the evening. For the clinical study they were combined into one. Given these changes, the question is whether or not the formula will still be considered the *amchi* family's invention.

Confronted with this question, Ngawang Dawa answered that in principle he was confident that he and his family were entitled to the intellectual property of their lineage. When I asked him whether the drug's registration number would belong to him or to the research institute, he said: 'That registration number will be mine. This medicine comes from our ancestors. Therefore we will get the registration number first. According to the law, we have a right to get the number. If a person is the first one to make a thing then he has the right'. Seeing that he had not fully dispelled my scepticism, Ngawang Dawa added that he knew how cunning 'the Chinese' could be and that he would not be surprised if their partners tried to outwit them. In Ngawang Dawa's view, the main aim of his partners was to earn money from the medicine. 'But we don't have this aim', he reasserted. Nevertheless, the looming question whether his family would finally profit from the endeavour or not bothered him.

The Knowledge Commodity

Over the course of our conversations Ngawang Dawa provided me with more details about the agreement between the research institute and his family. The initial proposition was that 60 per cent of the revenues would go to the family and 40 per cent to the research institute. However, this proposition had been abandoned. Now the research institute insisted on equal shares. In addition, it was claimed that the government's 'investment' would have to be paid back in full before the family received its share. The new plan was to sell the formula to a major pharmaceutical corporation once it had passed drug registration. Ngawang Dawa mentioned an envisioned sales price of 30 million yuan ($4.4 million). He said that the government would help to find a buyer and set up such the deal.

The moral argument that bringing Langchenata to the market would benefit a greater number of patients was no longer Ngawang Dawa's most urgent concern. He knew that this was beyond his control. He emphasised that now all depended on the research institute. If they were going to sell the formula and give him his share then he would have no problem with that.

Is the Langchenata project just another instance of what Nandy (1994: 7) identifies as colonialism disguised in a development agenda, an example of science in the service of authoritarianism? Or will it stand for an *amchi* lineage successfully finding their way and making claims in contemporary China? Despite my suspicion that the first is more likely than the latter, it is too early to pronounce a verdict. It remains to be seen if Langchenata will succeed in the clinical trial and finally become a patented drug with an exclusive registration number, if a major company will buy the rights, if the family will get its share, and if Langchenata will become accessible to a larger circle of patients.

What is clear, however, is the fact that at the conjuncture of intellectual property regimes and the apparatus of drug administration, knowledge is being transformed. Its distinct use value as a secret formula of a locally well-respected lineage has vanished and the formula has become a potential commodity with an exchange value yet to be defined. Whereas the value of the formula as such remains difficult to assess, its 'refinement' in the form of scientific evidence has a visible price tag: 1.8 million yuan and counting. As a result, the value of the formula now stems from being scientifically confirmed and thereby conforming to the requirements of industrial production and intellectual property protection.

The 'inventive step', the 'human intervention' – necessary preconditions for patentability – lie in the formula's description and not in its actual invention. In Oguamanam's words: 'When the same knowledge is presented 'scientifically', it ... becomes entitled to protection' (Oguamanam 2006: 161). Despite the rhetoric that intellectual property rights are meant to protect inventions, a Langchenata patent or exclusive drug registration number would not protect the invention as such but the possibility of its industrial application and the investment that was necessary to make it a marketable commodity.

Following Kopytoff, commodification – or 'commoditization' in his terms – is best looked at 'as a process of becoming rather than as an all-or-none state of being' (1986: 73). An object can enter and exit one or more commodity phases during its life span. In the present case, the same can be said for Langchenata as an object of knowledge: only through the process of filtration does it become a marketable commodity. More precisely, the process of filtration objectifies Langchenata as intellectual property. Following Appadurai (1986: 13–16), Langchenata is not yet a commodity but merely a 'commodity candidate'. It may subsequently acquire an exchange value and become a commodity, but only if the prospects are good that a new use value will result from the exchange. Commodification marks a crucial turning point in the biography of things, according to the Appadurai and Kopytoff. Applied to the present case this means that the process of becoming a commodity alters Langchenata's biography and social life – the ways it is valued, the field of its possible application, the locus of its further development, and the power relations in which it is embedded.

Decoupling Forms of Knowledge

In his analysis of agricultural change in India, Appadurai (1990) notes that the critical fact about commercialisation was that it 'decoupled' practical, technological knowledge from its primary cultural settings and inserted it into new cultural settings. This resulted in a division of practical, technical knowledge (*techne* in Appadurai's terms, but equivalent to Scott's *mētis*) from its larger epistemological context. The emergence of an 'agronomic episteme' (which Scott would call a *techne*) divorced from agrarian discourse on the ground rendered practical knowledge obsolete, according to Appadurai.[9]

The same could be argued for the scientific episteme to which both drug administration and intellectual property regimes refer. Ngawang Dawa's knowledge is no longer required in the new cultural setting of a hospital and laboratory in Jiangsu province. The practical knowledge of his lineage – not only the formula itself but also how it is produced and employed in clinical practice – is 'decoupled' from the scientific knowledge that is being manufactured in the clinical trial. In short, the image that emerges is the following: practical knowledge is being filtered, appropriated and finally rendered obsolete. Or in Scott's terms: *mētis* is being replaced by *techne*.

This is undeniably a facet in the Langchenata case. However, we have seen in Chapter 3 in relation to GMP that the problem was not that a 'foreign' *techne* superseded the practical knowledge of medicine production; *techne* is sometimes either ignored or it simply does not extend to the level of practice. In the domain of production, I argued that the real conflict stemmed from the side effects of the way GMP was introduced. The question is if the same can be said for the filtration of practical knowledge in the case of Langchenata. The short answer is: no.

Comparing GMP introduction with the filtration of knowledge, a crucial difference comes to light. In the first case, GMP as a global form was recontextualised in the social and cultural milieu of Tibet where, as we have seen, it met with various forms of tactical resistance. In the Langchenata case, however, Tibetan knowledge is exported into a new cultural setting outside Tibet and consequently also outside the reach of tactical manoeuvres by Tibetan practitioners. The decoupling effect is arguably much stronger in this context.

Property, Knowledge

Let me review the argument at this point. This chapter began with an admittedly rhetorical question: to whom does Sowa Rigpa belong? Given the fact that it is practised not only by Tibetans but by a variety of groups in a variety of settings and states, there can be no simple answer. The question itself, however, points to an even more fundamental issue: asking to whom it belongs entails a perspective on Sowa Rigpa which no longer regards it primarily as a system of knowledge but as a pool of intellectual property.

This shift, I suggested, has to be seen in the light of global biopiracy, which has given rise to a heightened awareness about intellectual property rights vis-à-vis traditional knowledge. The debate found its way into several international agreements, including the Biodiversity Convention. At the same time, intellectual property rights have also become a central issue of economic globalisation as they touch on vital aspects of transnational corporations. Binding treaties, first and foremost the WTO's TRIPS agreement, aim at a harmonisation of intellectual property regimes in order to protect industrial interests and, at a more general level, to make knowledge a globally tradable commodity.

I argued that both the fear of biopiracy and China's WTO membership have shaped the PRC's approaches to intellectual property rights regarding traditional knowledge. Forms of administrative protection were set up as an alternative to patents. However, regardless of the intentions behind these protection regimes, they proved their capacity to reconfigure local power relations, as demonstrated with the case of Tibetan companies losing their right to produce certain high-value *rinchen rilbu* under the pretext of a regime originally established to protect traditional knowledge. However, as the authorities are aware of the problems with the current protection system, and the protection periods are about to run out, the situation may change in the future.

Global debates about biopiracy, national approaches to the protection of traditional knowledge, company interests, development agendas, and the apparatus of drug administration – these factors together form the nexus in which the question of how intellectual property regimes can be adjusted to suit the needs of traditional knowledge becomes superseded by the question of how traditional knowledge can be rendered malleable to the needs of intellectual property regimes. In this context, evidence-based medicine joins forces with intellectual property regimes to make RCTs the only acceptable approach to the documentation (or filtration) of knowledge.

The case of Langchenata sheds light on the effects of these forces in turning an old lineage formula into registered and protected knowledge. This process entails much more than simply a study to corroborate an old formula's efficacy and safety. It profoundly changes the entire context of knowledge, including its value characteristics, its application, the locus of its production, and the power relations in which it is embedded.

Despite having secured the necessary funds, the research institute developing the formula had to contract a partner in Jiangsu about the clinical trial because of a lack of experienced researchers, insufficient infrastructure, and the simple fact that there were 'not enough patients' in Tibet. In this respect, the harsh criticism voiced in exile that Sowa Rigpa is being appropriated by non-Tibetans appears justified. Be it simply for practical reasons such as patient numbers and infrastructures, the future development of Sowa Rigpa as a system of knowledge may well take place outside Tibet and beyond the control of Tibetans.

In general, this means that turning knowledge into a form of property changes the property of that knowledge – its locus and value characteristics, its social life and the power relations of its holders. Ngawang Dawa was well aware of his position in this context. The course of events was no longer in his hands. As there was not much he could do apart from await the results of the RCT, his energy shifted to other endeavours. He opened a small studio dedicated to the production of video clips for local bands. Before we parted, however, Ngawang Dawa asked me if I knew a reliable partner in Switzerland or America to develop another of the family's secret formulas.

Notes

1. Other prominent cases in India involved patent disputes concerning basmati rice (Randeria 2007: 11) and turmeric (Marshall and Bagla 1997).
2. See Merlan (2009) for an inspiring discussion of the term 'indigeneity', local and global.
3. Both the granting and revoking of the patent for neem were based on this provision in US patent law. It was granted because W.R. Grace and Co. claimed that there was no documented evidence in India, and it was revoked because Jeremy Rifkin presented several hundred journal articles that showed that the extraction of azadirachtin had indeed been widely described and therefore could not be counted as W.R. Grace's invention.
4. Around the same time, rumours that South Korea was in the process of seeking world-intangible-cultural-heritage status for Korean medicine evoked a public outcry in China. Korean medicine is closely related to TCM and a vague report on the internet was enough to trigger the fear that South Korea might try to appropriate Chinese traditional knowledge under the pretext of the UNESCO conventions. China's State Administration of Traditional Chinese Medicine (SATCM) has also been seeking UNESCO world heritage status since 2003 and, as mentioned in Chapter 3, *tsothal* and Rinchen Drangjor were listed as intangible cultural heritage in 2006. SATCM looked into the Korea case but found no indication that the Korean government was indeed seeking intangible heritage status for 'Korean medicine' (C-Med 2006; *Legal Daily* 2006).
5. According to the patent database of the State Intellectual Property Organisation (SIPO), Jigme Phuntsog holds nine and Cheezheng's Lei Jufang forty-six patents. See www.sipo.gov.cn/sipo_English (accessed 5 February 2010).
6. In this vein, Ashis Nandy critically remarks, 'while the scientific worldview cannot be judged by other worldviews, the other worldviews can be judged and indeed should be judged by science' (Nandy 1997: 10).
7. See Banerjee (2009: 251–68) for an extensive discussion of regulatory frameworks in the EU and USA, including their effect on the international market for Ayurvedic medicines.
8. In addition, China's drug regulations call for a Phase IV 'new drug postmarketing study' after the drug has been successfully registered in order to assess its therapeutic effectiveness and possible adverse reactions when used widely.
9. Regarding the terminology in use here, Appadurai follows Marglin's (1990) usage of the terms *techne* and episteme. In short, Scott's oppositon of *mētis* and *techne* is equivalent to Marglin's and Appadurai's distinction between *techne* and episteme.

Chapter 6
The Aesthetic Enterprise

The elements of the assemblage so far discussed include techniques of production, laws and regulations, machines and factory premises, raw materials and different forms of knowledge. These elements condition and enable industrial production. What has not been examined so far is the output the factories produce and the aesthetic reasoning behind the manufacturing of Tibetan medicines.

The study of aesthetics, in the original sense of the term, is concerned with the question of beauty, taste, style and artistic quality. My interest in the aesthetic, visual and material dimensions of the Tibetan medicine industry, however, is of a different kind. In this chapter I will explore the use of aesthetic expressions for strategic, social purposes and, at the same time, inquire how the things and images companies produce, and the things they are composed of, shape the modes in which the industry operates.

In the introduction I mentioned Todorov's argument that industry in the Soviet Union was largely an allegorical figure of communist modernity, which resulted in a deficit of goods and an overproduction of symbolic meaning (Todorov 1995: 10). Although in the present case one can hardly speak of a deficit of goods, the production of symbolic meaning remains essential. Symbolic meaning, I intend to show, has a strong aesthetic component.

As the production of Tibetan medicine lies at the crossroads of various agendas for Tibet's future, each embedded in its own symbolic universe, the aesthetic expressions produced in the context of the industry are diverse and cover much of the visual territory of contemporary Tibet. The companies present themselves simultaneously as modern, scientific, GMP-compliant, loyal to the party-state as well as Tibetan, mystical and in harmony with nature. In other words, while the industry remains an allegorical figure of Tibet's march towards modernisation (IOSC 2001), Sowa Rigpa also stands for an enchanted Tibet. It is this enchanted Sowa Rigpa on which many patients – Westerners and, more importantly in our case, Chinese – cast their hopes when seeking an antidote to the illnesses of a disenchanted modern world.

Disenchantment, Enchantment

The disenchantment of the world as a corollary of industrial modernity was famously proposed by Max Weber (2002). Weber's argument, however, is more subtle. He contends that the advancing intellectualisation and rationalisation that accompany industrial modernity do not imply an increasing general knowledge about the conditions one's life is shaped by: 'They rather imply a knowledge about or a belief that such knowledge *could*, if *desired*, be gained at any time; that consequently there are no arcane and unpredictable powers, and that therefore everything is – in principle – controllable by *rational calculation*. This, however, means: the disenchantment of the world [*die Entzauberung der Welt*]' (ibid.: 488). Weber's grand critique of occidental industrial modernity, voiced in a lecture more than ninety years ago, holds an insight applicable to the present case: it is not necessarily scientific knowledge as such but rather the promise implied in the scientific project, the imagination of a scientific rationality, that is the enemy of enchanted, arcane powers.

The overall strategic movement portrayed in the preceding chapters – the introduction of GMP, the border regimes governing the transition of herbs and traders between spheres, the commodification and filtration of knowledge – can be described as one of disenchantment. As incomplete and challenged by tactical manoeuvres as they may be, science and development remain the overarching framework under which the integration of Sowa Rigpa into modern Tibet is pursued. Magic and enchantment do not figure in this vision. On the other hand, equally strong counter-currents cannot be overlooked. The portrayal of Sowa Rigpa as a product of magical Tibet represents a movement in the opposite direction – towards an enchantment or, perhaps, a re-enchantment of Tibetan medicine for commercial purposes. Capitalism, as Jean and John Comaroff suggest, 'has always been shot through with its own magicalities and forms of enchantment' (Comaroff and Comaroff 1992: 6).

Here is a simple, provisional hypothesis: enchantment and disenchantment denote two opposite directions of the aesthetic enterprise. However, they are intrinsically linked. As much as an enchanted Tibetan medicine looks towards scientific disenchantment to consolidate its position, a disenchanted Tibetan medicine industry uses strategies[1] to re-enchant its products. Two examples will serve as point of departure for an exploration of the disjuncture and reunion of enchantment and disenchantment.

Mendrup

The first example is a consecration ritual known as *mendrup* (*sman sgrub*). The ritual is meant to endow a medicine with spiritual powers and thereby enhance its efficacy. The Tibetan term consists of *men* (*sman*), 'medicine', and *drup* (*sgrub*), 'to accomplish, achieve or perfect'. The main ritual manual for *mendrup* as practised today is the *Yuthog Heart Essence* (*g.yu thog snying thig*), a corpus of texts attributed to the twelfth century Yuthog Yonten Gonpo the Younger and his disciples (Yuthog 2005). The *Yuthog Heart Essence* shares many techniques and theories with *chülen* (*bcud len*), the alchemical transmutation of substances into *dütsi* (*bdud rtsi*), 'nectar' or 'elixir' (Garrett 2009, 2010; Craig 2010). *Mendrup* aims at bringing out the nectar-like qualities of medicines. It is meant to complete the metamorphosis of products from nature into potent elixir. The ritual consists of recitations over the course of many days accompanied by a series of burnt offerings (*sbyin sreg*) and the creation and destruction of a mandala. It is often combined with *tsebang* (*tshe dbang*), a public longevity ritual (see Gerke 2008).[2]

Frances Garret attended and filmed a week-long *mendrup* ritual at the TAR Tibetan Medicine Factory in Lhasa in 2001. The yearly ritual was performed by senior Mentsikhang physicians in possession of the necessary initiations; it was led by Tsultrim Gyeltsen, a renowned *amchi* and lama. Garret writes: 'Attended by large numbers of lay people, the event joined medical, religious and lay communities and interests. Many lay people and physicians asserted that the efficacy of the factory's medicines would be enhanced by this ritual performance' (Garrett 2009: 208). Agreement about the purpose and efficacy of performing *mendrup*, however, is not universal among Tibetans. Adams notes (2001: 562), for example, that during her fieldwork in the late 1990s the director of the TAR Tibetan

167

Medicine Factory argued against the need for it and regarded it as mere superstition. According to Theresia Hofer (2009a: 183), there was a ban on the performance of the ritual in 1995. The doctors and staff of the Mentsikhang hospital, however, were still strongly in favour of consecrating the medicines they were using.

Describing a similar tension, Craig (2006: 281–96, 2010) recounts the discussions surrounding the question of whether to perform a *mendrup* ritual or not for drugs used in a clinical trial and whether both placebo and medicines should receive the same treatment. Members of the study's project team finally decided to perform the ritual secretly, without the knowledge of scientifically oriented project leaders. Of course, there was no scientific study trying to prove that the ritual was not effective – just as was the case with the validation requirement discussed at the end of Chapter 3. Much as in Weber's sense, it is not science that is opposed to magic but the tutelary myth of science.

In addition to being difficult to reconcile with a scientific epistemology, *mendrup* is also politically sensitive. In 2007 and 2008, for example, no *mendrup* rituals were held at the TAR Tibetan Medicine Factory in Lhasa. The ritual and especially its public component were regarded as too delicate a matter I was told by one of the doctors who would usually participate. Remarkably, in the eyes of the authorities, the alchemical Buddhist *mendrup* ritual poses a greater safety threat than the similarly alchemical *tsothal* practice, which involves the purification of mercury. The 'magic' of *mendrup*, on the other hand, served as a theme in a recent television commercial produced by the very same TAR Tibetan Medicine Factory, as we will see.

Despite these sensitivities and the overall belief in the scientific enterprise in which magic and ritual have no place, *mendrup* continues to be performed in many GMP-certified Tibetan medicine factories throughout Tibet. Some companies follow the Mentsikhang's example and invite a high lama once a year to consecrate a factory's yearly output; others organise *mendrup* rituals more regularly for each batch of medicines.

One could assume that *mendrup* is a residue of a formerly 'enchanted' Sowa Rigpa, threatened but not yet displaced by the gradual process of disenchantment. In general, however, there is no evidence that the importance attributed to *mendrup* has decreased with the creation of the Tibetan medicine industry. On the contrary,

while *mendrup* is performed in many of the bigger companies in Tibet, it is often forgone by the smaller, private manufacturers, who,
at the same time, criticise the larger companies for not following
traditional Tibetan ways.

In short, evidence suggests that *mendrup* is as much a contemporary phenomenon as it is a well-established centuries-old practice.
It might even have become more important recently – not only as
a ritual to increase the medicine's efficacy but also as a marker of
Tibetanness, as a means to re-enchant what is seen to be threatened
by the disenchanting effects of industry. In other words, the *mendrup*
ritual serves as what Alfred Gell (1988, 1992) termed a 'technology
of enchantment'. Gell's term is meant to emphasise the strategic side
of artistic or aesthetic expressions, including painting, music, ritual
and rhetoric. The aim of a technology of enchantment, according
to Gell, is to make the counterpart perceive social reality 'in a way
favourable to the social interests of the enchanter' (Gell 1988: 7).

In Gell's approach, the term 'magic' is closely related to technology
and enchantment. Gell suggests that magic consists of a 'symbolic
commentary' on technical strategies (ibid.: 8). To illustrate his case,
he calls to mind Malinowski's classic *Coral Gardens and their Magic*
(1935). A Trobriand gardener calls upon spiritual powers to let his
crop be plentiful. His magic spells thereby refer to an ideal garden,
'the garden to end all gardens, in which everything occurs absolutely
as it should in the best of all possible worlds. The pests which
inhabit the soil will rise up, and, of their own accord, commit mass
suicide in the sea. Yam roots will strike down into the soil with the
swiftness of a green parrot in flight, and the foliage above will dance
and weave like dolphins playing in the surf' (Gell 1988: 8).

Magic, in this sense, is an 'ideal' technology, after which the real
garden, meticulously laid out and weeded with utmost care, is modelled. But as much as the magic, imaginary, ideal garden provides a
model for the construction of real gardens, the real gardens (with
their productivity) sustain the magic. Only because non-magical
technology is effective, the ideal technology embodied in magical
discourse is so compelling. While technology sustains magic, magic
inspires fresh technical efforts, according to Gell's argument. As an
'ideal' technology, magic 'orients practical technology and codifies
technical procedures at the cognitive-symbolic level' (ibid.: 9).

From this perspective, the *Yuthog Heart Essence* can be seen as the 'magic', the 'symbolic commentary' on a technical strategy of production. It represents an ideal technology by which medicines are effortlessly transformed into perfect nectar. As a technology of enchantment the ritual employs aesthetic expressions to this end – the creation of a mandala, the sound of chanting, the smoke of burnt offerings.

Admittedly, such a description may depart quite substantially from how a Tibetan *amchi* would describe *mendrup*. After all, the explicit purpose of *mendrup* is not to enchant a counterpart to perceive social reality in a particular way, but to enhance the potency of the medicine regardless of the social context in which it is used. Reducing the *Yuthog Heart Essence* to a symbolic commentary resonates with what Adams aptly describes as the 'rational-but-still-wrong' school of thought (Adams 2002: 99) – an essentially functionalist perspective that regards belief as rational and logical but empirically still untrue. My intention here is not to claim that the *mendrup* ritual serves exclusively as a technology of enchantment; the point I seek to make is rather that, in the context of industrial production, the ritual automatically acquires an additional layer of meaning, as it endows – or re-enchants – the industry with the aesthetics and power of tantric Buddhism.

Rituals of GMP

Gell's reflections on enchantment, technology and symbolic commentary also provide a perspective on the aesthetics and performance of GMP production. Visiting a GMP factory always starts with the same ritualised entry procedure, which typically takes place in a windowless room equipped with a few lockers, a green floor and a knee-high barrier covered with shining chromium steel. Sitting on the barrier one slips into protective footwear covers, balancing carefully and trying neither to touch the barrier's surface nor the floor on the other side with one's dirty shoes. The barrier demarcates the entry to the factory's clean inner realms.

In an adjacent room hooded overalls and face masks are donned. In the next room hands are washed and disinfected. Plastic-laminated signs describe the procedures of washing and disinfecting hands in detail, one of many 'standard operating procedures' (SOP) that govern GMP production. The booths always feature sealed doors and serve as air gates to maintain the required pressure differential between the outside and the clean area of the factory.

Finally, one enters the main corridor of the clean area. White doors in aluminium frames lead to a series of booths to the left and right, each equipped with a single machine made of stainless steel – a grinder, a mixer, a dryer, and so forth. These booths are also equipped with signs detailing the respective SOP to be followed. If a machine is running, the process is usually supervised by one, sometimes two workers. The noise of the machines is muted by the sealed windows between the main corridor and the booths.

The door to each booth as well as each machine features a coloured label showing its current status: a machine or room that is cleaned and ready to be used again carries a green label; a machine or room yet to be cleaned carries a red one. The labels include detailed information about when and by whom the cabinet was cleaned and the time frame in which it has to be used again before another round of cleaning becomes necessary. Labelling and documentation of each step of production are cornerstones of GMP's quality philosophy, and the colour codes are consistently used throughout the industry for this purpose. Bags of raw materials, for instance, are first given a red label; after testing is completed they obtain a green label.

Whereas humans have to don overalls and face-masks, wash their hands and proceed through a series of rooms with sealed doors, the raw materials have their own entry procedure, guarded by the mandatory (but usually unused) microwave ovens. From the microwave booth the herbs usually pass through an air gate into an empty room with a sealed, ground-level door, where they are packed on trolleys and brought to intermediate storage facilities. Only after the raw materials have completed their transformation into medicines and have been packed in at least one layer of air-tight material are they allowed to leave the factory's inner realms again through the same kind of air gate.

The visual appearance of GMP factories across the industry is strikingly similar: sealed cabinets, white doors in aluminium frames, usually green floors, white and slightly glossy synthetic walls, and rounded aluminium skirting boards. This is partly due to the fact that most manufacturing plants were built at roughly the same time (between 2002 and 2004) and often designed by the same architects; partly it is because of the abundant regulations which are manifest in various details of factory design; and partly it is simply the result of aesthetic decisions inspired by conventions about what a medicine factory should look like. The green and white colours of walls and floors, the white, blue, or green overalls, and the labels following the same colour scheme are aesthetic decisions made outside GMP regulations.

The acquisition of certain machinery that is never used nor even required by the regulations themselves can be taken as a hint that a general vision of how a modern and scientific Tibetan medicine industry should look was a crucial aspect of the endeavour. James Scott (1998: 82) has noted in this respect that modernist schemes are often not based on the scientifically grounded insights they claim to be but more on aesthetic visions of a final outcome – their own 'ideal garden', so to speak.

The particular aesthetics of factory design, the strict segregation of space, the colour codes, rounded skirting boards, sealed windows, hooded overalls and face-masks – each detail meaningful in its context – set the stage on which GMP production is carried out. The entry procedures for humans and herbs, the SOPs that guide almost every action of the employees, and the requirement of meticulous documentation provide the script for GMP production. The resulting activity is a ritual performance guided by a liturgy of SOPs – precisely in the sense of symbolic commentaries on technical strategies.

In this respect, contrary to Weber's prediction, ritual and magic have not disappeared in the age of industry but rather changed their appearance. Coming back to Weber's and Scott's insights, one can argue that precisely because it is not science as such but the imaginary of science that calls magic into question, the aura of science and the aura of religion are not fundamentally different. Ritual 'disenchantment', then, is very close to enchantment in disguise. When GMP as mindful performance is used in advertisement side by side with the magic of *mendrup* (as we will see shortly), it becomes a technology of enchantment in its own right. When commodities are inserted into a mythologised universe, all possibilities are open, Gell remarks (1988: 9).

Both the *mendrup* ritual and GMP production do not stand for themselves. They are enmeshed in a larger context of representation where they acquire additional layers of meaning and purpose and where their distinct aesthetics are put to use as technologies of enchantment. The coexistence, and sometimes even the fusion, of such radically different worlds as found in a Buddhist ritual and a pharmaceutical factory are characteristic of the Tibetan medicine industry.

The resulting aesthetics between enchantment and disenchantment, or re-enchantment in disguise, are even more apparent when looking at packaging and advertising, the visual expressions meant to situate a company in public.

Packaging Remedies

We have seen that one of the major shifts that occurred with the emergence of an industry producing commodities for a nationwide market was the separation of production from medical practice. Tibetan drugs are increasingly bought over the counter and consumed without consultation. The potency of a formula is no longer directly linked to the skill of an *amchi* as a doctor-pharmacist, who diagnoses disease, makes and prescribes medicines, gives dietary recommendations, and possibly spiritual advice. Whereas this may be perceived of as a lack, is also has a specific 'charm', as Sjaak van der Geest and Susan Whyte argue: 'Pharmaceuticals objectify the healing art of physicians and make it into some-*thing* that can be used by anyone. Pharmaceuticals break the hegemony of professionals and enable people to help themselves. Medicines, therefore, have a "liberating" power' (van der Geest and Whyte 1989: 348). This argument, made with regard to synthetic, biomedical drugs, is also applicable to packaged Tibetan medicines. With their name and indication printed on boxes and leaflets they are less tied to an individual prescription for a specific condition. Their appearance suggests that they can easily be transferred from one context to another, stored away and given to a friend with similar symptoms later. In this sense, packaging is more than simply a result of industrialised production. The rise of packaged Tibetan medicines has the potency to reconfigure the entire practice of Sowa Rigpa.

As mentioned in the preceding chapter, Igor Kopytoff argues that commodification is best looked at as a process of becoming rather than as a state of being (Kopytoff 1986: 73). A piece of clothing, for example, becomes a commodity when it leaves the factory. Once it is bought, it ceases to be a commodity and becomes a personal item, a 'singularity' in Kopytoff's terms. At a later stage the same piece of clothing may enter the commodity phase again when its owner

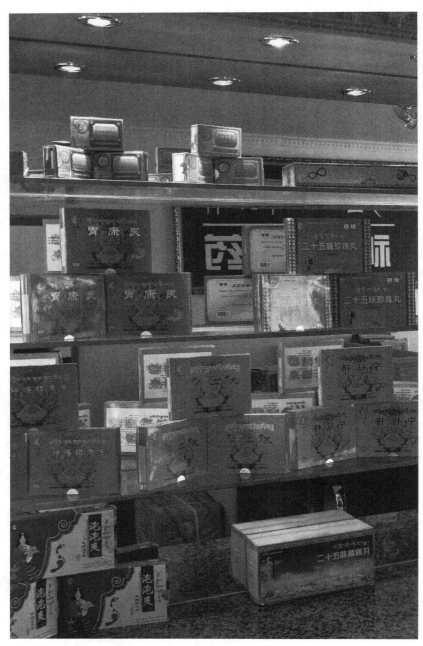

Figure 6.1: Boxed Tibetan medicines.

decides to sell it in a second-hand shop. Following Kopytoff's suggestion, three exemplary biographies of Tibetan medicines can be identified.

First, a Tibetan medicine may remain a singularity and never enter a commodity phase. When a rural *amchi* collects herbs, compounds them into a formulation, which he directly administers to a patient without demanding payment, the formulation remains singular throughout its life. The medicine has the character of a personal gift, for which the patient, in return, may choose to give a donation.

Second, a Tibetan medicine may be prescribed for a specific condition of an individual patient. When the patient buys the prescribed medicine from a doctor, clinic, or pharmacy it is clearly a commodity. However, being purchased, it undergoes a radical singularisation, which is not meant to be reversed because the medicine is efficacious only for a specific condition and patient. Its commodity phase can be called 'terminal', according to Kopytoff (1986).

Third, an industrially produced, packaged Tibetan medicine potentially passes through several phases of commodification and singularisation. A box of 'precious pills' *(rinchen rilbu)* bought in Dharamsala as a gift for a relative in Tibet, for example, may be stored away and given as a present to somebody else, who – short of cash – may then decide to sell it on the black market in Lhasa's old town. Packaged Tibetan medicines are the most 'mobile' of all; they are less tied to clinics and doctors. As a result, the separation of medical practice from production – one of the preconditions for industrial manufacturing – is further amplified by the industry's products themselves.

Van der Geest and Whyte argue that 'one of the "charms" of medicines is that, even removed from their medical context, they retain a potential connection to it' (van der Geest and Whyte 1989: 359). The authors speak of a metonymic relation between medicines and their producers. A drug bought over the counter without the help of a doctor is still linked to its origins: it stands for the factory that produced it and maybe a famous physician associated with it. It is against this background of the metonymic connections of medicines that we may understand the extreme importance of appearance and packaging. The immediately apparent form of a medicinal commodity has the potential for suggesting such connections (ibid.: 360).

Two aspects need to be looked at in this respect: the graphic design of boxes and pouches as well as the materiality of packaging itself.

Design

As opposed to the brown pills in an *amchi*'s ward, the industry's commodities are branded products, their smell and looks hidden from the world by one or more layers of packaging. With packaging, forging a metonymic relation between producer and product is thus a matter of visual communication.

At first sight, the design of boxes and pouches is strikingly similar across the industry: the medicine's Chinese name features prominently on a simple background, mostly in monochrome. Sometimes Tibetan ornaments overlay the background or adorn the edges. Photographic images are usually absent. The medicine's Chinese name is often accompanied by its Tibetan and sometimes its English counterpart, which is set in smaller type. The company name, in both Chinese and Tibetan, is typically placed at the bottom, the drug's registration number at the top. The company logo mostly features in the upper left or right corner. On the back, manufacturing date, shelf life, batch number and some brief patient information can be found, including a list of ingredients, indications, suggested dosage and instructions for taking the drug.

The inscriptions on a pouch or box are officially called the 'drug label' (Kuwahara and Li 2007: Annex I, §6). The design of drug labels is tightly regulated. GMP requires that 'the content, format, and wording of labels and direction inserts shall be approved by the drug regulatory department' before being released (ibid.: Article 46). The SFDA's Provisions for Drug Insert Sheets and Labels further details these requirements (SFDA 2006a).

Here, the concept of the official 'adopted name in China' comes into play. The concept of the adopted name has to be seen in relation to imported drugs and the need for a consistent, official Chinese name. The adopted name is therefore by definition Chinese and has to be printed in 'standardised Chinese characters published by the National Language Commission' (ibid.: Article 7). The rules also stipulate that should the drug have another name then this must be no more conspicuous than the adopted name in China and the size of the type in which it is set should be less than half that of the adopted name (ibid.: Article 26).

These rules directly affect the appearance of Tibetan medicines, as they give prominence to the adopted Chinese over the well-established Tibetan one. This was sometimes a matter of regret in the conversations I had on the topic, but generally it was also accepted as a logical precondition for access to the market of inland China. Other specific requirements for the layout of the drug labels are as follows.

The adopted name in China shall be conspicuous and prominent, and its typeface, size and colour shall be consistent, and meet the following requirements: (1) for horizontal labels, the adopted name in China shall appear in a prominent position within the area of the upper third of the label; for vertical labels, it shall appear in a prominent position within the area of the right third of the label; (2) no illegible typefaces using cursive and seal characters shall be used, and no format such as italics, margining and shading shall be used to modify the typefaces; (3) the font colour of the adopted name in China shall be black or white, in sharp contrast to the light-coloured or dark-coloured background respectively; (4) writing in separate lines shall be avoided unless limited by the packaging size (ibid.: Article 25).

Unlike other rules and regulations, these requirements appear to be strictly enforced. Several people involved in packaging design told me that the authorities frequently found fault with this or that detail of the drafts they submitted to them. In one case, the authorities even objected to the photograph of a stupa as a background image on the box of one product. A manager of the company suggested that it was probably considered to be too religious, although it might just have been in contradiction with the requirement of a plain light or dark background to guarantee the legibility of the medicine's adopted name. An image of the Potala, on the other hand, seems to be no problem. Be that as it may, the fact is that references to Tibetan Buddhism, and more generally to companies' Tibetanness, are generally not emphasised in the design of boxes, pouches and leaflets.

For the company logos, however, no such rules exist. The logos are therefore all the more important as a means of invoking the metonymic relation between a company and its commodities. To this end, logos often provide a condensed aesthetic vision of a company's perspectives and endeavours. The logo of the TAR Tibetan Medicine Factory, for example, depicts three streams originating in the Himalayas. The three streams meet and empty into the ocean, where a pair of leaves hold a myrobalan fruit, the paramount *arura*. According to the company this iconic depiction of nature should also be understood in a symbolic way: the left and the right rivers symbolise the Indian Ayurvedic and traditional Chinese influences, the middle stream represents Tibetan medicine, and the ocean stands for the profundity of Sowa Rigpa as a system of knowledge.

The logo is usually accompanied by the inscription '1696' – the year the famous monastic Chagpori medical school in Lhasa was founded. This is a noteworthy detail because the TAR Tibetan Medicine Factory originated from, and is still linked to, the Mentsikhang. The Mentsikhang, however, was founded in the early twentieth century with the goal of reforming the old-style monastic Sowa Rigpa education epitomised by the Chagpori. By admitting lay students, the Mentsikhang sought to distinguish itself from monastic Sowa Rigpa education. Nonetheless, by declaring 1696 as its founding year, the TAR Tibetan Medicine Factory claims the heritage of the Chagpori, which was destroyed during the 1959 Lhasa uprising. As the major Tibetan medicine producer in the TAR, the company sees its role as the guardian of Sowa Rigpa.

The TAR Tibetan Medicine Factory's logo bears many similarities to the logos of two other producers mentioned earlier. The Tibetan Medicine College Factory in Lhasa and Aku Jinpa's private pharmacy both use the same motifs – mountains, water and *arura*, the myrobalan fruit. In the case of the College Factory, the same three streams coming from the Himalayas meet in the plains. Instead of two leaves, it is a bowl that holds the fruit of *arura*. On Aku Jinpa's logo, three mountains are depicted but no rivers. The myrobalan floats in a bowl on the open water.

Besides giving a condensed vision of a firm's outlook and endeavours, some logos also provide an insight into a company's distinctive culture. Jigme Phuntsog's logo, for example, depicts Jigme Phuntsog himself. The logo appears in two variations: one portrays the master in monk's robes, one shows him wearing a gown and a mortarboard. The two varieties pay tribute to the different roles Jigme plays in the company.

When I first visited Jigme Phuntsog, half a dozen Tibetans were waiting in front of his office. My friend and I were called in. The walls in Jigme's generous office were decorated with the numerous awards he had received, amidst monastic drapery and religious objects. A large heater provided warmth and comfort. Jigme was engaged in intense discussion with one of his employees about a new requirement that the factory needed to implement. It obviously upset him greatly. After a while he turned to us and his mood changed. During the interview two of the Tibetans whom I had seen waiting outside the office, an elderly woman and her son, knocked on the door and entered. Jigme excused himself and turned to them. For a short time, the office became a doctor's clinic. Jigme took the woman's pulse, asked a few questions, and finally wrote a prescription.

Within twenty minutes Jigme switched from being an entrepreneur navigating his company through turbulence to a host and helpful informant of a Western researcher, then to being a traditional *amchi*, and back again. Jigme's office was the indisputable centre of the company where all threads came together. The two versions of the logo highlight the many aspects unified in his personality: the monk's robe refers to his origins as a monastically trained *amchi* and underscores the importance of Buddhist heritage to his company; the gown and mortarboard stand for scientific innovation, official recognition and his involvement in international exchange.

By contrast, Arura's logo neither depicts the myrobalan fruit nor the Group's paramount leader. The logo consists of a simple encircled ཨ – the Tibetan letter *a*, which stands for *arura*. Tibetan, but elegant and sleek, the logo is perfectly adaptable to the Arura Group's various endeavours. It is consistently used by the Group, marking the factory's products and the research centre's publications as well as the entrance doors to the museum, the hospital, and the lecture rooms at the medical college.

The Arura Group's headquarters are located just across the street from Jigme's factory. The cultures and aesthetics of the two companies are markedly different. The spacious, open-plan offices of Arura's headquarters impress one with their almost austere simplicity. The white walls are sparsely decorated; no awards, religious objects or company products can be seen (they are all on display in the headquarters' showroom and the new museum, to which I will return). The office of the factory's managing director follows the same style and features the same furniture as the other offices.

When I had an appointment one day with a senior manager responsible for production, one of his assistants, a graduate from the medical college, received me. The manager I was meant to meet had not yet come back from Beijing, I was informed. But his assistant was ready to replace him, answer my questions, and show me around. Here, the corporation is the centre. A senior manager who had to reschedule his business trip could easily be replaced by somebody else. The emphasis lies on professional management and shared responsibility. On the bookshelves of one of the company's vice directors I noticed a copy of *The Toyota Way*, the handbook of the famous management philosophy put forward by the Toyota corporation. Arura's logo, the style of its premises and its approach to management speak the language of an internationally oriented corporation that could easily be located in London, Shanghai or Tokyo.

Materiality

Apart from positioning a company's products in the market and forging a metonymic relationship between product and producer, there is a concrete pragmatic reason for packaging Tibetan drugs. Pills and powders sold in inland China are much more susceptible to mould and fungal attack, and so they need to be protected from the humid climate of the lowlands. State-of-the-art packaging thereby employs several layers: pills are sealed in blisters, the blisters are wrapped in airtight plastic-aluminium pouches, and the pouches are finally packed in boxes.

Whereas pouching and boxing are relatively straightforward procedures, blistering poses a technical challenge. A blister's top piece consists of a transparent thermoplastic film moulded to accommodate the product. Blistering machines are geared towards pressed, relatively flat tablets and not round Tibetan pills. Consequently, the moulds for round pills must be much deeper than usual. As more material is needed for the extrusion, the tops of the extruded moulds become fragile and thin. A thicker film has to be used, which not all blow-moulding machines can handle.

In addition, differences in altitude have to be taken into account. Blisters filled at high altitudes tend to implode when brought to the lowlands. The factory in Nyalam, for example, located at around 3,800 metres above sea level, faces frequent problems with blistering. The technicians needed to repair and fine-tune the machines have to be brought from inland China and a good solution to the problem has not yet been found. It is no surprise that some companies on the Tibetan Plateau have given up on the idea altogether and their expensive blister packaging machines remain unused.

Moreover, the laborious process of multilayer packaging makes medicines considerably more expensive. Many customers in Tibet are neither able nor willing to bear these added costs, as the following excerpt from an interview with a Mentsikhang doctor in Lhasa suggests:

> Packaging is very expensive. Local people cannot afford it. It looks nice. The package is nice for a gift. Very nice. But the patients cannot buy it. So it is better for them to buy from our pharmacy. Very cheap. One pill of Ratna Samphel costs 11.7 yuan [$1.7]. Elsewhere, one pill may be twenty or thirty yuan. The pills are exactly the same quality.

Given the local patients' reluctance to pay more, most pharmacies and factory outlets in Tibet have resorted to selling their products in two ways: in composite plastic-aluminium pouches and in boxes containing pouched and/or blistered pills. Some medicine shops started charging an extra eight to ten yuan for the box. In addition, the pouches-only approach has the benefit that smaller quantities can be sold, which many customers prefer.

The boxed versions have a different purpose, as the Mentsikhang doctor's comments indicate: apart from being remedies they can also serve as expensive gifts. This is especially true for precious pills like Ratna Samphel, Rinchen Mangjor and Rinchen Drangjor, which account for a considerable part of the industry's revenue. Geared towards the inland Chinese market, they come in lavish boxes similar to the packaging of jewellery or expensive watches. In this sense one could say that while packaging represents a crucial step in facilitating a medicine's entry into a commodity phase, it also opens the door to a specific form of its singularisation, namely its suitability as a gift.[3]

Legally, only a limited number of Tibetan medicines are licensed to be sold over the counter (OTC). For all other Tibetan drugs, including precious pills, a prescription is required. The distinction between OTC and prescription drugs is part of the SFDA's strategy to establish 'good supply practices' (GSP) along with GMP. However, in practice this distinction is largely ignored. Tibetan medicines that technically require a prescription are readily available over the counter – as is the case with synthetic, biomedical prescription drugs.

Both OTC and prescription medicines have to include an information leaflet for patients, which details the drug's indications and usage. These leaflets are by definition in Chinese and their content has to follow the published descriptions in the *Tibetan Drug Standards* of the *Chinese Pharmacopoeia*. This poses a set of problems, especially for the market in inland China, as Rinchen Wangdu points out:

> For some leaflets we have a Tibetan indication. But that raises another problem ... You know, at the beginning when people made the *[Chinese] Pharmacopoeia*, for some medicines they used the Tibetan terms, for some they just used the biomedical or even the traditional Chinese indications. So, the medicines for which they used the biomedical or the TCM indications – they sell very well. But for those where they used the Tibetan terms – you can sell them, but ... [t]he distributors who sell these medicines sometimes just provide the patients with another leaflet, explaining, for example, that *lung* [*rlung*, wind disorder] means this kind of disease. So when Chinese patients look at the leaflet [they] will know what kind of disease this medicine is good for ... The distributors do these things. But basically it is illegal ... If you want to change [the content of the information leaflet] you have to obtain permission from the SFDA.

Generally, leaflets are only included in the boxed version of a drug and do not come with medicines sold in simple pouches over the counter in Tibet. The pouches usually just feature a brief outline of ingredients and indications.[4]

Leaving all exceptions aside, a clear tendency can be made out: boxed medicines suitable as gifts for the inland market, pouches for Tibetan patients. In fact, the composite plastic-aluminium pouches have become the most common form in which Tibetan medicines are sold in Tibet today. Even medicines meant for hospital patients and not for the market are increasingly packaged in these pouches.

In summary we can say that industrial production of Tibetan medicine goes hand in hand with a radical change in the material and visual appearance of the medicines produced. This change was neither fully planned nor envisioned. It was triggered by regulations, facilitated by new machines, espoused by pragmatic considerations, and tempered by technical difficulties or local patients' reluctance to pay for expensive boxes. Nevertheless, packaging affects the biographies of medicines: mobility inspires new usages, and the fragile metonymic relations between product and producer need to be constantly invoked.

Advertising

In his reflections on magic and technology, Gell argues that magic has not disappeared in the modern world; it has only become more difficult to identify: 'One form it takes, as Malinowski himself suggested, is advertising. The flattering images of commodities purveyed in advertising coincide exactly with the equally flattering images with which magic invests its objects' (Gell 1988: 9). Indeed, advertising strategies frequently emphasise ideal technology. Highlighting a company's mastery in the domain of production, advertising relies on what Gell would call the enchantment of technology, namely, 'the power that technical processes have of casting a spell over us so that we see the real world in an enchanted form' (Gell 1992: 44). Let me explain by means of three advertising campaigns: two television commercials and one poster. These campaigns provide an overview of the strategies and visual themes employed to promote Tibetan pharmaceuticals in contemporary China.

Three Campaigns

The first is a television commercial by the TAR Tibetan Medicine Factory in Lhasa. It opens with two monks blowing *dungchen* (*dung chen*), long bass trumpets, on the roof of a monastery. The deep sound of the trumpets announces the beginning of a ceremonial metamorphosis. A view of green Tibetan grasslands and blue skies is presented. White clouds pass by in quick motion and flowers miraculously emerge and populate the plains. The next shot shows a statue of a sage with a beard and a topknot, presumably Yuthog Yonten Gonpo the Elder.

The sage is holding a Tibetan book in his left hand. His right hand glides over the text as if he was absorbing it. The flowers from the previous shot orbit the sage until he opens his right hand where, lured by the gesture, they spontaneously gather. The sage closes his right hand, rays of bright light emerge, and on opening his hand again an instant later the flowers have completed their magical transformation into a potent elixir: brown, round Tibetan pills hover over the palm of the sage's hand.

183

A sonorous voice proclaims, 'An epic history, its origins in the Land of Snows, a crystal of wisdom'. An image of the Potala appears and the company logo emerges in the sky above. The final shot depicts an old man with a white beard, very much like the statue of the sage. He resides in front of an ornamented bookshelf holding the *Kangyur* (*bka' 'gyur*) and *Tengyur* (*bstan 'gyur*), the canon of Tibetan Buddhism. He smiles as the company logo descends on him. The narration continues, 'The brand of the people, a medicine coming from the ancestors: Ganlu Tibetan medicine'.[5]

The second advert is a television commercial by Shongpalhachu. It follows a markedly different strategy. The commercial begins with a master shot of the factory in its surroundings, followed by a sequence of images of GMP production. Very much in the sense of GMP as mindful performance, workers in green and blue overalls are shown walking through white corridors and supervising grinding, mixing and packaging. A narrator explains that these specialists are in the course of producing, selecting and distributing a pure Tibetan medicine derived from a sophisticated culture. A short glimpse of the company's assembly hall, decorated with elaborate thangkas (Tibetan-style paintings), is intercut to illustrate this claim. The narrator continues that here traditional manufacturing techniques are combined with scientific understanding and modern standards. A laboratory technician is shown at work, followed by a series of awards the company has received for its achievements. Finally Shongpalhachu's logo is displayed, together with the company's slogan: 'Tibetan medicine made with divine waters, honouring the great medical knowledge, spreading the soul of health'.

While the TAR Tibetan Medicine Factory's television commercial portrays the technical process of manufacturing Tibetan pills as a magical transformation from nature into medicine – a condensed visual trope of a *mendrup* ritual – Shongpalhachu's spot depicts Tibetan medicine production primarily as being enfolded in a scientific aura.

Both commercials were aired by Xizang TV, the local broadcaster in the TAR, before each episode of a Tibetan-language television series. The target audience was clearly Tibetan. However, both commercials were in Mandarin and they may have also been shown on Chinese national television. The TAR Tibetan Medicine Factory's commercial in particular is technically and visually very sophisticated and would certainly be suitable for larger audiences in inland China.

The two television commercials do not advertise specific products but rather the companies' brands. This has to be seen in relation to current regulations stipulating that only OTC drugs can be advertised publicly. Adverts for prescription drugs are confined to publications for a specialist audience, such as trade magazines or medical journals. This rule has seen strict enforcement. As a result most of the well-known Tibetan formulas, including precious pills, can no longer be advertised publicly.[6]

The third example is a poster for Cheezheng's pain relief plaster, the best selling Tibetan OTC formula in China. The campaign has been running for many years and has acquired almost iconic status. Everybody in Tibet is familiar with the poster, and it has also been used several times in academic publications and conference presentations (cf. TIN 2004).

The poster shows a young, beautiful Tibetan woman wearing a pink blouse. The sleeves of a nomad's winter *chuba* (*chu ba*), a robe lined with fur, are tied around her waist. Her hair is arranged in many thin braids in the style preferred by nomad women from some areas of Kham and Amdo. She wears Tibetan jewellery and her child-like face is full of youth, light-heartedness and the purity of the Tibetan grasslands. In the palms of her open hands she holds, like an offering, a box of Cheezheng's pain relief plasters.

Cheezheng's advertisement is definitely made to reach a nationwide audience. It speaks the language of the gift (Anagnost 1997: 57–62) and its message is clear and to the point: the pureness of the Tibetan plateau, captured in the company's product and endowed with Tibetan beauty, is offered to the big family of the People's Republic of China.

Visual Themes

The principal visual themes employed by these three campaigns are nature (the grasslands and flowers), Tibetanness (the monks blowing *dungchen*, the Tibetan nomad girl, the sage, the scripture), and modern science/technology (the GMP production line, the laboratory). These three visual themes underpin most advertising efforts in the industry. Following van der Geest, Whyte and Hardon's suggestion that pharmaceuticals 'constitute a perfect opportunity for the study of the relation between symbols and political economy' (van der Geest, Whyte and Hardon 1996: 170), I will take these three visual themes and analyse them in terms of their capacity to produce symbolic meaning in the context of contemporary Tibet.

Of the three themes, nature is the most frequently used. Many companies have produced lavish brochures, which can be handed out to customers in pharmacies and factory outlets. Most of these brochures are in standard Chinese and Tibetan and follow a very similar design and structure. The main part of a typical brochure consists of a display of the company's products, both OTC and prescription medicines. The medicine boxes are usually shown against the background of Tibetan landscapes – grasslands, snowy mountains and rivers. The potency of Tibetan medicines is presented as being directly derived from pristine, wild and beautiful Tibetan nature.[7]

The relation between Tibet's environment and the company's products is often spelled out in the brochure's text, emphasising, for example, that precious Tibetan medicinal herbs only grow 'on the roof of the world'. The brochures portray the companies as environmentally conscious; references to plant cultivation projects are made and images of excursions showing experienced *amchi* teaching factory employees about medicinal plants suggest a mindful attitude towards nature.

The Tibetan Plateau's ecology plays an increasingly important part in Chinese imaginaries of Tibet. On the one hand, Tibet is perceived and promoted as a realm of pristine natural beauty. On the other hand, concerns about the fragility of this natural environment have entered public discourse and official policies. This can be seen in the partial logging ban imposed in Eastern Tibet, the efforts to stop the degradation of Tibetan rangelands that is threatening inland China's water supplies, and the protection of endangered animal species like the Tibetan antelope (see IOSC 2003). In this sense, the emphasis on nature and conservation found in the industry's advertising materials mirrors the importance Tibet's ecology has gained over recent years in official and public discourse.

Concern for Tibet's fragile ecosystem is also a cornerstone of Tibetan self-representations in exile. Toni Huber (1997) coined the term 'Green Tibetans' to describe essentialist representations of Tibetan people that posit them as being in harmony with nature and refraining from exploitation. Such representations started entering exile agendas in the mid 1980s. Drawing a direct relation between Tibetan Buddhism and Tibetans' 'traditional' environmental consciousness, these representations are cast against a view of Chinese rule as exploitative and destructive. The party-state's portrayal of its concern for Tibet's ecology is also to be seen in relation to this criticism voiced in exile and among Tibet support groups around the globe.

Similar essentialist representations also characterise Chinese discourse on ethnic minorities and their relationship with nature (Heberer 2001). However, instead of casting these representations against the state's exploitive demeanour, they are embedded in images of the large 'family' of multiethnic China living together in harmony under the leadership of this Communist Party.

This brings us to the second visual theme: the representation of Tibetanness. The young nomad woman in the Cheezheng's advert resonates with both the theme of nature and the theme of China as a harmonious big 'family' of nationalities (*minzu*). Offering pain relief to this grand 'family' presents the Tibetan *minzu* as a joyful and devoted member of this 'family' – a powerful image and a clever move.

In contrast to the nomad girl on Cheezheng's poster, the TAR Tibetan Medicine Factory's commercial showing the magical transformation of nature into medicine suggests a different vision of the Tibetan people's role vis-à-vis China. It is not exotic beauty that is employed to bring the potency of Tibetan nature to inland China but powerful knowledge embodied in the figure of a sage. However, the sage – presumably Yuthog, the founding father of Sowa Rigpa – is one of the few important Buddhist figures traditionally not depicted as a Tibetan Buddhist monk but rather with a beard and a topknot. The image of the sage in the advert corresponds quite closely, whether intentionally or not, to the depiction of Confucius and some of the Daoist sages. Arguably, the sage is therefore not necessarily understood as standing for Tibetan Buddhist knowledge. What can be read as a symbolic commentary on a technical strategy (*mendrup, tsothal*) can also be read as a generic vision of China's ancient wisdom – 'a medicine from the ancestors', as the narrator says.

In summary, the first two visual themes – nature and Tibetanness – are closely intertwined both in the discourse on minorities and in the notion of China as a big 'family' of nationalities. Both expressions of Tibetanness – the nomad girl and the sage as statue – produce symbolic value related to the political imagination of China as a multiethnic nation. The themes of nature and Tibetanness – or more generically ethnicity – are employed in a way that promises at once to enchant potential customers and to offer the allure of the industry's dutiful efforts in contributing to the party-state's agendas.

The third visual theme employed in advertising is exemplified by Shongpalhachu's commercial. The party-state's agenda for the Tibetan medicine industry was, initially at least, predominantly couched in notions of modernisation, science and technology. Shongpalhachu's television commercial portrays the company's ventures as an effortless combination of technology, modern science and age-old wisdom. It does so by showing images of GMP production intercut with the factory's almost monastic assembly hall, combined with a narration that declares a perfect harmony between Sowa Rigpa and GMP.

The predominance of the three main visual themes employed in advertising — nature, Tibetanness, and technology/science — also means that other possible themes are relatively absent. Most prominent among them is Tibetan Buddhism. When images of Buddhism are used, they tend to be general allegorical figures of Tibetan culture (monks in red robes, the Potala, scriptures) rather than expressions of the deep concern for the Buddhist roots of Sowa Rigpa, which many of the professionals working in the industry share. It is remarkable, for example, that in all the company brochures I have collected there is not one single depiction of the Medicine Buddha. Visual expressions of Tibetan Buddhism are considered sensitive. They either tend to be confined to certain contexts such as museums and exhibition halls where religion can be read as culture, or else they find their expression as spirituality in new ventures not recognisable as Tibetan Buddhist at first sight.

The Buddhist Company

Yuthog

One of the most interesting cases in regard to Buddhism is Cheezheng, the largest Tibetan medicine company.[8] Cheezheng is in several ways atypical of the industry. The company's headquarters are in Lanzhou, outside the Tibetan areas. It operates three manufacturing plants, one of them in the town of Bayi (Nyingtri, eastern TAR). Moreover, Cheezheng's main product is neither one of the highly valued *rinchen rilbu* nor another famous Tibetan formula but the pain-relief plaster encountered in the advert above. The plaster is well known throughout China and is also one of the few Tibetan medicine products exported in large quantities abroad.[9]

Unlike the majority of companies, Cheezheng did not emerge from the nexus of a hospital pharmacy but was established as a private company as early as 1993 by a certain Lei Jufang. Madame Lei, as I will call her, is unusual not only because she is Chinese but also because she is a woman in an otherwise male-dominated industry. Generally, women are much more prominent in Cheezheng than in other companies. The director of Cheezheng's cultural affairs department, for example, is a Chinese woman, and during my visit in 2008 Madame Lei's closest assistants were two young, inland-educated, Tibetan women. Most importantly, however, Madame Lei is a devout Buddhist. In an interview with *China Daily* she openly admitted that her biggest joy in life was worshipping in a Tibetan monastery (*China Daily* 2008).

The first thing a visitor catches sight of when entering Cheezheng's GMP manufacturing plant in Bayi is a white statue of Yuthog the Elder, the founding father of Sowa Rigpa. The entry hall of Cheezheng's factory has a temple-like air. Yuthog resides in the middle of the foyer beneath a monastic baldachin and textile drapery. Four thangkas, one of them showing Sangye Menla (*sangs rgyas sman lha*), the Medicine Buddha, are displayed behind the statue. Fresh flowers adorn the scene and make clear that this statue is not just a piece of art but an object of active veneration.

Dorjie, the young Tibetan manager who had welcomed us with a white *khatag* (*kha btags*), a ceremonial scarf, told us that local people often came here to worship. He pointed towards a lump on Yuthog's forehead and explained that it had spontaneously grown since the statue was brought here. *Rang chung* (*rang byung*), 'spontaneous, natural emergence', is a common motif in Tibetan Buddhism and seen as an extremely auspicious sign. The statue of Yuthog had miraculously come to life in the entry hall of a GMP factory, of all places. The statue was the very first thing we were shown on our tour through the factory. It endowed the company with spiritual, metaphysical acceptance and gave it a place in the moral universe of Tibetan Buddhism.

The company's envisioned location in Tibetan space and history is even more evident in the murals adorning the entry hall of

Cheezheng's main factory on the outskirts of Lanzhou. All three of the company's manufacturing plants as well as its Lhasa offices are depicted as monastic edifices on a stylised map of Tibet. The factory in Bayi is shown at the foot of the hill with the cave where Yuthog the Elder meditated. The company's Lhasa branch is depicted in close proximity to the right of the Potala Palace. This auspicious location takes into account that the left side of the Potala is already occupied, physically and metaphorically, by Chagpori Hill on which the famous Chagpori medical school was situated. Behind the compound the grasslands start. Yaks and sheep can be seen grazing between black and festive white tents.

One feature of the murals attracted my attention: a white four-wheel-drive SUV, which reminded me of the brand new, luxurious company Land Rover in which we travelled during our visit to Lanzhou. The white SUV is depicted several times in the murals, mostly in close proximity to the company's edifices. Features of contemporary life, such as cars, roads, and tourists, have found their ways into a number of thangkas and murals throughout the Tibetan world. The white car's prominent presence is therefore not entirely novel. However, it points to the fact that other signs of contemporary life and industrial production are absent. No machines are depicted, and neither are GMP manufacturing plants, drug stores or packaged pills. They simply do not belong in the map of Cheezheng's location in the Tibetan universe.

I did not have a chance to verify Dorjie's claim and witness the stream of pilgrims coming to worship Yuthog at the company's Bayi factory. However, it is not my aim here to question the credibility of his account. Nor would I want to suggest that the statue and the murals merely served as a marketing strategy to enchant the occasional outside visitor. The murals and the statue of Yuthog are meant as gestures of veneration. As we will see in the next chapter, Madame Lei's moral engagement with Tibetan Buddhism extends far beyond the factory's entrance hall and includes many grassroots projects aimed at supporting local Tibetan communities.

Spiritual Spa

Madame Lei's vision of her company's duty as the largest Tibetan medicine producer, however, also includes making the benefits of Tibetan medicine available throughout contemporary China – not only in the form of physical pain relief but also, I dare say, in a spiritual way. What this looks like aesthetically can be seen in the company's new spa centre in downtown Lanzhou.

Medicinal baths are an integral part of the wide palette of Sowa Rigpa treatment, and several Tibetan hospitals also include spa sections. However, Cheezheng's vision of Tibetan spas takes them to a new level in terms of luxury and aesthetics. Cheezheng's spa caters to the taste of wealthy customers in search of a Tibetan well-being experience.

The spa's ground floor houses a hotel-style reception and a spacious lobby with voluptuous fauteuils made of heavy wooden frames covered with thick, square, crimson pillows. The walls are panelled with light-coloured wood (the same kind as that used for the frames of the fauteuils) and feature rich carvings. Buddhist iconography, although present in some of the carvings – a protector deity here, one of the eight auspicious signs there – is not particularly emphasised. Tibetan drapery lines the ceiling, but instead of the intense and saturated colours normally used for such drapery, apricot was chosen to fit the colour palette of the furnishings.

The interior design follows a distinct style of its own, heedful of every little detail. The bathtubs, for example, are made of the same

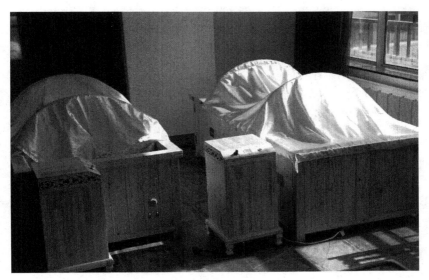

Figure 6.2: Bath tubs in Cheezheng's Lanzhou spa.

carved wood as the wall panels. The Tibetan doctors' white robes are braided with varicoloured woollen ribbons, matching the inlays of the fauteuils' pillows. Without being overtly Buddhist, the ambience of the centre is remarkably different from any other site I have seen in Tibet: it blends spirituality with well-being and luxury. A Chinese architect from Beijing was responsible for the design; but most ideas, I was assured, came personally from Madame Lei. The spa centre is designed to be an experience – an aesthetic experience of Tibetan medicine's quest for the well-being of body and soul.

Madame Lei, Cheezheng's founder and director, invited us for dinner in the spa centre's own vegetarian restaurant, located on the top floor. We declined the offer of being picked up at our hotel, took a taxi, got stuck in Lanzhou's early-evening traffic jam and were, to our great embarrassment, half an hour late. Madame Lei and her two Tibetan assistants were waiting for us in one of the restaurant's private booths. Madame Lei, a woman in her fifties, did not seem to be impatient or angry. An aura of utmost calm surrounded her and during the whole evening she did not let any unnecessary movement or gesture negate my initial impression. She wore an Indian-style embroidered jacket; not a traditional Indian piece of clothing, more the upmarket reincarnation of what Western hippies consider to be Indian – an elegant, somehow alternative and certainly unconventional outfit for a successful Chinese businesswoman.

The five of us – Madame Lei, her two Tibetan assistants, my Tibetan friend and I – were sitting at a round table in heavy chairs placed at perfectly equal distances from one another, as if somebody had measured them. In the middle of the table an elaborate stand had been placed – a bouquet of five silver flowers holding five *amuse-gueules* wrapped in salad leaves. During our conversation Madame Lei voiced strong concerns about the ecological implications of the burgeoning Tibetan medicine industry. She stressed that the first thing one had to do when thinking about the production of Tibetan medicines for a large market was the selection of suitable formulas for such an enterprise. It made no sense, she said, to start producing a famous formula if it was based on rare herbs. In fact, Cheezheng's pain-relief plaster does not use rare ingredients.

Madame Lei's concerns for Tibet's ecology were more than just rhetoric to please a Western researcher. Before she started Cheezheng, Madame Lei, a trained physicist and engineer holding an assistant professorship at Lanzhou University, left her position to set up her own research institution focusing on the treatment of industrial pollution. The company, established in 1987, did not get off the ground. 'A mistake committed by a foolish idealist', she said in an interview (*China Daily* 2008). 'I think it is important to waste less and improve the environment', she continues, 'but nobody else wanted that at that time'.

While we talked, a lavish banquet comprising around thirty different delicacies was served. All the dishes were vegetarian, a reference to the ethics of a new kind of Tibetan Buddhism that frowns upon the very Tibetan habits of eating meat and drinking alcohol, both in ample quantities. Instead of beer we were served tea. Each glass was embellished with a dried flower of a different kind. A hostess made sure that our table was always brimful and in perfect order. While we were talking, she would come and go silently, opening and closing the door almost inaudibly as if a child, sleeping lightly, might be disturbed. The entire arrangement, from the porcelain tea cups and dishes to Madame Lei's outfit and calm attentiveness, created an atmosphere of luxurious serenity, very unlike the usually loud and jolly Chinese or Tibetan banquets.

Back in the unheated room of our business hotel near the train station, with my friend smoking on the bed, watching TV and fighting off the receptionist's calls advertising local prostitutes, a line of Baudelaire's poem 'L'invitation au voyage' (Baudelaire 1857: LIII) came to mind:

> Là, tout n'est qu'ordre et beauté, luxe, calme et volupté.[10]

Madame Lei's spa centre was indeed, I thought, an invitation to a journey – an invitation to a small but growing stratum of wealthy people in search of a healthy, spiritual life; a technology of enchantment in which a new kind of Tibetan medicine and the style and ethics of a new kind of Buddhism converge – perfection in every little detail, spirituality reincarnated in design, aesthetics as a token of mindfulness.

Arura's Museum

No less ambitious than Cheezheng's spa, albeit in a radically different fashion, is the Arura Group's recent move to showcase the Tibetan and Buddhist heritage of Sowa Rigpa. As one of the major

Tibetan medicine companies in Qinghai province, the Arura Group is a prime example of the varied entanglements between state and business in the context of contemporary Tibet. Apart from a privatised, for-profit factory, the Arura Group also operates a state-owned Tibetan medicine hospital, a research unit, and a Tibetan department at Xining's medical college.

Arura's headquarters and factory are situated in Xining's Biotech Zone, a designated industrial area on the outskirts of the city. Among the fifty-odd companies in the Biotech Zone are a few other Tibetan medicine factories, among them Jigme Phuntsog's Jiumei Tibetan Medicine Co. Ltd. When new GMP-compliant factories had to be built between 2002 and 2004, many companies moved to the Biotech Zone, where they were offered cheap deals on land and the prospect of ten years' tax exemption (Bhaskara 2004).

Broad, empty boulevards lined by young trees emphasise the newness and planned character of this industrial zone. Amidst these empty boulevards and mundane factory buildings, an eye-catching new landmark has recently been erected: Arura's Tibetan Medicine Museum of China. The museum, opened in September 2006, is an imposing structure. It is surrounded by a vast and usually empty parking lot, surrounded by patches of well-kept lawn and flower beds lined with the same young trees as the broad boulevards. Inspired by Tibetan monastic and contemporary Chinese architectural styles, the museum has a temple-like air. The sheer size of the building and the enormous glass façades around the entrances give it an imposing appearance, something of an up-scaled Tibetan monastery on steroids. An investment of 120 million yuan ($17.6 million) – about double the cost of Arura's new GMP factory (*China Daily* 2006) – the museum is not meant to be a display of modesty. It is built to present Tibetan medicine and culture at its best.

The entire upper floor gives prominence to the world's largest thangka – six hundred metres long and worth an entry in the *Guinness Book of Records*. The ground floor houses a collection of artefacts and tools related to the history of Tibetan medicine, an exhibition of Tibetan *materia medica*, as well as a group of stuffed animals from the Tibetan Plateau. The basement features a lavish sales area where young Tibetan women in meticulous dresses, harmonised with the colours of the shop's interior design, sell Arura's products in an atmosphere similar to that of luxurious airport boutiques.

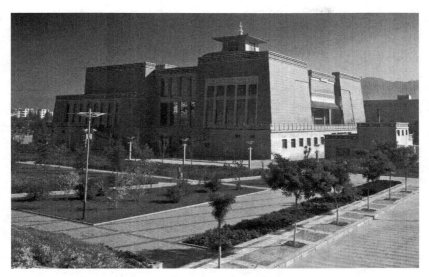

Figure 6.3: Arura's Tibetan Medicine Museum of China in Xining.

The initiative to build the museum came from Dr Ao Tsochen, director of the Arura Group. Initially, everybody on the Group's board was against Ao's museum plans. The project was considered to be too expensive, given that there was no obvious way to make it profitable. The other museum in the centre of Xining, the Japanese-sponsored Qinghai Museum, did not receive many visitors. The governor of Qinghai province, who had to be consulted on the matter, did not approve either. In her view, the project was too ambitious and the planned structure too prodigious. She urged the Arura Group to scale down the initial project, which had featured an even bigger structure. But Dr Ao finally convinced the board and governor, and construction started with Arura's own funds and a bank loan. Considering the museum's location in Xining's Biotech Zone, hardly a tourist attraction, this was a significant risk.

The museum's showpiece, the world-record thangka, was not Arura's idea; Tsunchi Rajie, a well-known thangka painter, had been the driving force behind the masterpiece. The story, unverified but related to me by a friend of his who had been following the thangka's odyssey for the previous seventeen years, goes as follows.

For more than twenty years Tsunchi Rajie had been thinking about the idea of combining the cosmos of Tibetan iconography in one magnum opus. Secure the necessary permissions and funds for such an enterprise proved to be extremely difficult, but he finally managed to secure a loan of 5 million yuan ($730,000) with which he started the project. Hundreds of artists in six different groups worked for four years to complete the thangka. The result is an extraordinary work of very high quality.

The thangka was shown in exhibitions in Beijing, Lhasa, South Korea and Xining. But financially, the enterprise turned into a disaster for Tsunchi Rajie. 'The banks literally hunted him', his friend told me. At this point Dr Ao Tsochen, Arura's paramount leader, approached him with an offer to buy the thangka for 15 million yuan ($2.2 million); a fair price, not only paying the painter's debts but also remunerating him for his immense accomplishment. The idea was to dedicate a whole storey of the planned museum to a permanent exhibition of the thangka.

The thangka depicts the entire universe of Tibetan history and Buddhism – kings, deities, lineages of important religious figures, including portraits of the first thirteen Dalai Lamas. Except for the missing fourteenth Dalai Lama, the thangka makes no compromise and presents itself as religious art. In the context of a museum (and, at that, as a world record) Tibetan Buddhism becomes part of the nation's diverse cultural heritage and ceases to be a sensitive domain. On the contrary, the entire universe of Tibetan religion and culture condensed in an art object perfectly fits with the officially sanctioned idea of the conservation and development of Tibetan culture.

Arura's decision to build the museum and buy the thangka proved to be a far-sighted one. The Qinghai government, which had initially shown little interest in the museum, soon changed their attitude. China's western development campaign (*xibu da kaifa*), formally initiated in 2000 and aimed at an increased pace of development in China's western regions (Dezhu 2000; Lai 2002), often brings delegations of high-ranking Beijing officials to Xining. As these delegations became regular visitors to the museum, the provincial authorities began to realise what an invaluable asset it was.

Arura's museum provides the provincial authorities with a showcase for their achievements – material evidence not only of the economic success of Arura as a company but also of the development of Tibetan culture. During his visit, China's foreign minister expressed his utmost delight: 'We always try to explain to the world that we actively do something good for Tibetan culture. But they never believe us. But here you have built something concrete, something material to prove our commitment to developing Tibetan culture. This is a great achievement'.[11]

For Arura as a company and for the different levels of government, the museum serves multiple purposes. First, it provides the local authorities with the means to present their accomplishments in a favourable light to the central government, which strengthens their position in the national arena. Second, the Communist Party headquarters in Beijing are given a welcome opportunity to showcase their achievements in 'developing Tibetan culture' to the world. Arura is an exemplary case: a Tibetan company making patriotic use (yet with a Tibetan flavour) of the freedom it is given under the 'socialist market economy' – a fine case of good governance on all levels and a visible effort in the building of national harmony. And third, Arura as a company benefits as well. Good and close relations with all levels of the state, including contacts with Beijing's Party elite, provide Arura with a good position and bargaining power in times when important decisions about the industry are increasingly taken in the capital. This easily translates into economic advantages. 'We are a good company, you know', one of Arura's senior managers told me, meaning: a good company in the eyes of the successfully enchanted government.

Furthermore, the museum has received ample attention in the Chinese press (CTIC 2006a, 2006d, 2008a), which leads to steadily increasing visitor numbers. When I came back to Xining in August 2009, the parking lot was no longer as empty as it had once been. A visit to the museum was now on the standard itinerary of Chinese tour groups, which benefited Xining's appeal as a tourist destination and made the museum's shop even more profitable. Within a year the number of guides employed rose from half a dozen to over thirty.

Enchanting Whom?

My aim in this chapter has been to analyse both the use of aesthetics for social and strategic purposes and the ways the world created by such aesthetic endeavours reciprocally affects the modes in which the Tibetan medicine industry operates. I suggested two broad orientations – disenchantment and enchantment (or re-enchantment)

– in order to categorise the variety of aesthetic endeavours found in the context of industrial Tibetan medicine. The hypothesis put forward was that the two were intrinsically linked, because Sowa Rigpa in the contemporary People's Republic of China had, at once, to conform to images of the scientifically disenchanted, modern as well as the enchanted, 'magic' Tibet.

The spiritual, aesthetic take on Tibetan spas, the museum housing a world-record thangka, the television commercial depicting the magical transformation of nature into medicine, and the *mendrup* ritual providing the inspiration for it – all these can be seen as movements towards enchantment or re-enchantment. The tightly regulated packaging designs and the television commercial showing GMP production as mindful performance, however, are more difficult to categorise. On the one hand, their aim is clearly to remove Sowa Rigpa from the realm of magic and 'superstition' and to position it in the field of technology and science. Therefore, they can be described as strategies of disenchantment. On the other hand, as Weber noted, not technology and science as such, but imaginaries of their omnipotence are what drive the disenchantment of the world. These imaginaries form no less a mythologised universe than the world they seek to replace. They are often based on an aesthetic vision of a final outcome rather than scientific scrutiny. Aesthetic expressions used as social strategies in the name of disenchantment thereby acquire the characteristics of technologies of enchantment in disguise.

The aesthetic visions of what 'modern' Tibetan medicine should look like and their actual outcomes – the GMP-certified manufacturing plants, the blisters, boxes and their design – stand in contrast with similarly aesthetic visions of what 'magic' Tibet should look like – monks blowing *dungchen*, grasslands with beautiful girls and potent herbs. This intersection of differing visions accounts for the immense heterogeneity of aesthetics found within the industry.

The images and things produced in this context, the aesthetic output of Tibetan medicine enterprises, are part of an aesthetic enterprise writ large: the remaking of Sowa Rigpa ties in with the remaking of Tibet. The resulting visualities and materialities – the colours and rites of GMP depicted in advertising, the packaged pills equipped with the charm of mobility, the spiritual and vegetarian spa, the lavish museum – all leave their imprints. As facts, objects, and images of everyday life they give rise to new perceptions of Tibet and its medicine. The question, however, remains: who are the technologies of enchantment/re-enchantment directed at?

In the park surrounding Cheezheng's factory in Bayi, 50 metres from the venerated statue of Yuthog, another symbol of Madame Lei's vision of mindful eco-Buddhism can be seen: a monument in the form of a knotted, twisted saw. The monument is clearly inspired by the twisted gun, the famous anti-war memorial at the UN headquarters in New York. Just as the knot in the gun's barrel disables its capacity to kill and stands for peace, the twist in the saw renders it unusable for cutting wood and continuing the deforestation of Eastern Tibet.[12] Would such an open criticism of China's Tibet policies be tolerated if it came from a Tibetan company or leader? As a highly successful Chinese company, Cheezheng enjoys certain freedoms and acts in ways Tibetan companies are careful to avoid. Cheezheng does not have to demonstrate its loyalty to the party-state in the same way as Tibetan-owned-and-managed companies. On the other hand, there is arguably a greater need for Cheezheng to emphasise its Tibetanness in the eyes of Tibetans. Consequently, different expressions of Tibetanness do not necessarily follow the lines of ethnic identity. We see that in addition to moving between enchantment and disenchantment, a 'magic' and a 'modern' vision of Tibet, the aesthetic enterprise oscillates between two other poles: its capacity to prove loyalty to the party-state and its capacity to inspire trust in the authenticity of the commodities at stake. Then, the question is not *what* but *whom* to enchant: A wealthy stratum of spiritual-well-being seekers? The visiting Party elite? An imagined collective of potential donors and Tibet-savers from outside China? Or the people living in Tibet who look for reliable, affordable medicines? This spectre defines not only a political and economic but also a moral space, a space in which Tibetanness is the good of a moral economy at large.

Notes

1. In the previous chapters, following de Certeau (1988), I often posited companies' endeavours as tactical in relation to the strategies of the state. Companies' aesthetic enterprises, however, clearly have a strategic nature in de Certeau's sense.

2. *Mendrup* can also take the form of a public ritual in which small blessed pills, usually referred to as *mani rilbu* (*ma ni ril bu*), are made and consecrated. Marietta Kind provides an ethnographic account of such a ritual in a Bon community in Dolpo, Nepal (Kind 2002). These small, blessed pills are not meant to treat a specific condition defined in the system of Sowa Rigpa, and their benefit is more general than specific. See Kloos (2010) for a discussion of the political and moral aspects of *mani rilbu* and *mendrup* in exile.

3. Hofer argues that *rinchen rilbu* are not commonly used in the rural practice of Tibetan medicine because even without packaging they are simply too expensive (Hofer 2009a: 179–80).

4. Whether and how these indications are taken into consideration by Tibetan patients falls outside the scope of my inquiry. However, how leaflets and written indications affect patient behaviour would be a worthy study of its own.

5. Ganlu is the brand name under which the TAR Tibetan Medicine Factory markets its products.

6. The enforcement of these regulations is a recent phenomenon; according to Theresia Hofer (2009a), public advertising for several non-OTC medicines was still common in Lhasa in 2006.

7. The fact that a considerable number of ingredients used in Tibetan medicine come from Nepal and India is never mentioned in advertising.

8. The company name is sometimes also spelt Qizheng; *qi* means 'wonderful', *zheng* can be translated as 'principle'.

9. In 2003, Cheezheng brokered a deal with the American retail giant Wal-Mart (Yi 2003) to distribute its pain-relief plaster. It is important to note that despite its unusual appearance in a world of round, brown pills, the plaster is actually based on an old formula associated with Jampa Trinley, a famous Tibetan physician and long-term director of the Mentsikhang in Lhasa. Externally applied remedies, often in the form of medicinal butters, have otherwise lost importance in the age of industrially produced pills and powders.

10. 'There, all is order and beauty, luxury, peace and pleasure.'

11. This is my paraphrase of the foreign minister's remarks based on how they were recounted to me.

12. Although logging officially stopped in many parts of Eastern Tibet after the devastating floods of 1998 (Wang et al. 2007), it still continues to some extent in Kongpo.

Chapter 7
The Moral Economy of Tibetanness

Tibetanness generates value. Consider Cheezheng's spiritual and vegetarian take on Tibetan spas, Arura's record-breaking museum, the magic sage in the TV commercial, or Aku Jinpa's school mentioned in the Introduction (the one not meant to be profitable but 'good for Tibetan culture') – be it as a product or service to be sold, as a technology of enchantment in advertising, or in Aku Jinpa's case as the basis for a successful fundraising application submitted to an American NGO – Tibetanness serves as a commodity or asset in each of these cases. All the actors engage, willingly or not, in the economy of Tibetanness.

The use of ethnic identity for commercial purposes is a worldwide, and by no means a uniquely Tibetan, phenomenon. The Tibetanness economy has to be seen in relation to what Jean and John Comaroff identify as the global rise of 'identity economies' and 'ethnicity industries' (Comaroff and Comaroff 2009). However, what may appear to be simply an extension of capitalist commodity fetishism in the domain of ethnicity produces more nuanced outcomes. Commodification and marketisation of ethnic identity create unprecedented opportunities for generating value of various kinds – also for those who are less well-positioned, the authors suggest. Following Swain (1990), Chambers (2000), Xie (2003), Geismar (2005) and others, the Comaroffs argue that any number of minority populations around the globe have 'enhanced their autonomy, their political presence, and their material circumstances by adroitly managing their tourist potential – and all that it has come to connote' (Comaroff and Comaroff 2009: 24). In short, the moniker 'Ethnicity, Inc.' can stand for unfettered exploitation as well as tactical 'ethno-preneuralism' (ibid.: 27) serving local economic and political agendas.

Aku Jinpa's school and factory, for example, can be seen from this angle. They would probably not have been funded by the NGO had they not alluded to the idea of safeguarding an 'authentic', traditional Tibetan medicine.

'Authenticity' and the economy of cultural identity are intrinsically linked. Charles Lindholm remarks in this respect that aid agencies around the globe tend to support the projects and people they regard as the most authentic. In southern Africa, for example, it is not the majority of the landless 'real San' working as impoverished labourers on farms who benefit most from international aid, but those who conform to popular stereotypes of authentic Bushmen – tracking animals, wearing loincloths, and eating nuts and berries (Lindholm 2008: 131). The notion of authenticity, he argues, touches on an increasingly wide range of human experience.

The tactical use of ethnicity and authenticity in the political economy of international aid is a figure of thought that may apply to Aku Jinpa's fundraising success. However, it would not represent the full picture. Branding Aku Jinpa's morality merely a clever tactical move would not do justice to the sincerity of his endeavour. Similarly, Arura's and Cheezheng's engagement in the Tibetanness economy cannot be characterised as merely strategic. Neither is Madame Lei's spiritual take on Tibetan spas just a clever marketing strategy, nor is Arura's investment in the thangka simply a device to strengthen the company's bargaining position vis-à-vis local and central government offices. To regard these efforts as exclusively informed by economic and/or political rationality would be to deny their integrity and fail to capture the complex relations between morality, authenticity, economy, and politics.

Following Polanyi (1957), Thompson (1971) and Scott (1976), I suggested earlier that the notion of moral economy is a useful means of approaching the issue – not the moral economy of traditional peasant societies but a contemporary version of it. I argued that unlike the cases analysed in classic moral economy scholarship, its main commodity was neither grain nor livestock but Tibetanness – objectified in herbs, pills, knowledge and aesthetic expressions of culture.

The term moral economy is not meant to describe a closed community untouched by national or global forces. On the contrary, a moral economy emerges when a community or society is confronted with a strong outside force that triggers a crisis of subsistence and threatens a well-established way of life. The response is one of self-protection, often couched in moral terms. Aku Jinpa's efforts to defend (or re-establish) a Tibetan medicine unencumbered by the logic of industry, capital, and markets can be understood as self-protective in this sense. However, unlike the worlds described by Polanyi, Thompson and Scott, the subsistence crisis in the present case is a crisis of cultural more than material subsistence. This crisis takes place amidst His Holiness the Dalai Lama's statement about ongoing 'cultural genocide' in Tibet (Coonan 2008; Eimer and Chamberlain 2008) as well as unprecedented efforts by the party-state to prove him wrong (IOSC 2008).

The positions of Aku Jinpa, the American NGO, the Tibetan government in exile, companies like Arura or Cheezheng, as well as the Chinese leadership have one thing in common: they all attribute great importance to Tibetan medicine as a part of Tibetan culture, and they all subscribe to the moral obligation that it needs to be preserved. Just as, in Thompson's case, the English working class emphasised well-established moral principles that were believed to be shared across class boundaries (Thompson 1964: 62–76; Thompson 1991: 188), the morality underpinning the Tibetanness economy claims universality – despite the fact that the meanings and agendas linked to it often stand in contradiction with one another. Moral understandings of local phenomena are couched in the same terms as global issues of social justice and human rights. Even Aku Jinpa's Buddhist ethics is connected to a global form of morality (cf. Calabrese 2005).

Finally, as the market for Tibetanness is not bound to a locality, the 'confrontations in the market-place', which Thompson defined as characteristic of a moral economy, naturally take a different shape (Edelman 2005). The resulting incarnation of a moral economy is therefore not a local one but rather a moral economy at large.

My aim in this chapter is to trace the threads of the moral economy of Tibetanness: the commodification of culture and the preservation of cultural heritage, conflicting perceptions of Tibet's past and present, and competing visions for its future, authenticity and morality. I begin by positioning the Tibetanness economy against the background of a larger economy of ethnicity in the People's Republic of China (PRC). I then look at relations between authenticity and morality and discuss what this means for companies involved in the industrial manufacturing of Tibetan remedies.

The Tibetanness Economy

Preservation and Development

One of the reasons why Arura's museum appeals to official China is the fact that it epitomises a vision of Tibet and Tibetan medicine that embraces both the preservation of culture *and* development. At first sight, preservation and development could be seen as conflicting agendas. Evidently, the state's overall strategy for Tibetan medicine is based on notions of progress, modernisation, standardisation and development. It is meant to align Sowa Rigpa with the needs of modern China and its primary goal is certainly not to preserve Tibetan medicine in its 'traditional' state.

However, the concept of the preservation of culture has become a central focus of the party-state's policies on Tibet. From this official perspective development and the preservation of culture are not seen as irreconcilable. On the contrary, government publications frequently mention the two notions together. A recent White Paper on Tibet, for instance, is titled *Protection and Development of Tibetan Culture* (IOSC 2008). We learn that Tibetan medicine is a 'unique part of traditional Tibetan culture', which itself is 'a lustrous pearl of Chinese culture as well as a precious part of world culture'. It is argued that 'accelerated development' has fuelled the 'old science' of Sowa Rigpa with 'vigour and vitality'. Impressive numbers of clinics, doctors, factories and publications in both Tibetan and Mandarin are given to substantiate the claim (ibid.: 1, 13).

The fusion of the preservation and development of culture is not unique to the PRC. It is part of a global trend reflected in the concept of 'intangible cultural heritage' – a centrepiece of UNESCO's strategy. Unlike the organisation's previous emphasis on identifying and protecting world heritage sites, this new approach extends the UNESCO strategy into the domain of non-material expressions of culture. The concept has fallen on fertile ground in the PRC. In

2003, the UNESCO conference in Paris adopted the Convention for the Safeguarding of the Intangible Cultural Heritage (UNESCO 2003) and China was among the first countries to ratify it in 2004. The convention defines intangible cultural heritage as: 'the practices, representations, expressions, knowledge, skills – as well as the instruments, objects, artefacts and cultural spaces associated therewith – that communities, groups and, in some cases, individuals recognize as part of their cultural heritage' (ibid.: Article 2.1). As the convention's title suggests, this intangible cultural heritage needs to be safeguarded. Safeguarding includes: 'measures aimed at ensuring the viability of the intangible cultural heritage, including the identification, documentation, research, preservation, protection, promotion, enhancement, transmission, particularly through formal and non-formal education, as well as the revitalization of the various aspects of such heritage' (ibid.: Article 2.3).

Note that the convention not only calls for identification, documentation, research and protection but also for the promotion, enhancement and transmission of cultural heritage. This falls perfectly in line with the approaches adopted by the PRC to protect *and* develop cultural heritage, or in the present case: Tibetan culture and medicine.

China has set up and is steadily expanding a catalogue of its intangible cultural heritage. In the case of Tibet, committees were established in the Tibet Autonomous Region (TAR) and Tibetan prefectures in other provinces to investigate and identify suitable items for the list. Sixty-one Tibetan 'reference works', including the Gesar epic, and thirty-one eminent people have since been listed (IOSC 2008: 11). Rinchen Drangjor, one of the famous precious pills, and the *tsothal* practice were included in 2006 (C-Med 2006). Tibetan medicine is always prominently mentioned when explaining the combined approach of the preservation and development of cultural heritage (CTIC 2007d; IOSC 2008: ii, 2009a: vi).

Civilisation, Culture

This positive view of 'cultural heritage' stands in stark contrast to the hostility against 'old traditions' that characterised the Mao era. What happened? How can the revival of 'ethnic culture' and 'ancient tradition' be explained? How is it that the display of ethnic customs and the wearing of local dress became not only acceptable again but also, for certain occasions, explicitly advocated by the PRC's leadership?[1] Ann Anagnost (1997) offers one explanation: in the course of the post-Mao reforms the notions of class and class struggle as organising figures of a national imaginary were superimposed on the notion of *wenming*, 'civilisation' or 'civility'. *Wenming* covers a range of meanings. It can denote Chinese civilisation (*zhongguo wenming*) as the nation's glorious past, but also a dreamed-of 'modernity' (*xiandaihua*). The notion of *wenming* 'encapsulates what has been called the "Janus-facedness" of the national imaginary, looking toward the past to face the future', she argues (ibid.: 164).

Whereas revolutionary discourse portrayed the past as something to be overcome at all cost in order to create a better future, the post-Mao reform period has been characterised by a multifaceted reflection on *wenming* and its relation to *wenhua*, 'culture'. It was questioned, for example, whether Chinese culture was responsible for the country's 'backward' status in the global community or whether *wenhua* was, on the contrary, the key to economic success and the new rise of China in the world; discussions took place about whether the revival of Confucianism might serve as the basis for an alternative modernity characterised by Chinese ethics, and whether Confucian values could simply help maintain factory discipline (Dirlik 1995; Ong 1996; Shue 2006; Tu 1996; DuBois 2010: 354–56).

The demise of class and the rise of culture and civilisation as guiding figures of political discourse had a direct impact on China's ethnic minorities. The PRC officially encompasses fifty-six nationalities (*minzu*), including the Han majority. This inclusion, Dru Gladney (2004: 35) notes, points to the fact that the notion of *minzu* is intimately connected with the construction of China as a harmonious, orderly, civilised, multi-*minzu* 'family'. Robert Shepherd remarks in this respect that the original world heritage site application for the Potala Palace in Lhasa argues for its inclusion because it 'embodies the outstanding skills of the Tibetan, Han, Mongol, Man, and other nationalities' (UNESCO 1993, cited in Shepherd 2006: 250).

Very often, the fifty-five minorities are presented, or actively present themselves, as 'living ancestors' that provide a glimpse into one's own past (Scott 2009: ix), as living fossils of ancient times (Oakes 1998: 188, 2000: 681) – much in the same way as the statue of the sage in the TV commercial discussed in Chapter 6 stands for 'a medicine coming from the ancestors'.

Theme Parks: Manufacturing Minzu

Together with rising household incomes and a burgeoning domestic tourism industry, cultural and 'ethnic' destinations have seen an unprecedented boom over the last two decades. This new interest in the past has led to the extensive construction of 'old towns' and theme parks throughout the country (Anagnost 1997: 161–76; Oakes 1998: 42–59; Gladney 2004: 32–48). National past times became a national pastime, to take the title and thesis of Anagnost's (1997) book.

The most famous and successful 'ethnic' destination is probably Lijiang, the capital of Naxi culture in Yunnan province. Lijiang is considered an enormous success in the tourism industry (Duang 2000). Annual visitor numbers reached an estimated six million by 2009, the large majority being domestic tourists (White 2010: 143). In a recent survey on the popularity of destinations among domestic tourists, Lijiang came second, right after the beaches of Hainan and before the Olympic city of Beijing (*China Daily* 2009).

Lijiang's old town, a prime example of Naxi architecture, suffered severe damage in an earthquake in 1996. A year later, ironically, the old town was listed as a UNESCO World Heritage Site and was

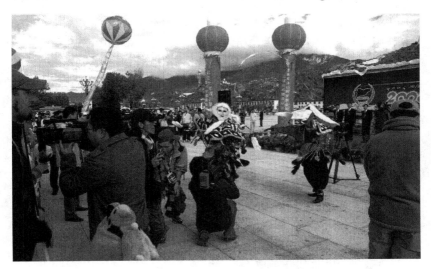

Figure 7.1: Masked dancers, media and tourists on Potala Square: the opening ceremony of the Namtso Hiking Convention, 2008. See also www.theotherimage.com/norway-for-namtso/.

completely reconstructed. The Naxi-style façades were retained but virtually every house was converted into a shop or restaurant to cater for tourists. Most Naxi families moved to the new part of Lijiang city. Outside Lijiang, a model Naxi village was set up where tourists can experience Naxi village life, including crafts, shamans at work, and folk dances on the hour.

With respect to ethnic tourism destinations such as Lijiang, Tim Oakes speaks of a veritable manufacturing of *minzu* culture (Oakes 1998: 140–48). He argues that this process follows two interlinked ideologies. On the one hand, the preservation of culture provides both the 'ideological glue to build a national community' and a means for minorities to participate in this larger project; on the other hand, the preservation of culture is pursued in the name of rural poverty alleviation. As a consequence, Oakes contends, '*minzu* traditions' are only preserved if they promise to accommodate commercial interests (ibid.: 149).

The combination of ethnic tourism and a revived fascination with *minzu* culture has also reached Tibet. Lijiang's success, for instance, inspired developments in Gyalthang (or Zhongdian in Chinese). The town and county of Gyalthang, located about 150 kilometres from Lijiang and marking the beginning of the Tibetan world, was officially renamed Shangri-la in 2001. Awarding the place the official name and title of James Hilton's hidden paradise[2] heralded the promotion of tourism in the region (Maconi 2007; Kolås 2008).[3] The airport nearby and the local Tibetan medicine factory inherited the precious brand name. A new road from Lijiang has been completed and now provides easy access for tour groups.

Other Tibetan examples of ethnic tourist destinations include the famous 'nine villages' – Dzitsa Degu or Jiuzhaigou – in Ngaba prefecture (Sichuan province) with an estimated three million mostly domestic visitors per year (DIIR 2007: 205), as well as an increasing number of smaller theme park-style sites throughout Tibet. In Lhasa, the construction of an 'intangible cultural heritage park' has recently started. With a planned reception capacity of 800,000 visitors per year and 1,000 staff, the park is envisioned as becoming 'the largest scale one-stop comprehensive cultural tourism destination in Lhasa' once it opens in 2014 (CTIC 2010).

The impact of these developments reveals a mixed picture. A Tibetan travel agent in Shangri-la will have a different view from, for example, a Tibetan nomad living in the vicinity of a tourist village on the shores of Qinghai lake, as the recent documentary *Kokonor* by the acclaimed Tibetan filmmaker Dorje Tsering Chenaktsang impressively demonstrates.[4] The film shows the grim side of theme park culture. Chinese tourists enjoy themselves riding yaks and taking pictures of beautifully dressed Tibetan nomad girls, who earn 1 yuan per photo. The owners of the site, however, have started charging increasingly high 'entrance fees' for those 'working' inside the fenced area – an area which above all was illegally established on the sacred communal land of the local nomads. When they raised their voice against these issues their settlement was raided and their leaders imprisoned.

The ramifications of mass tourism, however, lie beyond the topic of the present inquiry. It is sufficient to say that research on and the preservation and promotion of culture produce a variety of outcomes in different places. The point I seek to make is a different one. The booming interest in minorities, including their tourism potential, gave rise to a pronounced shift in how Tibet is conceived in China. The images of barbarian customs and feudal cruelty that previously dominated the discourse of Maoist liberation have given way to much more positive images of Tibet as a realm of unspoilt nature and as a 'lustrous pearl of Chinese culture'. It is this shift that enabled the emergence of a Tibetanness economy.

Exhibiting Sowa Rigpa and a Farewell to GMP

The question is, then, what the Tibetanness economy means for the practice of Sowa Rigpa. How is this space, created by the official endorsement of cultural preservation and development, used? How are conflicting notions of Tibetanness and authenticity dealt with? The following examples mark two ends of the spectrum.

The Mentsikhang in Lhasa has recently been granted funds for the reconstruction of its outpatient department and a new medicine factory. The latter is remarkable because the Mentsikhang actually has a factory – the well-known Mentsikhang factory, which was renamed the TAR Tibetan Medicine Factory in the course of its transition to a fully fledged industry. As mentioned in Chapter 2, neither the Mentsikhang hospital nor the TAR Tibetan Medicine Factory are very happy with the state of affairs. The hospital complains that the quality of medicines has decreased since GMP was introduced while for the TAR Tibetan Medicine Factory producing hospital medicines is a loss-making business.

I was proudly told at the Mentsikhang that, according to the TAR government's explicit wish, the new factory is to be built in a traditional Tibetan style. Furthermore, it would *not* be a GMP factory. As the factory's entire production is intended for the hospital and not for sale on the market, GMP is technically not a requirement. It remains to be seen how these plans will finally play out. By August 2009 a plot of land had been bought east of Lhasa but construction had not yet started.

In this case, 'Tibetan style' and 'traditional' seem to have gained the upper hand over GMP and the wish to create a 'pillar industry' for modern Tibet – at least at the present stage of planning. This was well received and acknowledged with a sense of satisfaction by the Mentsikhang staff I interviewed. The plans for a new non-GMP Mentsikhang factory can therefore be taken as an example of how the discourse of cultural heritage has created opportunities that were certainly not present before. Cultural heritage provides a legitimate framework for an initiative that is regarded as genuinely Tibetan.

The second example, marking the other end of the spectrum, is an exhibition at the Tibetan Medicine College in Lhasa. When I arrived in Lhasa in early September 2007 it had just been closed. Nevertheless, the exhibition had been such an annoyance that the topic kept coming up in conversations. Pieced together from several accounts this is approximately what happened: A Chinese entrepreneur had rented a space in the college for an exhibition on Tibetan medicine, tailored to Chinese as well as Western tour groups. The exhibition was actively advertised. Visitors to Lhasa were issued with appropriate leaflets on arrival at the airport, while travel agents received financial incentives for every person they brought to the premises. Tibetan medicine, in one form or another, features on standard tour programmes of most travel agencies, and the exhibition attracted a huge number of people.

'During summer the college looked like a tourist place', a former student at the Medical College told me. He used to work as a guide at the exhibition. One day he had a Portuguese tour group:

That day, the wife of the Chinese entrepreneur who ran the exhibition was also present. She insisted on doing most of the talking. But as she was not very knowledgeable about Sowa Rigpa, I sometimes added my thoughts when the things she said were not accurate. Of course, she did not like that at all. At the end of the tour the tourists were always supposed to buy herbs. There was a cabinet with a Tibetan doctor who, in fact, was Chinese and not an *amchi* at all. I tried to speak with him in Tibetan but he did not understand. There was an elderly man in my group. He was advised to buy some *yartsagunbu* to tackle his weight problem. But *yartsagunbu* is not good for overweight people! So I intervened again. The leader's wife got very angry and told me to mind my own business. A very unfortunate experience.

The story of the College exhibition caused widespread anger and a feeling that 'the Chinese' – not the government, simply 'the Chinese' (*rgya mi*) as a collectivity – were capitalising on Tibetan heritage. Students and teachers were utterly upset about the whole affair and launched a complaint to the relevant government office. It was argued that having a fake *amchi* was not helping the cause of Sowa Rigpa. Apparently, they were told not to speak about the issue. But when the entrepreneur's contract ran out it was not renewed and the exhibition closed.

Whereas in the case of the Mentsikhang's planned new factory the official emphasis on the preservation of cultural heritage offered a welcome opportunity to return to an older mode of production considered to be more authentic, the exhibition with its fake *amchi* was seen as an example of ruthless Chinese business culture which had nothing to do with real Tibetan medicine. After all, Tibetan medicine was not just about exhibiting Tibetan culture but helping people. Sowa Rigpa turned into an aesthetic theme park for tourists would certainly defeat its purpose.

Morality and Spectacles of Authenticity

Real and Fake

Those relying on Tibetan medicine for their health-care needs are naturally concerned with the question of authenticity. My conversations with Tibetans, medical professionals as well as patients, frequently centred around the notions of 'fake' and 'real', *dziima* (*rdzus ma*) and *ngoma* (*ngo ma*). Not only can an *amchi* in an exhibition be fake, but so too can precious raw materials, such as musk or sandalwood, be counterfeit (Harris 2009: 104–11), or the Tibetan pills and powders bought in the pharmacies of Lhasa or Xining. The latter, indeed, is a problem I experienced myself.

A friend of mine asked me to bring him from Lhasa a certain Tibetan medicine he had not been able to find in Xining. It was produced by a company called Retong, based in Chamdo and led by a famous Tibetan physician. The Retong brand was highly valued by several people I knew, and they expressed great confidence in the efficacy of their medicines. However, none of the bigger pharmacies had them in stock. Finally, I was advised to look for the factory's own store on the Barkor. I did so and indeed found a small pharmacy where I bought the medicines. On my way back home, however, I stumbled across a tiny dispensary, hidden beneath the Dicos fast-food restaurant. Its sign read Retong Tibetan Medicine Factory. A middle-aged Khampa woman welcomed me. Seeing the pouches I still held in my hand she immediately exclaimed: 'These are fake! Where did you buy them?' She showed me the original products to prove her case. The pouches were identical, but the size of the pills was clearly not. She explained that they had had many problems with fake drugs recently and that I should be very careful where I bought them. Later, I compared the real and the fake pills. They were indeed vastly different, not only in size but also in colour and taste.

Many companies have experienced problems with counterfeit products. One director told me that his company had even tracked counterfeits back to its own sales agent in inland China. The smaller companies often rely on sales contractors for distribution in inland China. In this case, one of the contractors apparently managed to order the factory's original packaging materials, which he filled with cheaper pills from another manufacturer in order to raise his profit margin. One Chinese-run company in Xining was well-known for being part of such schemes. It even came under investigation at one point but allegedly managed to bribe its way out. The company is still in business.

Both the fake *amchi* in the college exhibition and the fake medicines bought in a pharmacy in Lhasa point to the fact that authenticity is a practical as well as a moral question, especially in the domain of medicine. However, the issue of authenticity goes beyond counterfeit drugs and fake *amchi*. Relations between Tibetanness, morality and authenticity are more complex than these examples would suggest.

Profit and the Ethics of Being a Doctor

The Gyüshi's Second Treatise ends with a chapter in which ethical guidelines for Tibetan medical practice are laid out. It is stated that the prerequisites for being a doctor include intelligence, altruism, honour, knowledge in practice, diligence and being well-versed in social mores. Those who lack these qualities are 'like a fox in charge of [a lion's] kingdom'; they are 'neither honored nor respected by anyone' (Clark 1995: 223, 229). With regard to the exhibition's fake *amchi* we learn that one who 'out of desire [for material gain merely] assumes the guise (of a physician) is a destroyer of life' (ibid.: 229).

These principles correspond to the ethical code of many medical traditions, including Ayurveda, TCM and biomedicine. However, they also have to be understood in a Tibetan Buddhist way. The notion of *sampa karwa* (*bsam pa dkar ba*), which, following Clark, was simply translated as altruism above, literally means a 'white mind' or a 'pure, virtuous motivation'. In the Buddhist context it is often translated as a compassionate attitude. The Gyüshi defines *sampa karwa* as having faith in the 'three jewels' – Buddha, *dharma* (the teachings) and *sangha* (the community) – by means of aspiring to even-mindedness rather than clinging to moral notions of good and bad. 'By having such an attitude', the Gyüshi promises, 'the patients will become easier to treat, many will recover and become one's friends' (ibid.: 224).

Whether for an individual doctor or a industrial manufacturer of Tibetan pharmaceuticals, the ideal of Sowa Rigpa is inseparable from the principles of the Buddhist path because successful healing is linked to aspiring enlightenment – not simply for one's own benefit but for the sake of all sentient beings. Just as authenticity is tied to morality, morality is tied to efficacy.

Traditionally, Tibetan doctors would not ask for payment when they treated patients but would accept whatever donations their patients chose to give them. The idea that altruism and compassion are the basis of accomplished Sowa Rigpa practice, and that commerce and profit are fundamentally contradictory to this end is deeply rooted in Tibetan thinking. People who would choose the most expensive biomedical treatment they can afford may still opt for a traditional *amchi* who offers his services for free – not to save money but because his attitude is taken as testimony of his expertise.

The Buddhist principles of altruism and compassion are reflected in company slogans. Arura, for example, 'cares about the health of all beings'. Virtue, humanity, concentration and altruism are listed as the cornerstones of its company philosophy. Jigme Phuntsog's company slogan is: *sman lha'i pho brang lus sems bde ster*, 'palace of the Medicine Buddha, bestowing well-being on body and mind'. Considering how Jigme Phuntsog treated the elderly nomad woman amidst the hustle of managing his company, this is clearly more than a mere advertising strategy.

Nevertheless, aligning business needs with these Buddhist notions remains problematic – even for the most traditional *amchi*. In her work on Sowa Rigpa practice in rural Namring county (TAR), Theresia Hofer shows how important it still is not to demand payment in return for treatment, even if the prices for pills and medical raw materials are increasing. For an *amchi* aspiring to the ideal of the accomplished doctor it can be difficult to eke out a living. While there are diverging opinions about whether doctors in the 'old society' also treated those who were unable to give something in return, Hofer maintains that many *amchi* find that living up to the image of a compassionate and altruistic healer-physician has become much harder in recent years (Hofer 2009a: 196–97, 2009b: 495–504).

The tension between Buddhist morality and the need to make a living from practising Sowa Rigpa is not confined to Tibet alone. Florian Besch's work on *amchi* practice in Spiti (Besch 2006: 102–10, 222–64) and Laurent Pordié's analysis of the role of religion in Tibetan medicine, based on his research in Ladakh (Pordié 2003), suggest a similar picture. Both authors discuss the dilemmas *amchi* face in the light of the present-day cash economy and long-standing expectations about the Buddhist ethics a good *amchi* should follow.

Stephan Kloos shows that notions of capitalism and business underwent a remarkable transformation in exile. He argues that in the early years of exile, making money was regarded as a necessary means to enable the preservation of Tibetan culture. Now, however, business and capitalism are seen as the biggest threats to cultural survival. The Men-Tsee-Khang in Dharamsala operates amidst these tensions (Kloos 2010: 152–92). Kloos cites Tsering Agloe Chukora, editor of *Tibetoday*, who suggested that greed and the commercialisation of Sowa Rigpa have the potential to do more harm than the 'ideological holocaust of Mao's China' in terms of preserving 'the authenticity and the professional expertise' of Sowa Rigpa (Chukora 2007: 14, cited in Kloos 2010: 157). Not only is business incompatible with Buddhist morality from this perspective, it also endangers Tibetan authenticity and professional expertise. Authenticity, morality and therapeutic quality are portrayed as intrinsically linked and directly opposed to business interests.

Again, the issue I am concerned with here is not whether Sowa Rigpa ethics are different from the moralities and ethical codes of other medical traditions in Asia, or whether Tibetans act and feel in a particular moral way that sets them apart from Han Chinese, for example. The point is simply that among Tibetans commercial interests and the industrial production of Tibetan pharmaceuticals are widely perceived as being contradictory to the ultimate end of Sowa Rigpa as well as the authenticity and therapeutic quality of its medicines. For the companies, this creates a problem of trust.

The Problem of Trust

The dilemma the Tibetan medicine industry is facing is the following: on the one hand, the 'socialist market economy', declining state subsidies for the health sector, and the construction of GMP-compliant factories demanded an orientation towards the logic of the market, capital and profit; on the other hand, the reputation of a company rests to a considerable extent on its perceived Tibetanness.

The companies I was in contact with still generated between 30 and 70 per cent of their revenues in Tibet. Building and maintaining consumer trust is crucial for economic success. This poses a tricky problem, especially since the metonymic relation between company and product has become more fragile in the age of packaged medicines, and the risk of counterfeited pills has increased.

A tour through the factory outlets and pharmacies in Lhasa makes clear which companies have a good reputation among Tibetans. The factory outlet of Shongpalhachu in Ramoche Road, for example, was always crowded whenever I dropped in. Shongpalhachu's products are held in high regard, and many Tibetans choose to rely on them. Shongpalhachu is considered to be a 'real' Tibetan company, with Tibetan management and Tibetan workers. The atmosphere in the Shongpalhachu shop was distinctly Tibetan – the staff were Tibetan and all the customers I encountered in the course of several visits were Tibetan, mostly elderly people who would come and sit on the bench inside the store for a while, chatting with other customers and waiting until they were served. Shongpalhachu's perceived Tibetanness serves as a token for the quality of its remedies.

On the other hand, the outlet of the Tibetan Medicine College Factory on the Barkor was usually empty when I passed by. The quality of the company's products was said to have been in decline since it had come under Chinese management. In the late 1990s, the College Factory had an excellent reputation. A friend of mine whose mother used to work there mentioned that in those days the factory's medicines were so highly valued and sought-after that there was a permanent shortage. At that time, the factory was regarded as very traditional. The herbs it used were said to be carefully collected by students under the supervision of experienced teachers during summer expeditions. After a new GMP manufacturing plant was constructed, the factory was leased out to a Chinese entrepreneur and its status dwindled rapidly.

Based on my own observations, there is little evidence of any direct connection between approaches to production and a factory's perceived Tibetanness. Practices considered to be at odds with traditional methods are routine in factories reputed to be very 'Tibetan', while big, profit-oriented companies are sometimes assiduous about following traditional ways. Moreover, Tibetanness does not protect a company from the problem of counterfeit drugs. On the contrary, the companies with the best reputation, such as Retong (mentioned above), are an obvious target for ruthless counterfeiters. In a certain sense, the most reputed companies tend to become victims of their own success.

This being said, a company's reputation still rests to a large degree on its perceived Tibetanness. If a company is Chinese-owned or run, that may not be to its advantage. This point was particularly emphasised by a manager of the TAR Tibetan Medicine Factory in Lhasa. Citing several cases of companies in decline since they had been taken over by Chinese management, he expressed his fear that the TAR Tibetan Medicine Factory, at the moment still under the roof of the Mentsikhang, may one day face the same fate. 'That would lead to the factory making a loss. [...] That's why we are worried', he argued in strictly economic terms. In short, the moral economy of Tibetanness is directly linked to economic success, at least in the Tibetan market.

Balancing Profit and Altruism

The need to be economically successful while meeting Tibetan expectations of morality requires profit to be counterbalanced by altruism in one form or another. To some extent, the link to a clinic or hospital can provide such a counterbalance. The Arura Group in Xining, for example, has managed to channel part of the revenue generated from selling shares during privatisation into the construction of a new, government-operated hospital (see Figure 2.2). The TAR Tibetan Medicine Factory in Lhasa, which continues to have an excellent reputation, is still seen as part of the Mentsikhang, and in the backyard of Jigme Phuntsog's GMP factory a brand new hospital opened in 2009.

Operating a clinic is one of many forms of engagement in the moral economy of Tibetanness. Other forms include hiring predominantly Tibetan workers, starting the work day with a short collective session of reading the Gyüshi, organising free health camps in remote areas, offering training classes for aspiring Tibetan doctors, or supporting local schools and festivals – in short, adopting the traditional role of a *jindak* (*sbyin bdag*), a patron or sponsor, in Tibetan society.

An interesting example once again is Cheezheng. In the interview with the *China Daily* mentioned in the Chapter 6, Cheezheng's director Lei Jufang confessed that she sometimes had qualms about whether her company's pursuit of profit was reconcilable with her Buddhist beliefs. 'I was told that as long as your motivation is good and you put your money to good use, it is fine', she concluded (*China Daily* 2008). The right motivation and the will to put one's money to good use are the perfect preconditions for a *jindak*. And indeed, Madame Lei's company is involved in many grassroots projects in Tibetan areas, including a private school providing Sowa Rigpa training. This school is located in Menling in the southeastern borderlands of the TAR. Menling is an important place in the sacred geography of Tibetan medicine inasmuch as it is associated with Yuthog Yonten Gonpo the Elder. The school is close to Yuthog the Elder's meditation cave and the place where he established the very first school of Tibetan medicine in the eighth century.

The simple, modest school Cheezheng has built reveals no marks of the company's involvement. No company logos can be seen, and the world of large-scale GMP production seems far away. The school's agenda is a traditional Sowa Rigpa education for local students. It bears more resemblance to Aku Jinpa's school than to the government-run Tibetan medicine colleges in Lhasa and Xining. In addition, Cheezheng has helped establish more than a hundred small, private clinics in rural areas. Some of the school's graduates have found employment in these. Others are offered jobs in Cheezheng's luxurious spa centres in Beijing and Lanzhou.

Cheezheng's involvement in such grassroots projects is certainly not meant to impress high officials from Beijing in the way Arura's museum does. In fact, Madame Lei's engagement in the moral economy of Tibetanness is at times in conflict with official agendas. The company has established an extensive plant conservation area around Yuthog's cave. Menling (*sman gling*), literally 'the medicine sanctuary', is a biodiversity hotspot and famous for its medicinal plants. The county's location at the southeastern edge of the Tibetan Plateau where the big rivers have carved deep canyons into the Himalayas on their way southwards to the ocean is marked by enormous differences in altitude and an abundance of different habitats. Cheezheng has not technically bought the land but has paid a large sum of money to the local government in order to set up the conservation area. However, Menling's tourism bureau (a branch of the TAR's tourism bureau) had its own ambitions for the place. Menling sees few foreign visitors (a military permit is needed to enter the county) but it attracts large numbers of Chinese tour groups. At the very site of Yuthog's first Sowa Rigpa school, an ethnic tourist village has been set up. The last remaining stones of the ancient school building have been used to construct a new 'traditional' Tibetan Monpa house.[5] Cheezheng's management was very unhappy with this turn of events. It was seen as the destruction, rather than the promotion, of cultural heritage. At the time of writing, no solution had been found for the problem.

Although I had all the necessary permits to visit the place, the local authorities were sceptical about my presence in the region. When we reported to the police in Menling's county town, a young officer was sent with us. Finally I was allowed to visit Cheezheng's school, but not Yuthog's cave or the tourist village. This, I was told, was reserved for domestic tourists.

Despite Cheezheng's highly profitable Tibetan medicine business, and despite the fact that Madame Lei is Chinese, she has gained a great deal of respect among Tibetans. People who know her only speak well of her. And the two young Tibetan women assistants I met referred to her as *mola* (*mo lags*), 'grandmother', in her absence, an honorific reserved for very few Chinese in Tibet.

Morality at Large

Morality, however, is not only derived from Buddhist ethics, it is also an instrument in the political conflict over Tibet. Sowa Rigpa, which has been described as a relatively apolitical and secure space for Tibetan initiatives, has become increasingly entrenched in the larger 'ethico-politics' (Rose 1999: 173, 188–96) surrounding the 'Tibet question'.

A few months after the unrest of March 2008 I met with the CEO of a certain company. At the end of our conversation he slipped a short poem into my pocket, requesting me to make it public outside China. The poem reads:

བོད་མིའི་སྙིང་གི་དད་པ་དེ།	Tibetan people's heart and faith
དཔལ་འབྱོར་སྟོབས་ཀྱིས་ཉོ་མི་ཐུབ	cannot be bought with the power of wealth
ཆབ་སྲིད་དབང་གིས་བསྒྱུར་མི་ཐུབ	cannot be changed by the force of government
རྫས་འཕྲུལ་མཚོན་ཆས་གཏོར་མི་ཐུབ	cannot be destroyed by nuclear weapons.

On one level, these lines, filled with rebellious defiance, instantiate the image of authentic Tibet as a moral antithesis to the party-state and its emphasis on developing trade and business. On another level – by slipping the poem into my pocket – the director of a successful company, a clever businessman himself, made a clear statement about what he really thought of the current situation. The instruction to distribute it outside China implied that the world should watch the resistance of Tibetans and their attempts at preventing the loss of their 'heart and faith'. Here, the morality brought into play no longer stems from Buddhist notions of altruism and compassion but from the assumption that people outside China will support the Tibetans' moral struggle to protect their 'heart and faith'.

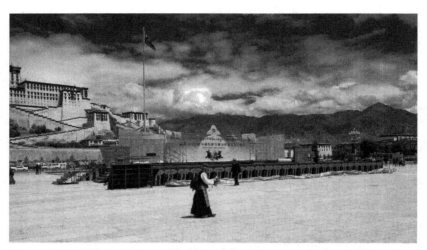

Figure 7.2: Building the stage for the opening ceremony of Lhasa's Shoton festival, August 2009.

The poem relates to Western and exile imaginaries of Tibet as a non-violent and peace-loving nation, threatened by the Chinese state. These imaginaries, which have been subjected to extensive debate in Tibetan studies (Calkowski 1997; Strøm 1997; Anand 2000; Barnett 2001b; Dodin and Räther 2001; Huber 2001; Dreyfus 2005), arguably define a similarly restrictive space for what Tibet can possibly be, as is the case with corresponding Chinese imaginaries (Barnett 2001b: 277, 2006b: 105; Heberer 2001; Kolås 2004, 2008). However, whether Western-cum-exile notions of Tibetan culture are more distorted than Chinese notions, or whether the figure of the Tibetan entrepreneur in Shangri-la is more adequate than Tibetans as 'prisoners of Shangri-la' (Lopez 1998) is not important here. What matters is that morality cannot be separated from the sphere of the global, political spectacle that surrounds the 'Tibet question'.

In her work on the Tibet support movement, Meg McLagan (2002) argues that the domains of politics and culture have become blurred, especially since public relations strategies have migrated from the entertainment industries to the organisation of political movements. 'The result has been a widening of the spaces in which politics can be conceived and performed', she concludes (ibid.: 91). The close links between morality, culture and political spectacle is true for the situation in Tibet as well as in exile, as Stephan Kloos's work on the Men-Tsee-Khang in Dharamsala shows (Kloos 2010). 'Subduing capitalism' and the 'business of altruism' (ibid.: 152–74) are similarly enmeshed in both Buddhist ethics and the political spectacle of cultural survival, for example when the Men-Tsee-Khang organises a medical camp in Kenya. Kloos cites one of his informants: 'It's about trying to use the positive impact of Tibetan medicine to earn the goodwill of the people in Africa. You know, if you look at the political aspect, the whole African continent has more than 40 countries, and we don't get a UN vote from a single one of them!' (ibid.: 132). As mentioned above, albeit in a slightly different context, the Gyüshi says: 'many will recover and become one's friends' (Clark 1995: 224).[6]

Building a Harmonious Society, Resisting Culture

Despite the obvious parallels between exile and Tibet, the situation is still more troublesome in the PRC. By and large, over the last decades the 'game' seemed to have followed a simple pattern: the world's sympathy with the Tibetans versus the political realities of a strong China; the 'soft power' of the Dalai Lama's moral authority versus the 'hard power' of economic interests and the PRC's security apparatus (see Barnett 2001b). Lately, however, matters have become more complex. In order to understand the nexus of the moral economy at large, a short detour away from Sowa Rigpa is necessary.

In 2005, Hu Jintao announced the need of 'building a socialist harmonious society' (Xinhua 2005). Whereas Deng Xiaoping's slogan – 'Let some get rich first, the others will follow' – emphasised private initiative and economic success as patriotic duties (a line that was more or less continued under Jiang Zemin), the fourth generation of the Chinese leadership proposes that the quest for harmony is patriotic: 'all people should co-exist harmoniously, love and help each other, encourage each other and make an effort to contribute to the building of a harmonious society' (*People's Daily* 2007). For the leadership under Hu Jintao, the 'harmonious society' is what the 'socialist market economy' was for Deng Xiaoping and what the 'three represents' was for Jiang Zemin – the key concept and label under which they imagined their political legacy.

Hu defined the 'harmonious society' as a comprehensive approach to development, 'which gives full play to modern ideas like democracy, rule of the law, fairness, justice, vitality, stability, orderliness and harmonious coexistence between ... humankind and nature' (ibid.). The notion of a 'harmonious society' (*hexie shehui*) has since become a guiding principle of policy-making in China. Party cadres were instructed to put it at the top of their agendas (See 2008).

The concept is closely linked to the notion of a 'scientific outlook on development' (*kexue fazhan guan*), which is defined as a coordinated and healthy approach to the development of 'material, political and spiritual civilizations' (*China Daily* 2007b). In his keynote address at the seventeenth Chinese Communist Party Congress in 2007, Hu Jintao explained that a 'scientific outlook on development' and social harmony were integral to each other and neither was possible without the other (Hu 2007).

The image of the 'harmonious society' was chosen in order to emphasise the need to balance economic growth with social responsibility.[7] Within three decades China has transformed itself from one of the most equitable countries to one of the most inequitable and its environment has suffered considerably (Ramo 2007: 30). The concept of the 'harmonious society' is a response to this growing inequality and the increasing display of dissent in relation to the social and environmental side effects of China's rapid economic development. In October 2006, guidelines entitled 'Resolution on Major Issues Regarding the Building of a Harmonious Socialist Society' were published. These guidelines outlined targets and tasks. The endeavour was clearly defined as a long-term project and the 'harmonious society' was described as a vision for the year of 2020 (Xinhua 2006a).

This being said, the 'harmonious society' is not only seen as a remedy for growing internal tensions but also as an instrument of current international diplomacy (Hu 2005; Wang 2008). In an insightful report titled *Brand China*, Joshua Cooper Ramo (2007) shows that the PRC's image of itself and other nations' views of it are increasingly diverging. While the Chinese have seen their country rapidly changing and their views account for the resulting ambivalences, in the eyes of the world China is often thought of as simultaneously humiliated and arrogant, while seeking to regain its status as a world power at any cost. Ramo argues that 'China's greatest strategic threat today is its national image' and that 'for a nation obsessed about territorial sovereignty, China has let its "image sovereignty" slip out of its control' (ibid.: 12–13).

The Chinese leadership is aware of this: Wu Jianmin, president of the China Foreign Affairs Institute, for instance, explained that foreigners were often biased against China. He argued that the concept of a 'harmonious society' would strengthen China's reputation in the international arena, 'thereby shrinking the market of China Threat' (Xinhua 2006b). Evidently, the 'harmonious society' is not only a vision for a better China in 2020; it is also seen as an asset for the PRC's contemporary efforts to reposition itself in the international community. However, as Ramo notes, 'until China becomes a more trusted nation, making her a more understood nation is a difficult task' (Ramo 2007: 17). In this context, authenticity and morality emerge as crucial questions once again, albeit on a different level.

The 2008 Beijing Olympics were regarded as a prime opportunity to mark the dawning of a new era in the PRC's international relations by showing the world the 'real' face of China. One episode during the Games' opening ceremony highlighted the problem particularly well: a choir of fifty-six children, one from each minority (*minzu*), performed a song together, a display of unity and harmony. Later, the Western media found out that actually all the children were Han Chinese. The discovery was taken as evidence that China's charm offensive was a fake, nothing but propaganda. The reaction of the official responsible in a television interview was simple and reasonable: 'It was a show', he said – a show for which the best performers were selected. The children were cast as actors; they were playing a role. They were not meant to be representatives of the fifty-six nationalities, but a representation of the ideal of multiethnic China as a harmonious 'family'.

By failing to see the show as a performance, the Western media took the episode as proof that it was all propaganda and lies and that there was no harmony in China. Tibet is often the focal point of this argument. Despite the scope of Chinese efforts to protect and promote Tibetan culture; despite the impressive numbers of Tibetan books published, monasteries rebuilt, Tibetan medicine clinics set up; despite extensive coverage by the Chinese media, the production of government White Papers,[8] films and brochures – despite all this, the whole endeavour has not attracted nearly as much international

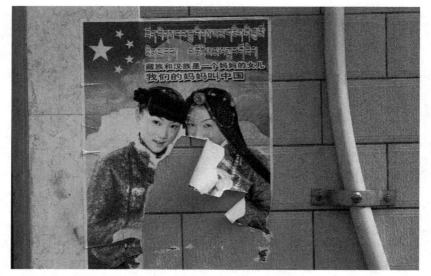

Figure 7.3: 'Tibetans and Chinese are the daughters of one mother. The name of our mother is China'. Propaganda poster in Lhasa, June 2008.

attention as the Dalai Lama's statements that 'cultural genocide' is going on in Tibet (Coonan 2008; Eimer and Chamberlain 2008), that China has turned Tibet into a 'hell on earth', and that 'the religion, culture, language and identity [of Tibetans], which successive generations of Tibetans have considered more precious than their lives, are nearing extinction' (Wong 2009).

In short, the 'cultural subsistence crisis' has taken centre stage on a global scale. The party-state's approach to the protection of Tibetan cultural heritage is not just embedded in the imaginary of a harmonious 'family' of multi-*minzu* China; it is tied to the problem of China's reputation in the world.

However, China is not just a victim of global misrepresentation. When it comes to Tibet, the official party line often undergoes subtle but remarkable transformations. Hu Jintao, for example, argued in October 2007: 'To maintain a harmonious and stable society is a prerequisite for the development of Tibet and the well-being of all ethnic groups living there' (Xinhua 2007). Note the inversion of the argument: what was meant to be a remedy to the side effects of rapid economic development, a vision for a better China in 2020, is now in the context of Tibet proclaimed a prerequisite for economic development. Here, the slogan 'building a harmonious society' holds a moral predicament rather than the promise of a better future. As a result, the 'harmonious society' acquires the taste of a cruel irony – not just for Western and exile observers, but also for the Tibetans living in Tibet.

One Tibetan reaction to this is to 'resist culture'. It started in 2006 with an episode sparked by the Dalai Lama's appeal to people to stop wearing festive fur-trimmed clothes, for which traditionally tiger, leopard, lynx, otter or fox pelts are used. When people throughout Tibet gathered to burn their festive robes, the authorities regarded it as an act of defiance – despite the fact that the Dalai Lama's appeal was very much in conformity with the PRC's wildlife protection laws. In 2007 people in Yushu were even ordered to wear their fur-trimmed robes for the annual horse-racing festival, which has become a tourist attraction. Not dressing in a traditional Tibetan manner meant being fined up to 3,000 yuan (Environment News Service 2006; Macartney 2007).

The figure of 'resisting culture' became even more pronounced in 2009 during the *losar* festival. Many Tibetans refused to celebrate *losar* (*lo sar*), the Tibetan New Year, as a silent protest against the current situation. This performance of Tibetanness by not celebrating the most important Tibetan festival of the year came to be seen as a threatening act of civil disobedience by the authorities. Woeser, a Tibetan writer known for her courage and outspokenness, wrote on 24 February 2009: '"Not to celebrate Losar" has been regarded as a serious "separatist" activity, so much so that some Tibetans have been accused of spreading "not to celebrate Losar" rumours and been arrested' (Woeser 2009). Official China blamed the matter on Dharamsala and the Tibetan Youth Congress, which had labelled 2009 a black year and called upon Tibetans around the world to follow their compatriots inside Tibet in not celebrating *losar* (TYC 2009).

Here, the story comes back to the Mentsikhang's involvement in all this. The Xinhua news agency cited a senior astrologer of the Lhasa Mentsikhang (after all, Mentsikhang literally means 'house of medicine and astrology') to prove the Tibetan Youth Congress wrong. Gongkar Rigzin, a 1957 graduate of the Mentsikhang who had been responsible for its calendar calculations for over thirty years, was quoted as saying that the coming year was by no means black but red, which was a sign that it would be 'festive and auspicious, but dry' (Xinhua 2009). In other words, the Tibetans in Tibet refused to play Tibetan, and China's governmental news agency cited a Tibetan expert to tell them that they were wrong and that one should not '"play politics" with Tibetan culture' (ibid.) – a remarkable development, given the Chinese Communist Party's history in fighting 'backward superstition'. Now, Tibetan astrology is used to create a moral truth about authentic Tibetanness. To make the argument waterproof, it was claimed that Gongkar Rigzin's calendar sold more than 100,000 copies per year, many of them exported to Nepal and India.

A few months earlier, delivering a lecture at the Indian Institute of Management in Ahmedabad, the Dalai Lama reiterated his claim to be a Marxist monk, 'because unlike capitalism, Marxism is more ethical' (Express News Service 2008). As one of his examples, not of Marxist ethics but of ruthless capitalist exploitation, he cited: the People's Republic of China. Just as the party-state has started criticising and even fining Tibetans for not being authentically Tibetan, the Dalai Lama blames the Chinese leadership for not being authentically communist.

The Moral Economy at Large

We have seen that Tibetanness, economy and morality are linked on multiple levels. First, among Tibetans, an orientation towards making a profit is depicted as incompatible with the path of an accomplished healer physician. On the one hand, this is what the Gyüshi says. On the other hand, the emphasis on the negative aspects of an overly economic orientation is also a response to what is perceived of as a world of lies and forgery, of propaganda and counterfeit Tibetan pills. In this sense, Buddhist morality is linked to the quality and efficacy of a treatment.

Second, this means that, in the context of industrial production, compassion and altruism are tied to economic questions by way of consumer trust. In order to mitigate the resulting dilemma and to counterbalance profit with altruism, Tibetan medicine companies often assume the role of a *jindak*. This does not mean, however, that the companies' motivations are purely economic. The point is that, while making economic sense, assuming the role of a *jindak* allows the companies and the people working for them to locate the industry within the moral realm of Tibetan Buddhism.

Third, morality and Tibetanness are linked in the figure of a harmonious 'family' of multi-*minzu* China, to which Tibetans are morally obliged to contribute, according to the party-state. The concept of a 'harmonious society' and the officially endorsed outlook on developing 'material, political and spiritual civilizations' provide a framework also for religious endeavours. After all, Chinese culture and Buddhist doctrine both value the concept of harmony, as the abbot of the renowned Shaolin temple Shi Yonxin explained: 'That's why Buddhism is popular in China … As a responsible country, China has had its own deep thoughts and a measure of foresight in the promotion of world harmony', he added wilily (Wang 2007).[9] However, the promotion of world harmony, which Hu Jintao himself claimed to be China's programme (Hu 2005), remains trapped by the political spectacle that is Tibet. In the global arena, Tibet often serves as the 'case' that challenges China's sincerity and moral authority. The 'natural' morality of Tibetanness as portrayed by Tibet support groups around the globe is equivalent to the image of China's immorality. The results are paradoxical: unlike reconstructed sections of the Great Wall, for example, which Western visitors may consider artificial or, at worst, a disappointing tourist trap, the preservation and development of Tibetan culture is a moral and political issue. The PRC's efforts to preserve Tibetan cultural heritage are no longer just a matter of creating an imagined multi-*minzu* China; they are also a matter of regaining 'image sovereignty'. This goes along with the party-state's attempt to define, in a moral way, what authentic Tibetanness is.

Fourth, the mode of 'resisting culture' – which Woeser calls 'non-violent non-cooperation with "Tibetan characteristics"' – consequently emerges as a new form of authentic Tibetanness amidst this global political spectacle. Remarkably, when Woeser writes about this mode of resistance, she explicitly refers to the 'weapons of the weak', the title of James Scott's famous analysis of subtle forms of resistance against state intervention and rapid technological change (Scott 1985). Anthropological analysis inspires political activism and Scott's writings come full circle. While Tibetanness is formulated as a question of contested authenticity, authenticity is formulated as a question of contested Tibetanness. In this context, Sowa Rigpa is increasingly dealt with as a problem of cultural heritage rather than medicine – or, in Rinchen Wangdu's words mentioned at the outset, as 'some kind of cultural thing', not to be taken seriously as medical knowledge.[10]

Amidst all of this, how are we to understand companies' engagements in the moral economy of Tibetanness?

My suggestion is that they are best looked at as tactical responses, as attempts to strike a fine balance between political statements, economic decisions and the different understandings of morality and authenticity. In this perspective, the moves of Arura, Cheezheng and Aku Jinpa, as different as they are, have something in common: they express a vision of Sowa Rigpa's purpose in the greater scheme of Tibet's future. Arura's museum displays Sowa Rigpa as national cultural heritage in order to help Tibet and the Tibetans gain the respect and appreciation they deserve; Cheezheng's spiritual spa is offered as a remedy against a disenchanted modern China; and both Madame Lei's and Aku Jinpa's schools are meant to foster Tibetan medicine for the benefit of local communities and as a realm of Buddhist morality.

Notes

1. In the case of Tibet this meant, for example, that the Tibetan leaders were instructed to resume wearing traditional Tibetan dress when Hu Yaobang announced a six-point programme of reform and liberalisation in 1980 (Barnett 2006a: 36). Similarly, the photographs exhibited in Arura's showroom depict Dr Ao Tsochen wearing Tibetan dress when receiving high-status guests from Beijing.
2. The term Shangri-la was coined by James Hilton in his famous novel *Lost Horizon* (Hilton 1933) to denote a hidden paradise somewhere in Tibet. Shangri-la has ever since fuelled mystical images of Tibet and has served as a name for countless hotels and businesses throughout the Himalayas.
3. Shangri-la has also served as a name for countless hotels and businesses throughout the Himalayas.
4. Kokonor (China 2005), by Jangbu (Dorje Tsering Chenaktsang), 51 minutes.
5. The Monpa (*mon pa*) are a local Tibetanised Tibeto-Burman group. China lists the Monpa as one of the fifty-six officially recognised *minzu*.
6. Tibetan medicine has a long history of gaining support from powerful elites by providing excellent medical care. See Saxer (2010) for a Russian example.
7. Dennis Driscoll, of Beijing University's Law School, estimated in 2007 that throughout China there was almost one workshop a day on the topic of corporate social responsibility (See 2008: 2). The numerous donation cer-

tificates in all major Tibetan medicine companies also have to be seen in this context.

8. See IOSC (2008, 2009a: vi, 2009b).

9. While such statements are possible in contemporary China, state re-education campaigns in Tibetan monasteries continue and the state has decreed guidelines to 'manage' the reincarnation of 'living Buddhas' (SARA 2007; see DuBois 2010: 352) – moral best practices of sorts for those intending to be reborn as a lama.

10. Meanwhile, TCM is being transformed into Chinese medicine and pharmacotherapy (CMP) and its nationalistic celebration as traditional Chinese science increasingly takes a back seat (Hsu 2009b: 113, 120).

Chapter 8
Conclusions

The wave of change that has accompanied Tibetan medicine's rapid industrialisation has not abated. While the outcome is still unfolding, chances are high that the creation of an industry will be looked at as a crucial turning point in the history of Sowa Rigpa in Tibet. I hope to have shown that the industry continues to reformulate much of the context in which Sowa Rigpa is pursued and conceived of today, ranging from manufacturing practices and the herb trade to the production of knowledge and Sowa Rigpa's new entanglements with the politics of cultural heritage.

However, the ways in which Tibetan medicine was affected (or left untouched) by the policies and regulations that triggered the process of industrialisation, and the ways the industry itself is shaping the context in which it is operating, turned out to be rather different from what I had presumed. Most of my tacit assumptions and initial working hypothesis were wrong, or at least overly simplistic. To start this concluding chapter I will revisit three of those assumptions that turned out to be fallacies.

Fallacies

One: Industry and Modernism

The creation of an industry, I assumed, was a matter of development agendas, market forces and capitalist interests. I saw Sowa Rigpa as the target of a radical modernisation project. I suspected that the industrialisation of Tibetan medicine was a high-modernist scheme as described by Scott (1998) – well-intentioned but prone to failure. Given the importance attributed to Tibetan medicine production as one of the region's 'pillar industries', I did not expect to hear complaints that the authorities regarded it as 'some kind of cultural thing' and therefore did not take it seriously; neither did I expect that the party-state would resort to the expertise of a Mentsikhang astrologer to define authentic Tibetanness. In short, I imagined the creation of an industry to be a thoroughly modern endeavour producing friction at its edges. What I encountered, however, was a pervasive moral economy of cultural identity.

In the same vein, I supposed 'good manufacturing practice' (GMP) and its accompanying regulations to be endorsing an evidence-based approach to quality control in which the production of Tibetan pharmaceuticals would be subjected to the scrutiny of hard science. Although I anticipated that GMP would encounter all forms of subtle resistance and reinterpretations, and therefore not arrive in Tibet unaltered, I was surprised to learn that the SFDA implemented GMP in a way that often contradicted the spirit and letter of the regulations themselves. The industry, I thought, was meant to spearhead the principles of science and evidence-based medicine in Sowa Rigpa. What I found, however, was at least as much an aesthetic as a scientific enterprise.

Two: Globalisation and Sinicisation

Furthermore, it seemed obvious that the industrialisation and commodification of Tibetan pharmaceuticals were meant to facilitate access to global markets and capital. However, the free flow of Tibetan medical goods in and out of China turned out to be an illusion. In terms of exports, the drug regulations in the West remain prohibitive and an international harmonisation of (national) GMPs does not seem to be a prospect for the near future. Some products like Cheezheng's pain-relief plaster may be exported in large quantities, but the primary market for Tibetan pharmaceuticals today is the People's Republic of China (PRC).

On the other hand, a considerable amount of the raw materials used in the industry originates from Nepal and India. Despite the PRC's membership of the World Trade Organisation (WTO), the improvement in transport links, and the official commitment to eliminating trade barriers and fostering cross-border business via the Friendship Highway that links Tibet and Nepal, the international trade in medicinal plants has become more difficult than it used to be. Contrary to the image of globalisation's free flows, newly established border regimes restrict and channel the transit of people and goods across the border.

I suspected that the industrialisation of Tibetan medicine would trigger a substantial influx of capital from inland China and thereby imply a shift of ownership and control away from Tibetans. Of course, private Chinese investors have entered the industry, but so have Tibetan investors and major banks. Moreover, the widespread idea (also among Tibetans) that the Han Chinese were better and tougher businessmen has partly been reversed with regard to the industry. Several companies run by Chinese managers are not doing very well, and the most successful Chinese-owned Tibetan medicine company does not conform to the image of Chinese business culture at all – it is run by a Chinese woman who is a devout follower of Tibetan Buddhism.

I also presumed that the creation of an industry would attract foreign investment. For a short while, this prospect may have been flirted with, but subsequent regulations, the overall political climate, and the prospect that it would be difficult to extract single active ingredients from complex multi-component Tibetan formulas resulted in the fact that no transnational pharmaceutical companies have become involved in the industry.

Three: Knowledge

I assumed that Tibetan medical knowledge would be at once sidelined and appropriated in the context of the industry. This has happened to a certain extent but not in the ways I hypothesised. I took it for granted that GMP and the well-established practices of making Tibetan medicines would stand in contradiction with each other, and that the creation of an industry would entail a clash of knowledge systems. Given the asymmetric power relations, I assumed that GMP as abstract, generalised knowledge (a global form, a *techne*) would supersede traditional Tibetan knowledge of pharmacy.[1] What I found, however, was that GMP and the Gyüshi mostly just have different outlooks. The widely lamented conflicts between the new regulations and well-established practices stem from the side effects of a hasty implementation rather than from a clash of Sowa Rigpa knowledge with a scientific episteme.

At the same time, I anticipated an increasing commodification of Tibetan medical knowledge. This has turned out to be true, but again not in the way I expected. The industrial era and the regulations that came with it have indeed affected access to and control over Tibetan medical knowledge. The requirement to carry out clinical trials in order to obtain drug registration for any 'new drug' means that undocumented Tibetan formulas will increasingly be processed and 'refined' outside Tibet, beyond the control of Tibetans. Furthermore, most Tibetan companies have lost their right to produce certain high-value *rinchen rilbu* (precious pills) in the course of recent developments. However, ironically, it was the state's attempt to protect traditional knowledge against illegitimate appropriation rather than a contrived patent system that excluded these companies from producing the formulas in question.

In brief, the industrialisation of Tibetan medicine does not conform to standard narratives of modernisation. This, one may argue, is a result of the vantage point from which the story was observed and told. Ethnography has always had an affinity with the unexpected and singular, for revealing the exception rather than the master narrative or grand theory. However, the creation of an industry on the Tibetan Plateau is not just a special case. It echoes, and even amplifies, a characteristic historical conjuncture of the early twenty-first century in the PRC and elsewhere – a conjuncture where global forms translate into an increasing range of practices and life worlds and meet tactical manoeuvring on the ground, a conjuncture where different versions of the modern project reverberate and produce at times unexpected outcomes. My aim in this concluding chapter is to localise this conjuncture conceptually in time and space. I will do so by revisiting the notion of assemblage.

Assemblage Revisited

The starting point of my inquiry was an attempt to understand the emerging Tibetan medicine industry as an assemblage of heterogeneous elements: people, technologies, histories, laws, regulations, factory architecture, products of nature, packaged medicines, knowledge, aesthetic expressions, and concepts of Tibetanness and morality. An assemblage has both a temporal and a spatial dimension because it aggregates ideas, techniques and materials from different epochs as well as different places. Just as the industry is contemporary by assemblage, as Michel Serres would say (Serres and Latour

233

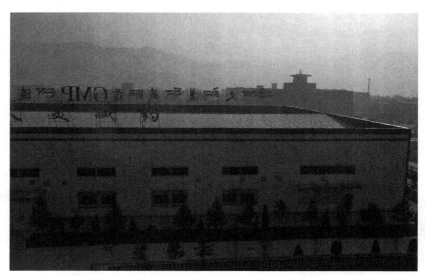

Figure 8.1: Layered histories, entangled spaces: Jigme Phuntsog's GMP factory, Arura's museum.

1995: 45), it is also territorial by assemblage, according to Ong and Collier (2005: 4). I will discuss both dimensions in turn.

Contemporary by Assemblage

Paul Rabinow suggests that assemblages are relatively ephemeral. They last years or decades rather than centuries; 'either a more structured apparatus emerges from them or they disaggregate' (Rabinow 2003: 56). According to Rabinow, assemblages 'stand in a dependent but contingent and unpredictable relationship to the grander problematizations', which tend to be more durable and often characterise an era. Following Foucault, Rabinow contends that a problematisation arises from a troubling event in which previous ways of understanding and acting no longer produce the intended result (Rabinow 2003: 15–20, 2005: 43–45). Such an event introduces uncertainty and a loss of familiarity. A problematisation, however, is more than just an ensemble of difficulties at a particular historical conjuncture. The 'diacritic marking' of a problematisation, as Rabinow puts it, is the play of 'true and false' that comes into view once a set of difficulties is constituted as a problematic object of thought (Rabinow 2003: 18–20). For Foucault and Rabinow, a problematisation emerges when these difficulties acquire the form of an articulated problem to which diverse solutions are proposed. These solutions often take the form of a strategic response (ibid.: 54) or, in Foucault's terms, an 'apparatus'.[2]

Five such problematisations and a bundle of related strategic responses frame the emergence of the industrial assemblage of the present case. They relate to the different visions or layers of modernity encountered throughout this monograph. I designate these five problematisations: 'lagging behind', 'culture and nation', 'opening up', 'side effects of rapid growth', and 'saving Tibet'.

'Lagging behind' is a figure of thought that has haunted China since at least the First Opium War of 1839 to 1842 (Ramo 2007: 7). When after more than a century of chaos the PRC was founded, the problem of 'lagging behind' served as the backdrop against which a radical and rapid modernisation and industrialisation was initiated. The topos of accelerated development guided a variety of strategic responses throughout the history of the PRC, reaching from the Great Leap Forward (accelerated collectivisation) to Deng Xiaoping's reform agenda (finally catching up with the world after ten lost years). On a lesser scale, the same notion informed strategies with regard to regions within the PRC: Tibet is seen as 'lagging behind' and therefore in need of accelerated development; so too is Tibetan medicine: it has to catch up with national and international standards of industrial production and quality control.

The second problematisation is 'culture and nation'. Chinese culture, and especially Confucianism, was often seen as the cause of China's 'lagging behind' (Anagnost 1997: 22, 84), resonating with Weber's thesis of world religions and industrialisation (Weber 1962). This view was epitomised in the explicit problematisation of culture during the Cultural Revolution, which sought to root out the 'four olds' and open the path to accelerated socialist development. Mao's China, however, was also a nationalist venture in which Chinese culture and knowledge played a crucial role. The creation of 'traditional Chinese medicine' (TCM) in the late 1950s and early 1960s can be seen as a result of this tension. Furthermore, when in the post-Mao era the notion of *wenming* (civilisation) started to stand in for the notion of class as an organising principle of the national imaginary, the discussion around culture (*wenhua*) was revived. The strategic response was to emphasise the safeguarding of cultural heritage, which in turn enabled the booming Tibetanness economy. Meanwhile, the problematisation of 'culture' took shape on a global scale as well, especially in the post-1989 era. It was constituted and responded to as 'ethnic conflict', 'indigeneity and human rights', 'integration of diasporas', or the infamous 'clash of civilisations' (Huntington 1993). Just as with their Chinese counterparts, these articulations and responses are freighted with the question of right and wrong. In this sense, the morality discussed in the previous chapter is caught between the problematisation of 'culture' in different spheres.

The third problematisation is 'opening up'. It is directly linked to Deng Xiaoping's reform programme and has been articulated as one of the most critical issues in post-Mao China. It includes active learning from other countries, openness to foreign investment, taking a prominent role in UN organisations such as the WHO and UNESCO, accession to the WTO (achieved in 2001), and events like the 2008 Beijing Olympics and the 2010 Shanghai World Expo. At the same time, 'opening up' remains problematic and informs a cautious attitude. Strategic responses to temper the potentially negative effects of opening up include a tight control of foreign NGOs (like the one sponsoring Aku Jinpa's school; see Introduction), a ban on foreign investment for certain strategically important sectors, a vast security apparatus, and the import regime for foreign drugs (described in Chapter 4).

The fourth and most recent problematisation can be labelled 'side effects of rapid growth'. These side effects include both social tensions and ecological threats. The strategic responses aimed at managing the negative consequences of China's economic success are being articulated under the slogan 'building a socialist harmonious society'. Working towards social harmony and ecological sustainability became patriotic duties and the apparatus emerging around the slogan influences the aesthetic enterprise (see Chapter 6) – the ways in which Tibetan medicine is represented and its stake in the visions of a future Tibet.

Finally, the fifth problematisation is 'saving Tibet'. It is linked to all four problematisations above, and has accordingly triggered a variety of strategic responses over time. The first was the 'liberation' of Tibet from 'feudal oppression'. It was followed by a strategy of non-interference under the Seventeen-point Agreement (in complete contradiction to liberation discourse). For Sowa Rigpa this meant being left untouched while the making of TCM went on in inland China. In the post-Mao era, 'saving Tibet' was sometimes considered as a variation of the 'lagging behind' problem and was dealt with in economic terms. Sometimes it was portrayed as protecting the Land of Snows from foreign imperialism and left to the security apparatus. More recently, 'saving Tibet' has centred around the problematisation of 'culture' and the emergent apparatus of safeguarding and promoting Tibet's cultural heritage. 'Saving Tibet' has also informed transnational responses, often combining a vision of saving Tibet from China with a vision of saving Tibet from poverty and backwardness. The different meanings of development and the preservation of culture fuel the spectacle surrounding the moral question of authenticity, of real and fake, truth and lie (cf. Adams 2004).

In summary, the temporal dimension of the industrial assemblage is characterised by the ebb and flow of these problematisations and strategic responses. While the problematisations are relatively stable, respective responses often overlap or contradict each other. As a result, their configuration remains dynamic and the context in which the industry operates is not at all stable. Consider the import regime that requires licences, permits and the testing of herbs: it was ignored for years but suddenly, in a particular constellation, it became highly relevant. As these constellations keep changing, the actors in the field continue to adjust their tactics and initiatives as well.

Territorial by Assemblage

Strategic responses increasingly take the shape of global forms. A typical pattern encountered throughout this monograph is that a global form – often linked to an acronym: GMP, RCT, CITES, TRIPS, WTO, UNESCO, and so on – is being articulated in a local context, or 'territorialised' in an assemblage (Ong and Collier 2005: 4).

This brings us to the spatial arrangements in which the industry is unfolding. I argue that this arrangement is marked by marginality, frontiers and border regimes: Sowa Rigpa is practised at the margin of two large nation-states. This spatial location at the margin of territories is doubled by a conceptual one: Sowa Rigpa is peripheral both as 'alternative' medicine vis-à-vis biomedicine and as a minority medicine vis-à-vis TCM.

This location at multiple peripheries implies proximity to multiple frontiers where spatial and conceptual borders tend to fall together. Such borders are often guarded by border regimes, as I suggested calling them (Chapter 4). Border regimes are characterised by their capacity to delineate conceptual as well as spatial spheres: the foreign and raw product of nature from the domestic and certified medicinal ingredient, for example. When global forms are territorialised in an assemblage, they rely on such border regimes to define and defend space.

Global forms reflect a specific type of knowledge: abstract, generalised *techne*. De Certeau argues that this type of knowledge is characteristic of strategies. Strategies are sustained and determined by the power to delimit space. Military or scientific institutions, de Certeau shows, 'have always been inaugurated through the constitution of their "own" areas' (Certeau 1984: 36) – autonomous cities and laboratories, for example – or in the present case: medicine factories, museums, theme parks and so forth.

In this sense, border regimes are not exclusive to national frontiers. Wherever the pathways between different conceptual and spatial spheres intersect, border regimes in one form or the other tend to be established in order to guard them and manage entry and exit procedures. Consider the demarcation of classified clean areas within a GMP factory, for example. The space of a clean area is defined by entry and exit procedures for humans and herbs. Demarcating conceptual as well as spatial spheres, these procedures constitute a border regime similar to that which manages the flow of herbs and people across the Sino-Nepalese border at the Friendship Bridge. Another case in point is the filtration of knowledge that is necessary to turn Ngawang Dawa's lineage formula into intellectual property (Chapter 5). The hospitals and laboratories equipped with the required infrastructure to transform an undocumented formula into a registered drug are guarded spaces to which a lineage *amchi* from Nagchu has no access.

The term 'border regime' hints at a paradox. On the one hand, the term denotes a regime in the sense of state power. The 'border', on the other hand, is a liminal space where state power is potentially rendered vulnerable. Penba's encounters at the border in Dram suggest that overambitious border regimes can only maintain the illusion of accomplishing their task if they tolerate a certain amount of tactical evasion. Enforced strictly, these regimes would lose their legitimacy and the people in charge of enforcing them their careers.

Ong and Collier suggest that global forms are restricted and defined by technical infrastructures, administrative apparatuses and value regimes, but not by 'the vagaries of a social or cultural field' (Ong and Collier 2005: 11). This is true for the global form as such. However, looking at border regimes in the service of global forms in the present case, it is exactly the vagaries of the cultural and social field that define and restrict them. These border regimes are penetrated but, paradoxically, also stabilised by tactical evasion. In this respect, the redundant microwave ovens protecting the clean area of a factory serve their purpose perfectly well. The guardians of the factory's inner realms were secretly subdued and now keep the GMP inspectors at bay instead of the microbes.

Nevertheless, global forms clearly affect the local practice of medicine production in a Tibetan factory – if not directly then through their side effects. These side effects, as we have seen, are often a consequence of Sowa Rigpa's location at multiple peripheries and the fact that recontextualisation typically consists of more than one step. A global form is first recontextualised in the national sphere. Once packaged in national policies and laws it is then recontextualised again within the industry of Tibetan medicine. Spatially, the flows still point from global to local, but via the national.

Less obvious is the opposite movement: the process of decontextualisation, or the question how global forms are being abstracted from experience. Decontextualisation would potentially point to flows in the opposite direction – from small to large, from Tibet to the PRC, and from both into the global sphere.

On the one hand, China has been lauded for its policies on traditional medicine by the international community and has certainly a voice in the international process of policy-making. WHO director Dr Margaret Chan is Hong Kong's former Director of Health, and Dr Xiaorui Zhang from the WHO's Department of Essential Drugs and Medicines Policy played a significant role in designing the organisation's traditional medicine strategy (WHO 2002, 2003, 2005a, 2006a, 2006b). There is good reason to believe that the experiences gained locally in the PRC constitute part of the material from which global forms are distilled. China has also been engaged in shaping other global forms, including UNESCO's approaches to cultural heritage. Between national and global spheres, the exchanges are definitely bidirectional.

On the other hand, the translation of experiences gained with the Tibetan medicine industry into national policies and laws remains limited. This was often cited as one of the major problems in the conversations I had with people in the industry. A case in point is the 1995 *Tibetan Drug Standards* (see Chapter 2), which have not been amended despite continuing efforts to convince the central authorities of the problem's urgency. In terms of medical regulations, Sowa Rigpa's marginal position vis-à-vis TCM, and more generally traditional medicine's marginal position vis-à-vis biomedicine, remains problematic. This may be one reason to posit the industry as a problem of 'culture' rather than health care. 'Culture' promises a better forum in which to be heard. Decontextualised from local experience, Tibetanness itself becomes a global form and gains the capacity to move across diverse social and cultural situations (cf. Ong and Collier 2005: 11).

The same can be said for the commodities the industry produces. The limited number of Tibetan pills that find their way through the administrative apparatuses of other countries do so either clandestinely or in disguise: as Tibetan food supplements or even as Tibetan talismans. Decontextualised from Sowa Rigpa practice they take the global form of a 'cultural' rather than a medical commodity.[3] However, there is a price to pay, namely that Sowa Rigpa becomes even more regarded as 'some kind of cultural thing' instead of what it strives to remain: the Tibetan science of healing.

What, then, is the position of the industry in time and space? And what does this mean for the future of Sowa Rigpa? Located at multiple peripheries, in close proximity to spatial as well as conceptual boundaries; located also amidst the fault zones of overlapping problematisations, the industry's position is delicate and characterised by quick and unpredictable change. Foretelling its future would be easier if the border regimes were less permeable, the power of interpretation over the rules and laws did not rest exclusively with an authority possessing limited knowledge about Sowa Rigpa, and the configuration of apparatuses pertaining to the industry remained stable for a while. Only in retrospect will one be able to tell in detail how the creation of an industry affected Sowa Rigpa as a system of knowledge and practice.

The ambitious project of industrialising Tibetan medicine may still fail. Practical knowledge in the sense of *mētis* may finally be pushed aside, border regimes become tighter, and the industry, one day, be regarded as yet another of Scott's failed schemes. It is also possible that global forms will continue to gain in importance, that an apparatus will emerge from the assemblage, and the industry will become as dominant a figure for Sowa Rigpa as the pharmaceutical industry is for biomedicine. Or, Sowa Rigpa may become even more entrenched in the political and moral spectacle of saving Tibetan culture. In the near future, however, chances are that the industry will remain a site for a variety of Tibetan initiatives yet to be imagined.

Notes

1. The terms *techne* and *mētis* are taken from Scott (1998). For a discussion of their relevance to the present study, see the Introduction.
2. The original French term is *dispositif* (Foucault 1977: 299).
3. J. Crow's Marketplace, for instance, offers Ratna Samphel on its website (www.jcrowsmarketplace.com) with the following disclaimer: 'Offered for sale only as a "talisman". We make no claims with respect to its efficacy for any purpose whatsoever'. With respect to industrially produced Chinese medicines and their usage in East Africa, Elisabeth Hsu argues that their disjuncture from TCM as a scholarly system amounts to a veritable folklorisation of Chinese medicine (Hsu 2009b: 114). Ironically, the industry as archetypal figure of scientific modern medicine may in fact give rise to its eternal alter ego – unscholarly, 'superstitious charlatanry'.

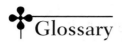 Glossary

amchi	*am chi*	Tibetan doctor
Amdo	*a mdo*	Northeastern Tibet, mostly incorporated in present-day Qinghai province
arnag	*ar nag*	Black Eaglewood, *Aquilaria agallocha*
aru	*a ru, a ru ra*	*Terminalia chebula*, Chelubic Myrobalan
Ayurveda		'The science of life'; one of the great Indian medical systems. Ayurveda and Tibetan medicine share many common concepts
bandh		A common form of general strike in Nepal
Barkor	*bar skor*	Literally, 'the middle circle'. The Route encircling the ➤Jokhang temple in central Lhasa
baru	*ba ru, ba ru ra*	Belleric Myrobalan, *Terminalia belerica*
beken	*bad kan*	Bile, one of the three ➤*nyepa*

243

bianzheng lunzhi		The method of pattern differentiation in Traditional Chinese Medicine
bömen sotra	*bod sman bzo grwa*	Tibetan medicine factory
bongkar	*bong dkar*	Aconite species with white tubers, most commonly identified as *Aconitum heterophyllum*
bongnag	*bong nag*	Aconite species with black tubers
bütog	*bul tog*	A water containing carbonate known as trona
Chagpori	*lcags po ri*	The famous medical school on the Chagpori hill in Lhasa, established by Desi Sangye Gyatso in 1696, destroyed during the Tibetan uprising in 1959
chimagyü	*phyi ma rgyud*	Subsequent Tantra, the fourth and last treatise of the ➤ Gyüshi
Chinnä Künchom	*mchin nad kun 'joms*	Jigme Phuntsog's famous liver drug
chuba	*phyu pa*	Tibetan robe
chumtsa	*lcum rtsa*	*Rheum palmatum*
dalu		Mainland, Mainland China
danwei		Work unit
dräbusum	*'bras bu gsum*	The three fruits: ➤ *aru, baru, kyuru*

dülwa	*'dul ba*	Literally: subjugation. The processing of mercury; also: monastic discipline
fang		Chinese for Formula
gangachung	*gang ga chung*	*Gentiana urnula*
gangkizhungchung	*gangs kyi zhun chung*	Synonym for *bongkar*
gangla metog	*gangs lha me tog*	Saussurea medusa/laniceps
Gelugpa	*dge lugs pa*	One of major schools of Tibetan Buddhism, also referred to as Yellow Hat sect
Great Leap Forward (GLF)		An episode in China's history (1958-1961) characterised by radical collectivisation of agriculture, social change, and a devastating famine
guanli		Chinese for 'management'
Guru Rinpoche	*gu ru rin po che*	Tibetan name for Padmasambhava, the Indian yogi associated with the eighth century introduction of Tantric Buddhism in Tibet
gyanag	*rgya nag*	China
Gyüshi	*rgyud bzhi*	The Fourfold Treatise, the foundational text of ➤ Sowa Rigpa
hexie shehui		Hu Jintao's concept of the 'Harmonious Society'

jihua		Chinese for 'planning'
Jokhang	*jo khang*	The central temple in Lhasa
kache gurgum	*kha che gur gum*	Saffron, see also ➤ *tsa gurgum*
Kashag	*bka' shag*	The council of ministers in Tibetan government (pre-1959 and in exile)
kexue fazhan guan		The concept of a 'Scientific Outlook on Development'
Kham	*khams*	Eastern Tibet, partly falling within the TAR, partly within Yunnan and Sichuan provinces
Khampa	*khams pa*	Man from ➤ Kham
kyuru	*skyu ru, skyu ru ra*	Emblic myrobalan, Emblica officinalis
latsi	*gla rtsi*	Musk
lhachen mahadeva	*lha chen ma ha de wa*	A secret name for mercury, a reference to Lord Shiva
losar	*lo sar*	Tibetan New Year
lung	*rlung*	wind, one of the three ➤ *nyepa* in Tibetan medicine
Maobadi		The Maoists in Nepal
Men-Tsee-Khang	*sman rtsi khang*	Spelling for ➤ Mentsikhang, used by the Tibetan Medical and Astro Institute in Dharamsala

menpa	*sman pa*	Tibetan doctor; literally 'medicine person'
menpa dratsang	*sman pa grwa tshang*	Medical college
Mentsikhang	*sman rtsi khang*	Literally: 'The House of Medicine and Astrology'. This spelling refers to the Mentsikhang in Lhasa
Nagchu	*nag chu*	Prefecture and county in the northern TAR
neidi		Inland, Inland China
ngochor	*sngo sbyor*	Name of chapter 12 of the ➤ Gyüshi's fourth Treatise, see ➤ *yänlagdün*
nyepa	*nyes pa*	The three 'faults' in Sowa Rigpa theory: wind (➤ *lung*), bile (➤ *tripa*), and phlegm (➤ *beken*)
pangpö	*spang spos*	Spikenard, *Nardostachys grandiflora/jatamansi*
precious pills		See ➤ *rinchen rilbu*
Ratna Samphel	*rat na bsam 'phel*	One of the most famous ➤ *rinchen rilbu* (precious pills), also known as Mutig 70
Rilkar	*ril dkar*	One of the precious pills (➤ *rinchen rilbu*)
Rinchen Drangjor	*rin chen sbrang sbyor*	Another famous ➤ *rinchen rilbu*

Rinchen Mangjor	*rin chen mang sbyor*	Yet another famous ➤ *rinchen rilbu*
rinchen rilbu	*rin chen ril bu*	Category of especially powerful Tibetan pharmaceuticals knows as 'precious pills'
Rinpoche	*rin po che*	Literally: 'the jewel', 'the precious one'; an honorific in Tibetan Buddhism
ruta	*ru rta*	Saussurea lappa
setru	*se 'bru*	Punica granatum, pomegranate seeds
shel phreng		Crystal Rosary, famous eighteenth century text by Deumar Geshe Tenzin Phuntsog
shingtudugme	*shin tu dug med*	Synonym for ➤ *bongkar*
Shongpalhachu	*gzhong pa lha chu*	Pilgrimage site west of Lhasa, name of a factory
solomarpo	*sro lo dmar po*	Rhodiola crenulata
sosordugme	*so sor dug med*	Synonym for ➤ *bongkar*
Sowa Rigpa	*gso ba rig pa*	Literally: 'the science of healing'; a general term for medicine, often used as a synonym for Tibetan medicine
sumchutigta	*sum chu tig ta*	A *Saxifraga* species
thangka	*thang ka*	Tibetan scroll-painting

tripa	*mkhris pa*	Bile, one of the three ➤ *nyepa*
Trisong Detsen	*khri srong lde btsan*	Emperor of Tibet in the eighth century
tsa gurgum	*rtsa gur gum*	Safflower, Carthamus tinctorius
Tsongkhapa		Founder of the ➤ Gelugpa school
tsothal	*btso thal*	Substance used for certain ➤ *rinchen rilbu*, contains purified mercury
Tsotru Dashel	*btso bkru zla shel*	One of the famous ➤ *rinchen rilbu*
xi zang		Chinese for 'Tibet'
xingzheng		Chinese for 'Administration'
yänlagdun	*yan lag bdun*	Seven Essential Limbs of Medicinal Plants, short: the Seven Limbs, included in chapter 12 of the Gyüshi's Subsequent Tantra
yao		Chinese term for 'medicine' or 'pharmaceuticals'
yartsagunbu	*dbyar rtswa dgun 'bu*	Ophiocordyceps sinensis, caterpillar fungus
Yothog Yonten Gonpo the Elder	*g.yu thog rnying ma yon tan mgon po*	eighth century founding father of ➤ Sowa Rigpa

Yothog Yonten Gonpo the Younger	*g.yu thog gsar ma yon tan mgon po*	twelfth century Tibetan, credited with the Yuthog Heart Essence (Yuthog 2005) and, according to some Tibetan historians, the ➤ Gyüshi itself
zang yao chang		Chinese for 'Tibetan medicine factory'
zang yi		Chinese term for 'Tibetan Medicine'
zhengfu zhineng zhuanbian		Chinese for 'the changing function of government'
zhili		Chinese for 'governance'
zhong guo		China, literally: 'middle kingdom' or 'central nation'
zizhi		Chinese for 'autonomy'

✣ References

Adams, V. 2001. 'Particularizing Modernity: Tibetan Medical Theorizing of Women's Health in Lhasa, Tibet', in L.H. Connor and S. Geoffrey (eds), *Healing Powers and Modernity: Traditional Medicine, Shamanism and Science in Asian Societies*. Westport, CT: Bergin and Garvey.

——— 2002. 'Randomized Controlled Crime. Postcolonial Sciences in Alternative Medicine Research', *Social Studies of Science* 32(5/6): 659–690.

——— 2004. 'Saving Tibet? An Inquiry into Modernity, Lies, Truths, and Beliefs', *Medical Anthropology* 24(1): 71–110.

——— 2008. 'Modernity and the Problem of Secular Morality in Tibet', in V. Houben and M. Schrempf (eds), *Figurations of Modernity: Global and Local Representations in Comparative Perspective*. Frankfurt am Main: Campus.

Adams, V., S. Miller, S. Craig, A. Samen, Nyima, Sonam, Droyoung, Lhakpen and M. Varner. 2005. 'The Challenge of Cross-cultural Clinical Trials Research: Case Report from the Tibetan Autonomous Region, People's Republic of China', *Medical Anthropology Quarterly* 19(3): 267–289.

Adams, V., M. Schrempf and S. Craig. 2010. 'Medicine in Translation between Science and Religion' in V. Adams, M. Schrempf and S. Craig (eds), *Medicine between Science and Religion: Explorations on Tibetan Grounds*. New York and Oxford: Berghahn.

Alonso–Zaldivar, R. 2008. 'Contaminated Heparin Made in China Related to More Than 62 Suspected Deaths', *Los Angeles Times*, http://articles.latimes.com/p/2008/apr/22/nation/na–heparin22 (accessed 5 May 2009).

Anagnost, A. 1997. *National Past-times: Narrative, Representation, and Power in Modern China*. Durham, NC: Duke University Press.

Anand, D. 2000. '(Re)Imagining Nationalism: Identity and Representation in the Tibetan Diaspora of South Asia', *Contemporary South Asia* 9(3): 271–287.

Appadurai, A. 1986. *The Social Life of Things: Commodities in Cultural Perspective*. Cambridge: Cambridge University Press.

——— 1990. 'Technology and the Reproduction of Values in Rural Western India', in F.A. Marglin and S.A. Marglin (eds), *Dominating Knowledge*. Oxford: Oxford University Press.

Arnason, J. P. 2000. 'Communism and Modernity', *Daedalus* 129(1): 61–90.

Arura. 2006. 'Development of the Tibetan Medicine', http://www.tibetanmd.com/english/tibetaninfo/view.asp?id=494 (accessed 6 July 2009).

251

Aschoff, J. C. and T. Y. Tashigang. 1997. 'On Mercury in Tibetan "Precious Pills"', *Journal of the European Ayurvedic Society* 5:129–35.

Aumeeruddy-Thomas, Y., and Y.C. Lama. 2008. 'Tibetan Medicine Today: Neo-traditionalism as an Analytical Lens and a Political Tool', in L. Pordié (ed.), *Tibetan Medicine in the Contemporary World: Global Politics of Medical Knowledge and Practice*. London: Routledge.

Balick, M.J., and P.A. Cox. 1996. *Plants, People, and Culture: The Science of Ethnobotany*. New York: Scientific American Library.

Banerjee, M. 2009. *Power, Knowledge, Medicine*. Hyderabad: Orient Blackswan.

Barnett, R. 1996. 'Cutting Off the Serpent's Head: Tightening Control in Tibet', *Human Rights Watch/UNHCR*, http://www.unhcr.org/refworld/publisher,HRW,,CHN,3ae6a82a0,0.html (accessed 22 September 2009).

——— 2001a. The Chinese Frontiersman and the Winter Worms: Chen Kui-yuan in the T.A.R. , 1992–2000', unpublished paper presented at the History of Tibet seminar, St Andrew's University, Scotland, August 2001.

——— 2001b. '"Violated Specialness": Western Political Representations of Tibet', in T. Dodin and H. Räther (eds), *Imagining Tibet: Perceptions, Projections, and Fantasies*. Boston: Wisdom Publications.

——— 2006a. 'Beyond the Collaborator-martyr Model: Strategies of Compliance, Opportunism, and Opposition within Tibet', in B. Sautman and J.T. Dreyer (eds), *Contemporary Tibet: Politics, Development, and Society in a Disputed Region*. New York: M.E. Sharpe.

——— 2006b. *Lhasa: Streets with Memories*. New York: Columbia University Press.

Baudelaire, C. 1857. *Les Fleurs du mal*. Paris: Poulet-Malasse et de Broise.

Beck, U. 2001. *Die Modernisierung Der Moderne*. Suhrkamp: Frankfurt.

Berman, M. 1982. *All That Is Solid Melts into Air: The Experience of Modernity*. London: Verso.

Besch, N.F. 2006. 'Tibetan Medicine off the Roads: Modernizing the Work of the Amchi in Spiti', PhD thesis, Ruprecht–Karls–Universität Heidelberg.

Bhaskara, H. 2004. 'Xining Builds Industrial Park Dedicated to Tibetan Plateau', *Jakarta Post*, http://www.thejakartapost.com/news/2004/12/15/xining–builds–industrial–park–dedicated–tibetan–plateau.html (accessed 6 July 2009).

Bode, M. 2004. 'Ayurvedic and Unani Health and Beauty Products', PhD thesis, University of Amsterdam.

Bourdieu, P. 1979. *La Distinction: critique sociale du jugement*. Paris: Minuit.

Bramall, C. 2000. 'Inequality, Land Reform and Agricultural Growth in China, 1952–55: A Preliminary Treatment', *Journal of Peasant Studies* 27(3): 30–54.

Brown, M.J. 2002. 'Local Government Agency: Manipulating Tujia Identity', *Modern China* 28(3): 362–395.

Brush, S.B., and D. Stabinsky. 1996. *Valuing Local Knowledge: Indigenous People and Intellectual Property Rights*. Washington, DC: Island Press.

Cai, Y. 2000. 'Between State and Peasant: Local Cadres and Statistical Reporting in Rural China', *China Quarterly* 163: 783–805.

Calabrese, A. 2005. 'Communication, Global Justice and the Moral Economy', *Global Media and Communication* 1(3): 301–315.

Calkowski, M.S. 1997. 'The Tibetan Diaspora and the Politics of Performance', in J. Korom (ed.), *Tibetan Culture in the Diaspora*. Vienna: Verlag der Österreichischen Akademie der Wissenschaften.

Certeau, M. de. 1984. *The Practice of Everyday Life*. Berkeley: University of California Press.

Chakrabarty, D. 1992. 'Postcoloniality and the Artifice of History: Who Speaks for "Indian" Pasts?', *Representations* 37: 1–26.

Chambers, E. 2000. *Native Tours: The Anthropology of Travel and Tourism*. Prospect Heights, IL: Waveland Press.

China Daily. 2006. 'Firm Preserves Ancient Cures', *China Daily*, http://chinadaily.cn/bizchina/2006–10/12/content_706519.htm (accessed 6 July 2009).

——— 2007a. 'Former SFDA Chief Executed for Corruption', *China Daily*, http://www.chinadaily.com.cn/china/2007–07/10/content_5424937.htm (accessed 23 June 2009).

——— 2007b. 'Scientific Outlook on Development', *China Daily*, http://www.chinadaily.cn/language_tips/2007–10/12/content_6170884.htm (accessed 15 June 2010).

——— 2008. 'Medicine Woman', *China Tibet Information Center*, http://eng.tibet.cn/news/today/200806/t20080630_409970.htm (accessed 11 September 2008).

——— 2009. 'Domestic Travel Poised for Takeoff', *People's Daily Online*, http://english. people. com. cn/90001/6576348. html (accessed 3 July 2009).

Chukora, T.A. 2007. 'The Sorig Revolution', *Tibetoday* 1(4): 14–18.

Clark, B. 1985. 'The Practice and Theory of Therapeutics in Tibetan Medicine', *Tibetan Medicine* 9:16–27.

——— 1995. *The Quintessence Tantras of Tibetan Medicine*. Ithaca, NY: Snow Lion Publications.

——— 2000. 'Problems in Identifying and Translating Materia Medica Used in Tibetan Medicine', *Ayur Vijnana* 7: 55–57.

C-Med. 2006. 'TCM Bids for Intangible Heritage Status', *Hong Kong Jockey Club Institute of Chinese Medicine*, http://www.hkjcicm.org/5news/2/3_e.asp (accessed 8 July 2009).

——— 2009. 'SFDA Guidelines on Protection of Traditional Chinese Medicines', *Hong Kong Jockey Club Institute of Chinese Medicine*, http://www.hkjcicm.org/5news/2/65_e.asp (accessed 8 July 2009).

Cohen, L. 1995. 'The Epistemological Carnival: Meditations on Disciplinary Intentionality and Ayurveda', in D.G. Bates (ed.), *Knowledge and the Scholarly Medical Tradition*. Cambridge: Cambridge University Press.

Comaroff, J.L., and J. Comaroff. 1992. *Ethnography and the Historical Imagination*. Boulder, CO: Westview Press.

——— 2009. *Ethnicity, Inc*. Chicago: University of Chicago Press.

Conner, V., and R. Barnett. 1997. *Leaders in Tibet*. London: Tibet Information Network.

Conrad, S. and S. Randeria. 2002. 'Geteilte Geschichten. Europa in Einer Post-kolonialen Welt' in S. Conrad and S. Randeria (eds), *Jenseits Des Eurozentrismus*. Frankfurt: Campus.

Coombe, R.J. 2005. 'Protecting Traditional Environmental Knowledge and New Social Movements in the Americas: Intellectual Property, Human Right, or Claims to An Alternative Form of Sustainable Development', *Florida Journal of International Law* 17: 115–135.

Coonan, C. 2008. 'Dalai Lama Attacks "Cultural Genocide"', *Independent*, http://www.independent.co.uk/news/world/asia/dalai–lama–attacks–cultural–genocide–796795.html (accessed 8 January 2010).

Cox, P.A., and M.J. Balick. 1994. 'The Ethnobotanical Approach to Drug Discovery', *Scientific American* 270(6): 60–65.

Craig, S. 2003. 'SARS on the Roof of the World', *Explorers Journal* (Summer), pp.20–21.

——— 2006. 'On the Science of Healing: Efficacy and the Metamorphosis of Tibetan Medicine', PhD thesis. Ithaca, NY: Cornell University.

——— 2007. 'A Crisis of Confidence. A Comparison Between Shifts in Tibetan Medical Education in Nepal and Tibet', in M. Schrempf (ed), *Tibetan Medicine: Proceedings From the 10th International Association of Tibetan Studies Meetings*. Amsterdam: Brill.

——— 2010. 'From Empowerments to Power Calculations: Notes on Efficacy, Value, and Method', in V. Adams, M. Schrempf and S. Craig (eds), *Medicine Between Science and Religion: Explorations on Tibetan Grounds*. New York and Oxford: Berghahn.

——— 2011. '"Good" Manufacturing by Whose Standards? Remaking Concepts of Quality, Safety and Value in the Production of Tibetan Medicines', *Anthropological Quarterly* 84(2): 331–378.

Craig, S., and V. Adams. 2009. 'Global Pharma in the Land of Snows: Tibetan Medicines, SARS and Identity Politics Across Nations', *Asian Medicine* 4: 1–28.

Croizier, R.C. 1976. 'The Ideology of Medical Revivalism in Modern China', in C. Leslie (ed.), *Asian Medical Systems: A Comparative Study*. Berkeley: University of California Press.

Crook, F.W. 1973. 'Chinese Communist Agricultural Incentive Systems and the Labor Productive Contracts to Households: 1956–1965', *Asian Survey* 13(5): 470–481.

CTIC. 2006a. 'Giant Tibetan Thangka Painting Appears in Xining', *China Tibet Information Center*, http://eng.tibet.cn/news/today/200801/t20080116_335871.htm (accessed 12 September 2008).

——— 2006b. 'Tibetan Medicinal Materials Planting Training Class in Mailing', *China Tibet Information Center*, http://eng.tibet.cn/news/tibet/200801/t20080115_312863.htm (accessed 12 September 2008).

———— 2006c. 'Tibetan Medicine Industry Develops Fast in Nyingchi', *China Tibet Information Center*, http://eng.tibet.cn/news/tibet/200801/t20080115_319950.htm (accessed 12 September 2008).

———— 2006d. 'Tibetan Medicine Museum Opens', *China Tibet Information Center*, http://eng.tibet.cn/news/tibet/200801/t20080115_318260.htm (accessed 12 September 2008).

———— 2006e. 'Tibetan Medicine Research Institute Sets Up', *China Tibet Information Center*, http://eng.tibet.cn/news/tibet/200801/t20080115_316746.htm (accessed 12 September 2008).

———— 2006f. 'Tibetan Medicine Sees Best Development Period', *China Tibet Information Center*, http://eng.tibet.cn/news/tibet/200801/t20080115_319143.htm (accessed 12 September 2008).

———— 2007a. 'Endangered Tibetan Herbal Medicine Successfully Planted', *China Tibet Information Center*, http://eng.tibet.cn/news/tibet/200801/t20080115_328960.htm (accessed 12 September 2008).

———— 2007b. 'Mailing County Strengthens Tibetan Medicinal Material Planting', *China Tibet Information Center*, http://eng.tibet.cn/news/today/200801/t20080116_338471.htm (accessed 12 September 2008).

———— 2007c. 'Tibetan Medicine Industry Rapidly Develop', *China Tibet Information Center*, http://eng.tibet.cn/news/tibet/200801/t20080115_323306.htm (accessed 12 September 2008).

———— 2007d. 'Tibetan Medicine to Declare World Intangible Culture Heritage', *China Tibet Information Center*, http://eng.tibet.cn/news/today/200801/t20080116_338749.htm (accessed 12 September 2008).

———— 2008a. 'Tibetan Medicine Museum to Build in Qinghai', *China Tibet Information Center*, http://eng.tibet.cn/news/china/200801/t20080116_348012.htm (accessed 9 April 2006).

———— 2008b. 'Tibetan Medicine Research Wins Support', *China Tibet Information Center*, http://eng.tibet.cn/news/today/200802/t20080218_368253.htm (accessed 12 September 2008).

———— 2010. 'First Intangible Cultural Heritage Park Starts Construction in Tibet', *People's Daily Online*, http://chinatibet.people.com.cn/7003946.html (accessed 28 June 2010).

Dash, B. 1988. *Formulary of Tibetan Medicine*. Delhi: Classics India Publications.

Dashiyev, D. 1999. 'Experiences with Comparative Studies of Tibetan Medical Formulae', *Ayur Vijnana* 6: 10–16.

Dawa. 2002. *A Clear Mirror of Tibetan Medicinal Plants*. Rome: Tibet Domani Association.

Dawa. 2004. *Key to the Revealed Secrets of the Practical Preparation of Sowa Rigpa's Formulae* [bod kyi gso ba rig pa las sman rdzas sbyor bzo'i lag len gsang sgo 'gyed pa'i lde mig]. Delhi: Rig Drag Publication.

Deng. 1994. *Selected Works of Deng Xiaoping*. Beijing: Foreign Language Press.

De'umar Geshe Tenzin Phuntsog. 1986[1727]. *Crystal Rosary/Shel Phreng* [Bdud nad 'joms pa'i gnyen po rtsi sman gyi nus pa rkyang bshad gsal ston dri med shel gong; Bdud rtsi sman gyi rnam dbyed ngo bo nus ming rgyas par bshad pa dri med shel phreng]. Beijing: Mi rigs dpe skrun khang.

Dezhu, L. 2000. 'Large Scale Development of Western China and China's Nationality Problem', *Qiushi* 11(1): 22–25.

DIIR. 2007. 'Tibet: A Human Development and Environment Report'. Dharamsala: Department of Information and International Relations of the Central Tibetan Administration, Tibetan Government in Exile.

Dirlik, A. 1995. 'Confucius in the Borderlands: Global Capitalism and the Reinvention of Confucianism', *Boundary* 22(3): 229–273.

Dodin, T. and H. Räther. 2001. *Imagining Tibet: Perceptions, Projections, and Fantasies*. Boston: Wisdom Publications.

Donden, Y. 1986. *Health Through Balance*. Ithaca, NY: Snow Lion Publications.

Dreyfus, G. 2005. 'Are We Prisoners of Shangrila? Orientalism, Nationalism, and the Study of Tibet', *Journal of the International Association of Tibetan Studies* 1(1): 1–21.

Drungtso, T.T. and T.D. Drungtso. 2005. *Tibetan–English Dictionary of Tibetan Medicine and Astrology* [bod lugs sman rtsis kyi tshig mdzod bod dbyin shan sbyar]. Dharamshala: Drungtso Publications.

Duang, S. 2000. *Cultural Heritage Management and Tourism: Models for Cooperation among Stakeholders – A Heritage Protection and Tourism Development Case Study of Lijiang Ancient Town China*. Bhaktapur: UNESCO Office of the Regional Advisor for Culture in Asia and the Pacific.

DuBois, T.D. 2010. 'Religion and the Chinese State: Three Crises and a Solution', *Australian Journal of International Affairs* 64(3): 344–358.

Dutfield, G. 2001. 'TRIPS-related Aspects of Traditional Knowledge', *Case Western Reserve Journal of International Law* 33: 233–275.

Dutta, R., and P. Jain. 2000. *CITES Listed Medicinal Plants of India: An Identification Guide*. New Delhi: TRAFFIC/WWF.

Edelman, M. 2005. 'Bringing the Moral Economy Back in . . . to the Study of 21st–Century Transnational Peasant Movements', *American Anthropologist* 107(3): 331–345.

Eimer, D., and G. Chamberlain. 2008. 'Dalai Lama Condemns China's "Cultural Genocide" of Tibet', *Daily Telegraph*, http://www.telegraph.co.uk/news/worldnews/1581875/Dalai–Lama–condemns–Chinas–cultural–genocide-of–Tibet.html (accessed 8 January 2010).

Eisenstadt, S. N. 2000. 'Multiple Modernities', *Daedalus* 129(1): 1-29.

Environment News Service. 2006. 'Tibetans Burn Endangered Animal Skins, Rousing Chinese Ire', http://www.ens–newswire. com/ens/feb2006/2006–02–24–01.asp (accessed 24 November 2009).

Epp, R. 2000. 'Review: Seeing Like a State, by James Scott', *Canadian Journal of Political Science* 33(1): 201–203.

Escobar, A. 1998. 'Whose Knowledge, Whose Nature? Biodiversity, Conservation, and the Political Ecology of Social Movements', *Journal of Political Ecology* 5(1): 53–82.

Etkin, N.L. 1992. '"Side Effects": Cultural Constructions and Reinterpretations of Western Pharmaceuticals', *Medical Anthropology Quarterly* 6(2): 99–113.

Express News Service. 2008. 'I Am a Marxist Monk: Dalai Lama', *Express News Service*, Ahmedabad, January 19.

Farnsworth, N.R. 1988. 'Screening Plants for New Medicines', in E.O. Wilson and P.M. Frances (eds), *Biodiversity*. Washington, DC: National Academy Press.

Farquhar, J. 1994. *Knowing Practice: The Clinical Encounter of Chinese Medicine*. Boulder, CO: Westview.

FDA. 1994. 'Dietary Supplement Health and Education Act', US Food and Drug Administration, http://www.fda.gov/food/dietarysupplements/default.htm (accessed 7 May 2010).

Fisher, J.F. 1986. *Trans-Himalayan Traders: Economy, Society, and Culture in Northwest Nepal*. Berkeley: University of California Press.

Foucault, M. 1991. 'Governmentality', in G. Burchell, C. Gordon and M. Miller (eds), *The Foucault Effect: Studies in Governmentality*. Chicago: University of Chicago Press.

——— 1994[1977]. 'Le Jeu de Michel Foucault', in *Dits et Ecrits: 1954–1988*. Paris: Gallimard.

——— 2005[1966]. *The Order of Things: An Archaeology of the Human Sciences* [Les mots et les choses]. reprinted, e-Library edition. London and New York: Taylor & Francis.

Frangville, V. 2009. 'Tibet in Debate: Narrative Construction and Misrepresentations in Seven Years in Tibet and Red River Valley', *Transtext(e)s Transcultures*, http://transtexts.revues.org/index289.html.

Fürer-Haimendorf, C. von. 1975. *Himalayan Traders: Life in Highland Nepal*. London: John Murray.

Gabe Dorji. 1995. *Khrungs Dpe Dri Med Shel Gyi Me Long* [The Stainless Crystal Mirror: Sources and Identification (of Tibetan Materia Medica)]. Lhasa: Mi rigs dpe skrun khang.

Gamaqupei, G. 1990. 'Method for Processing Traditional Tibetan Medicine (Zuotai Powder)', patent held by the Hospital of Traditional Tibetan Medicine, Tibet Autonomous Region. Publication Number 1038406.

Garrett, F. 2009. 'The Alchemy of Accomplishing Medicine (*sman sgrub*): Situating the *Yuthok Heart Essence* (G. *Yu Thog Snying Thig*) in Literature and History', *Journal of Indian Philosophy* 37(3): 207–230.

——— 2010. 'Tapping the Body's Nectar: Gastronomy and Incorporation in Tibetan Literature', *History of Religions* 49(3): 300–326.

Geismar, H. 2005. 'Copyright in Context: Carvings, Carvers, and Commodities in Vanuatu', *American Ethnologist* 32(3): 437–459.

Gell, A. 1988. 'Technology and Magic', *Anthropology Today* 4(2): 6–9.

——— 1992. 'The Enchantment of Technology and the Technology of Enchantment', in J. Coote and A. Shelton (eds), *Anthropology, Art, and Aesthetics*. Oxford: Clarendon Press.

Gerke, B. 2008. 'Time and Longevity: Concepts of the Life-span among Tibetans in the Darjeeling Hills, India', PhD thesis. Oxford: University of Oxford.

Germano, D. and N. Tournadre. 2003. 'THL Simplified Phonetic Transcription of Standard Tibetan', *The Tibetan & Himalayan Library*. http://www.thlib. org/reference/transliteration/#essay=/thl/phonetics/ (accessed 12 February 2010).

Ghimire, S.K., D. McKey and Y. Aumeeruddy-Thomas. 2005a. 'Conservation of Himalayan Medicinal Plants: Harvesting Patterns and Ecology of Two Threatened Species, Nardostachys Grandiflora DC. and Neopicrorhiza Scrophulariiflora (Pennell) Hong', *Biological Conservation* 124(4): 463–475.

——— 2005b. 'Heterogeneity in Ethnoecological Knowledge and Management of Medicinal Plants in the Himalayas of Nepal: Implications for Conservation', *Ecology and Society* 9(3): 6.

Giedion, S. 1975. *Mechanization Takes Command: A Contribution to Anonymous History.* New York: Norton.

Gladney, D.C. 2004. *Dislocating China: Reflections on Muslims, Minorities, and Other Subaltern Subjects.* Chicago: University of Chicago Press.

Glover, D.M. 2006. 'Tibetan Medicine in Gyalthang', *Tibet Journal* 30(4): 31–54.

Goldstein, M.C. 1991. 'The Dragon and the Snow Lion: The Tibet Question in the Twentieth Century' in A.J. Kane (ed), *China Briefing, 1990.* Boulder, CO: Westview Press.

——— 1994. 'Change, Conflict and Continuity among a Community of Nomadic Pastoralists: A Case Study From Western Tibet, 1950–1990', in R. Barnett and S. Akiner (eds), *Resistance and Reform in Tibet.* London: Hurst and Co.

——— 1999. *The Snow Lion and the Dragon: China, Tibet, and the Dalai Lama.* Berkeley: University of California Press.

Goldstein, M.C., and G. Rinpoche. 1989. *A History of Modern Tibet, 1913–1951.* Berkeley: University of California Press.

Government of China. 1984. 'Law of the People's Republic of China on the Administration of Drugs (First Drug Administration Law)', Government of China, Standing Committee of the People's Congress, http://www.asianlii.org/cgi-bin/disp.pl/cn/legis/cen/laws/lotprocotaod582/lotprocotaod582. html?query=traditional+medicine (accessed 8 July 2009).

——— 1993. 'Regulations on Protection of Traditional Chinese Medicines', Laws of the People's Republic of China, http://www.asianlii.org/cn/legis/cen/laws/ropotcm541/ (accessed 23 December 2009).

Gupta, A. 1999. 'Review: Seeing Like a State, by James Scott', *Journal of Asian Studies* 58(4): 1093–1095.

Gyatso, J. 2004. 'The Authority of Empiricism and the Empiricism of Authority: Medicine and Buddhism in Tibet on the Eve of Modernity', *Comparative Studies of South Asia, Africa and the Middle East* 24(2): 83–96.

Gyatso, Y. 1991. 'The Secrets of the Black Pill Formulation', *Tibetan Medicine* 13: 38–55.

———— 2006. 'Nyes Pa: A Brief Overview of Its English Translation', *Tibet Journal* 30(4): 109–118.

HAA. 2009. 'Sowa Rigpa (Amchi Medicine) Conservation Project (SCP)', project brochure. Kathmandu: Himalayan Amchi Association.

Hagen, T., and D. Thapa. 1998. *Toni Hagen's Nepal: The Kingdom in the Himalaya*, 4th edn. Lalitpur: Himal Books.

Harrington, A. 1997. *The Placebo Effect: An Interdisciplinary Exploration*. Cambridge, MA: Harvard University Press.

Harris, T. 2009. 'Silk Roads and Wool Routes: The Social Geography of Tibetan Trade', PhD thesis. New York: City University of New York.

Heberer, T. 2001. 'Old Tibet a Hell on Earth? The Myth of Tibet and Tibetans in Chinese Art and Propaganda', in T. Dodin and H. Räther (eds), *Imagining Tibet. Perceptions, Projections, and Fantasies*. Boston: Wisdom Publications.

Hilton, J. 1933. *Lost Horizon*. London: Macmillan.

Himalayan News Service. 2010. 'Smugglers Robbing Sindhupalchowk', *Himalayan Times, 29 May*. www.thehimalayantimes.com/fullNews.php?headline=Smugglers+robbing+Sindhupalchowk+dry&NewsID=245628 (accessed 2 July 2010).

Hobsbawm, E., and T. Ranger (eds). 1983. *The Invention of Tradition*. Cambridge University Press.

Hofer, T. 2009a. 'Socio-economic Dimensions of Tibetan Medicine in the Tibet Autonomous Region, China: Part One', *Asian Medicine* 4: 174–200.

———— 2009b. 'Socio-economic Dimensions of Tibetan Medicine in the Tibet Autonomous Region, China: Part Two', *Asian Medicine* 4: 492–514.

Hoffman, L.M. 2006. 'Autonomous Choices and Patriotic Professionalism: On Governmentality in Late-socialist China', *Economy and Society* 35(4): 550–570.

Houben, V., and M. Schrempf. 2008. *Figurations of Modernity: Global and Local Representations in Comparative Perspective*. Frankfurt am Main: Campus.

Hsu, E. 1996. 'The Polyglot Practitioner: Towards Acceptance of Different Approaches in Treatment Evaluation', in S.G. Olesen and E. Høg (eds), *Studies in Alternative Therapy*. Odense: Odense University Press.

———— 1998. 'Review: Knowing Practice, by Judith Farquhar', *Journal of the Royal Anthropological Institute* 4(1): 162–163.

———— 1999. *The Transmission of Chinese Medicine*. Cambridge: Cambridge University Press.

———— 2007. 'La Médicine chinoise traditionnelle en Républic Populaire de Chine: d'une "tradition inventée" a une "modernité alternative"', in A. Cheng (ed), *La Pensée en Chine aujourd'hui*. Paris: Gallimard.

———— 2009a. 'The History of Chinese Medicine in the People's Republic of China and Its Globalization', *East Asian Science, Technology and Society* 2(4): 465–484.

——— 2009b. 'Chinese Propriety Medicines: An "alternative Modernity?" the Case of the Anti-malarial Substance Artemisinin in East Africa', *Medical Anthropology* 28(2): 111–140.

Hu, J. 2005. 'Build Towards a Harmonious World of Lasting Peace and Common Prosperity', speech delivered to the High-level Plenary Meeting of the United Nations', 60th Session, http://www.fmprc.gov.cn/eng/wjdt/zyjh/t213091.htm (accessed 15 June 2010).

——— 2007. 'Hold High the Great Banner of Socialism with Chinese Characteristics and Strive for New Victories in Building a Moderately Prosperous Society in All Respects', http://www.chinadaily.com.cn/china/2007-10/25/content_6225977.htm (accessed 9 March 2008).

Hua, C. 2008. 'The Diffusion of Tibetan Medicine in China: A Descriptive Panorama', in L. Pordié (ed), *Tibetan Medicine in the Contemporary World: Global Politics of Medical Knowledge and Practice*. London: Routledge.

Huang, F. 2006. 'Traditional Inheritance and Modern Development of Tibetan Medicine', *China Tibet Information Center*, http://eng.tibet.cn/culture/book/200801/t20080117_356090.htm (accessed 12 September 2008).

Huber, T. 1997. 'Green Tibetans: A Brief Social History', in J. Korom (ed.), *Tibetan Culture in the Diaspora*. Vienna: Verlag der Österreichischen Akademie der Wissenschaften.

——— 2001. 'Shangri–La in Exile: Representations of Tibetan Identity and Transnational Culture', in T. Dodin and H. Räther (eds), *Imagining Tibet. Perceptions, Projections, and Fantasies*. Boston: Wisdom Publications.

Huntington, S.P. 1993. 'The Clash of Civilizations?' *Foreign Affairs* 72(3): 22–49.

ICH. n.d. 'History and Future of ICH', International Conference on Harmonisation of Technical Requirements for Registration of Pharmaceuticals for Human Use, http://www.ich.org/Main.jser?@_ID=524 (accessed 1 March 2010).

Immel, B. 2000. 'A Brief History of the GMPs', *BioPharm* August 2000:1–8.

IOSC. 2001. 'Tibet's March Toward Modernization', *Information Office of the State Council of the People's Republic of China*, Government White Papers, http://www.china.org.cn/e-white/20011108/index.htm (accessed 22 March 2010).

——— 2003. 'Ecological Improvement and Environmental Protection in Tibet', *Information Office of the State Council of the People's Republic of China*, Government White Papers, http://www.china–embassy.org/eng/zt/zfbps/t36547.htm (accessed 4 February 2007).

——— 2008. 'Protection and Development of Tibetan Culture', *Information Office of the State Council of the People's Republic of China*, Government White Papers, http://www.china.org.cn/government/whitepaper/node_7054682.htm (accessed 22 March 2010).

——— 2009a. 'China's Ethnic Policy and Common Prosperity and Development of All Ethnic Groups', *Information Office of the State Council of the People's Republic of China*, Government White Papers, http://www.china.

org.cn/government/whitepaper/node_7078073.htm (accessed 22 March 2010).

——— 2009b. 'Fifty Years of Democratic Reform in Tibet', *Information Office of the State Council of the People's Republic of China*, Government White Papers, http://www.china.org.cn/government/whitepaper/node_7062754.htm (accessed 22 March 2010).

Jampa Trinley. 2004. *The History of Tibetan Medicine* [gso rig lo rgyus]. Beijing: People's Publishing House.

Janes, C.R. 1995. 'The Transformations of Tibetan Medicine', *Medical Anthropology Quarterly* 9: 6–39.

——— 1999. 'The Health Transition, Global Modernity and the Crisis of Traditional Medicine: The Tibetan Case', *Social Science and Medicine* 48(12): 1803–1820.

——— 2002. 'Buddhism, Science, and Market: The Globalisation of Tibetan Medicine', *Anthropology and Medicine* 9(3): 267–289.

Jia, Q. 2005. 'Traditional Chinese Medicine Could Make "Health for One" True', *WHO CIPIH Studies*, http://www.who.int/intellectualproperty/studies/Jia.pdf (accessed 19 December 2009).

Kalden Nyima. 2006. 'Bod Sman Thon Skyed Las Rigs Kyis GMP Lag Bstar Brgyud Rim Khrod Kyi Gnad Don Dang Re Ba 'G' Zhig' [Some hopes and problems concerning the practical side of professional medicine production under GMP], in *Spyi Lo 2006 Lo'i Bod Kyi Gso Rig Rig Gzhung Spel Res Tshogs 'Du'i Dpyad Rtsom* [Proceedings of the 2006 [Lhasa] Conference on Tibetan Medicine]. Lhasa: Nyima. e.v.-PSTTM.

Kandiyoti, D. 2000. 'Modernisation Without the Market? The Case of the 'Soviet East" in A. Arce and N. Long (eds), *Anthropology, Development and Modernities: Exploring Discourses, Counter-Tendencies and Violence*. London: Routledge.

Kaptchuk, T.J. 1998. 'Intentional Ignorance: A History of Blind Assessment and Placebo Controls in Medicine', *Bulletin of the History of Medicine* 73(3): 389–433.

Karmay, S.G. 1994. 'Mountain Cult and National Identity' in R. Barnett and S. Akiner (eds), *Resistance and Reform in Tibet*. London: C. Hurst & Co.

——— 1996. 'The Tibetan Cult of Mountain Deities and Its Political Significance' in A. Blondeau and E. Steinkeller (eds), *Reflections of the Mountain. Essays on the History and Social Meaning of the Mountain Cult in Tibet and the Himalaya*. Wien: Verlag der Österreichischen Akademie der Wissenschaften.

Kind, M. 2002. *Mendrub: A Bonpo Ritual for the Benefit of All Living Beings and for the Empowerment of Medicine Performed in Tsho, Dolpo*. Kathmandu: WWF.

Kletter, C., and M. Kriechbaum. 2001. *Tibetan Medicinal Plants*. Stuttgart: Medpharm.

Kloos, S. 2010. 'Tibetan Medicine in Exile: The Ethics, Politics, and Science of Cultural Survival', PhD thesis. Berkeley: University of California.

References

Knauft, B. M. 2002. *Critically Modern. Alternatives, Alterities, Anthropologies.* Bloomington: Indiana University Press.
Kolås, Å. 2004. 'Ethnic Tourism in Shangrila: Representations of Place and Tibetan Identity', PhD thesis. Oslo: University of Oslo.
——— 2008. *Tourism and Tibetan Culture in Transition: A Place Called Shangrila.* New York: Routledge.
Kopytoff, I. 1986. 'The Cultural Biography of Things: Commoditization As Process', in A. Appadurai (ed.), *The Social Life of Things: Commodities in Cultural Perspective.* Cambridge: Cambridge University Press.
Kung, J., and L. Putterman. 1997. 'China's Collectivisation Puzzle: A New Resolution', *Journal of Development Studies* 33: 741–763.
Kuwahara, S.S., and S. Li. 2007. *Chinese Drug GMP: An Unofficial Translation.* Bethesda: PDA Books.
——— 2008. *Chinese GMP Inspection Standard Checklist.* Bethesda: PDA Books.
Lai, H.H. 2002. 'China's Western Development Program: Its Rationale, Implementation, and Prospects', *Modern China* 28(4): 432–466.
Langman, C.B. 2009. 'Melamine, Powdered Milk, and Nephrolithiasis in Chinese Infants', *New England Journal of Medicine* 360(11): 1139–1141.
Larsen, H.O., and P.D. Smith. 2004. 'Stakeholder Perspectives on Commercial Medicinal Plant Collection in Nepal: Poverty and Resource Degradation', *Mountain Research and Development* 24(2): 141–148.
Latour, B. 1993. *We Have Never Been Modern.* New York: Harvester Wheatsheaf.
Law, J. 2006. *Big Pharma: Exposing the Global Health Care Agenda.* New York: Carroll & Graff.
Law, W., and J. Salick. 2005. 'Human-induced Dwarfing of Himalayan Snow Lotus, Saussurea Laniceps (Asteraceae)', *Proceedings of the National Academy of Sciences of the United States of America* 102(29): 10218–10220.
Law, W., J. Salick and T.M. Knight. n.d. 'Comparative Population Ecologies and Sustainable Harvest of Tibetan Medicinal Snow Lotus', unpublished paper.
Lefort, C. 1986. *The Political Forms of Modern Society: Bureaucracy, Democracy, Totalitarianism*, trans. J.B. Thompson. Cambridge: MIT Press.
Legal Daily. 2006. 'Protection for Traditional Chinese Medicine to Be Reinforced', *Intellectual Property Protection in China.* http://www.chinaipr.gov.cn/Frontier/241295.shtml (accessed 19 December 2009).
Lei, S.H. 2002. 'How Did Chinese Medicine Become Experiential? The Political Epistemology of Jingyan', *Positions* 10(2): 333–364.
Lemke, T. 2001. '"The Birth of Bio-politics": Michel Foucault's Lecture at the Collège de France on Neo-liberal Governmentality', *Economy and Society* 30(2): 190–207.
Lin, J.Y. 1990. 'Collectivization and China's Agricultural Crisis in 1959–1961', *Journal of Political Economy* 98: 1228–1252.

Lindemann, G. 2002. *Die Grenzen Des Sozialen: Zur Sozio-technischen Konstruktion von Leben und Tod in der Intensivmedizin.* Munich: Wilhelm Fink Verlag.

———— 2009. 'Geselllschaftliche Grenzregime und Soziale Differenzierung', *Zeitschrift für Soziologie* 38(2): 94–112.

Lindholm, C. 2008. *Culture and Authenticity.* Malden, MA: Blackwell.

Lopez, D.S. 1998. *Prisoners of Shangri–La: Tibetan Buddhism and the West.* Chicago: University of Chicago Press.

Macartney, J. 2007. 'Festival-goers Ordered to Wear Fur or Face Fines as China Flouts Dalai Lama's Ruling', *Times Online*, http://www.timesonline.co.uk/tol/news/world/asia/article2148342.ece (accessed 24 November 2009).

Macartney, J., and S. Yu. 2009. 'Chinese Milk Powder Contaminated with Melamine Sickens 1,253 Babies', *Times Online*, http://www.timesonline.co.uk/tol/news/world/asia/article4758549.ece (accessed 8 January 2010).

MacDougall, D. 1999. 'Social Aesthetics and the Doon School', *Visual Anthropology Review* 15(1): 3–20.

McLagan, M. 2002. 'Spectacles of Difference: Cultural Activism and the Mass Mediation of Tibet', in F.D. Ginsburg, L. Abu-Lughod and B. Larkin (eds), *Media Worlds: Anthropology on New Terrain.* Berkeley: University of California Press.

Maconi, L. 2007. 'Contemporary Tibetan Literature From Shangri-La: Literary Life and Activities in Yunnan Tibetan Areas,1950–2002' in S.J. Venturino (ed.), *Contemporary Tibetan Literary Studies.* Leiden: Brill.

Majumder, S. 2003. 'The Philosophy of Privatisation in China', *The Hindu*, http://www.thehindubusinessline.com/2003/12/03/stories/2003120300120900.htm (accessed 22 May 2009).

Malinowski, B. 1935. *Coral Gardens and Their Magic: A Study of the Methods of Tilling the Soil and of Agricultural Rites in the Trobriand Islands.* London: Allen and Unwin.

Marglin, S.A. 1990. 'Loosing Touch: The Cultural Conditions of Worker Accomodation and Resistance' in F.A. Marglin and S.A. Marglin (eds), *Dominating Knowledge.* Oxford: Oxford University Press.

Marshall, E. and P. Bagla. 1997. 'India Applauds U.S. Patent Reversal', *Science* 277(5331): 1429.

Marx, K. 1872[1867]. *Das Kapital: Kritik der Politischen Ökonomie.* Hamburg: Otto Meissner,.

Marx, K., and F. Engels. 2002[1848]. *The Communist Manifesto*, ed. G. Stedman Jones. London: Penguin.

Men-Tsee-Khang. 2006. 'Inauguration of Cold Storage Rooms', *Men-Tsee-Khang Newsletter* 14(2), http://www.men-tsee-khang.org/newsletter/nov06/focus.htm (accessed 6 May 2009).

Merlan, F. 2009. 'Indigeneity: Global and Local', *Current Anthropology* 50(3): 303–333.

Meyer, F. 1981. *Gso-ba Rig-pa, Le Système Médical Tibétain.* Cahiers népalais. Paris: Editions du Centre national de la recherche scientifique.

——— 1992. 'The Medical Paintings of Tibet' in Y. Parfianovitch, F. Meyer and G. Dorje (eds), *Tibetan Medical Paintings. Illustrations of the Blue Beryl Treatise of Sangye Gyamtso (1653-1705)*. New York: Harry N. Abrams.

———. 1995. 'Theory and Practice of Tibetan Medicine' in J. Van Alphen and A. Aris (eds), *Oriental Medicine*. London: Serindia Publications.

Mgbeoji, I. 2006. *Global Biopiracy: Patents, Plants, and Indigenous Knowledge*. Vancouver: UBC Press.

Miller, S., P.V. Le, S. Craig, V. Adams, C. Tudor, Sonam, Nyima, et al. 2007. 'How to Make Consent Informed: Possible Lessons From Tibet', *IRB: Ethics and Human Research* 29(6): 7–14.

Ministry of Health. 1995. 'Drugs Standards of Ministry of Public Health of the People's Republic of China: Tibetan Medicine'. Xining: Ministry of Health of the PRC.

Moerman, D.E. 2002. *Meaning, Medicine, and the 'Placebo Effect'*. Cambridge: Cambridge University Press.

Moser, M. 2001. 'Warnung vor tibetischen Pillen', *Tages-Anzeiger*, July 7.

Moynihan, M. 2003. 'Tibetan Refugees in Nepal', in D. Bernstorff and H. Welck (eds), *Exile As Challenge: The Tibetan Diaspora*. Hyderabad: Orient Blackswan.

Nandy, A. 1994. 'Culture, Voice and Development: A Primer for the Unsuspecting', *Thesis Eleven* 39: 1–18.

——— 1997. 'Modern Science and Authoritarianism: From Objectivity to Objectification', *Bulletin of Science, Technology and Society* 17(1): 8–12.

Neue Zürcher Zeitung. 2002. 'Ungesunde Arznei: Die Gesundheitsdirektion warnt', *Neue Zürcher Zeitung*, 7 February: 44.

Neupane, T. 2010. 'Robbing Karnali', *Nepali Times*, 28 May, http://www.nepalitimes.com/issue/2010/05/28/Nation/17120 (accessed 2 July 2010).

Norbu, D. 2001. *China's Tibet Policy*. London: Routledge.

Nussbaum, M.C. 1986. *The Fragility of Goodness. Luck and Ethics in Greek Tragedy and Philosophy*. Cambridge: Cambridge University Press, 2001.

Oakes, T. 1998. *Tourism and Modernity in China*. London: Routledge.

——— 2000. 'China's Provincial Identities: Reviving Regionalism and Reinventing "Chineseness"', *Journal of Asian Studies* 59(3): 667–692.

Oguamanam, C. 2006. *International Law and Indigenous Knowledge: Intellectual Property, Plant Biodiversity, and Traditional Medicine*. Toronto: University of Toronto Press.

Olsen, C.S., and H.O. Larsen. 2003. 'Alpine Medicinal Plant Trade and Himalayan Mountain Livelihood Strategies', *Geographical Journal* 169(3): 243–254.

Ong, A. 1996. 'Anthropology, China and Modernities: The Geopolitics of Cultural Knowledge', in H.L. Moore (ed.), *The Future of Anthropological Knowledge*. London: Routledge.

Ong, A., and S.J. Collier. 2005. *Global Assemblages: Technology, Politics, and Ethics As Anthropological Problems*. Malden, MA: Blackwell.

Ong, A. and D. M. Nonini. 1997. 'Chinese Transnationalism As An Alternative Modernity (Introduction)' in A. Ong and D. M. Nonini (eds), *Ungrounded Empires*. London: Routledge.

Parfianovitch, Y., F. Meyer and G. Dorje. 1992. *Tibetan Medical Paintings. Illustrations of the Blue Beryl Treatise of Sangye Gyamtso (1653-1705)*. New York: Harry N. Abrams, Inc.

Patel, S.J. 1996. 'Can the Intellectual Property Rights System Serve the Interests of Indigenous Knowledge?' in S.B. Brush and D. Stabinsky (eds), *Valuing Local Knowledge: Indigenous People and Intellectual Property Rights*. Washington, DC: Island Press.

Patwardhan, B., D. Warude, P. Pushpangadan and N. Bhatt. 2005. 'Ayurveda and Traditional Chinese Medicine: A Comparative Overview', *Evidence Based, Complementary and Alternative Med* 2(4): 465–473.

People's Daily. 2001. 'Tibetans Make Up Majority of Officials in Tibet', http://www.china.org.cn/english/Tibet/13278.htm (accessed 8 January 2010).

——— 2007. 'Harmonious Society', *People's Daily Online*, http://english.peopledaily.com.cn/90002/92169/92211/6274973.html (accessed 11 November 2009).

——— 2008. 'Industrial Output of Traditional Chinese Medicine Reaches 177.2 Bln Yuan', http://english.people.com.cn/90001/90776/90785/6453231.html# (accessed 28 July 2008).

Petryna, A., A. Lakoff and A. Kleinman. 2006. 'The Pharmaceutical Nexus', in A. Petryna, A. Lakoff and A. Kleinman (eds), *Global Pharmaceuticals: Ethics, Markets, Practices*. Durham, NC: Duke University Press.

Phillips, B., C. Ball, D. Sackett, D. Badenoch, S. Straus, B. Haynes, M. Dawes and J. Howick. 1998. 'Levels of Evidence', *Centre for Evidence Based Medicine*, http://www.cebm.net/index.aspx?o=1025 (accessed 29 April 2010).

Polanyi, K. 1957. *The Great Transformation*. Boston: Beacon Press.

Pordié, L. 2003. *The Expression of Religion in Tibetan Medicine: Ideal Conceptions, Contemporary Practices, and Political Use*. Pondicherry: French Institute of Pondicherry.

——— 2008. *Tibetan Medicine in the Contemporary World: Global Politics of Medical Knowledge and Practice*. London: Routledge.

Posey, D.A., and G. Dutfield. 1996. *Beyond Intellectual Property: Toward Traditional Resource Rights for Indigenous Peoples and Local Communities*. Ottawa: International Development and Research Centre.

Qin, T. 2009. 'The Process of Legislation on Access and Benefit Sharing in China: A New Long March', in E.C. Kamau and G. Winter (eds), *Genetic Resources, Traditional Knowledge, and the Law: Solutions for Access and Benefit Sharing*. London: Earthscan.

Qiu, J. 2007. 'China Tightens Up', *Nature* 448(7154): 636–637.

Rabinow, P. 2003. *Anthropos Today: Reflections on Modern Equipment*. Princeton, NJ: Princeton University Press.

——— 2005. 'Midst Anthropology's Problems', in A. Ong and S. J. Collier (eds), *Global Assemblages: Technology, Politics, and Ethics As Anthropological Problems*. Malden, MA: Blackwell.

Ramo, J.C. 2007. *Brand China* (淡色中国). London: Foreign Policy Centre.

Randeria, S. 2002. 'Entangled Histories of Uneven Modernities. Civil Society, Caste Solidarities and Legal Pluralism in India' in Y. Elkana and S. Randeria (eds), *Unraveling Ties*. Frankfurt: Campus.

——— 2004. 'Konfigurationen der Moderne: Zur Einleitung', in S. Randeria, M. Fuchs and A. Linkenbach (eds), *Konfigurationen der Moderne: Diskurse zu Indien*. Baden-Baden: Nomos Verlag.

——— 2007. 'The State of Globalization. Legal Plurality, Overlapping Sovereignties and Ambiguous Alliances Between Civil Society and the Cunning State in India', *Theory, Culture & Society* 24(1): 1–33.

Rizvi, J. 2001. *Trans-Himalayan Caravans: Merchant Princes and Peasant Traders in Ladakh*. Oxford: Oxford University Press.

Rofel, L. 1997. 'Rethinking Modernity: Space and Factory Discipline in China' in A. Gupta and J. Ferguson (eds), *Culture, Power, Place. Explorations in Critical Anthropology*. Durham: Duke University Press.

Rose, N.S. 1999. *Powers of Freedom: Reframing Political Thought*. Cambridge: Cambridge University Press.

Ross, J.L. 1982. 'Adaptation to a Changing Salt Trade: The View from Humla', *Contributions to Nepalese Studies* 10(1/2): 43–49.

Rostow, W.W. 1959. 'The Stages of Economic Growth', *Economic History Review* 12: 1–16.

Rueschemeyer, D. 1999. 'Review: On Benign and Disastrous State Action', *International Studies Review* 1(1): 105–109.

Sahlins, M. 2000. 'What Is Anthropological Enlightenment? Some Lessons of the Twentieth Century' in M. Sahlins, *Culture in Practice. Selected Essays*. New York: Zone Books.

Sallon, S., Tenzin Namdul, Sonam Dolma, Pema Dorjee, Dawa Dolma, T. D. Sadutshang, P. Ever-Hadani, T. Bdolah-Abram, S. Apter and S. Almog. 2007. 'Mercury in Traditional Tibetan Medicine – Panacea or Problem?', *SMan-rTsis Journal* IV(1): 7–22.

Samuel, G. 2001. 'Tibetan Medicine in Contemporary India: Theory and Practice', in L.H. Connor and G. Samuel (eds), *Healing Powers and Modernity: Traditional Medicine, Shamanism and Science in Asian Societies*. Westport, CT: Bergin and Garvey.

——— 2010. 'A Short History of Indo-Tibetan Alchemy', in S. Craig, M. Cuomo, F. Garrett and M. Schrempf (eds), *Studies of Medical Pluralism in Tibetan History and Society*. Halle: International Institute for Tibetan and Buddhist Studies GmbH.

SARA, State Administration of Religious Affairs. 2007. 'Management of the Reincarnation of Living Buddhas in Tibetan Buddhism', *State Religious Affairs Bureau Order No. 5*. http://www.sara.gov.cn/gb/zcfg/gz/89522ff7-409d-11-dc-bafe-93180af1bb1a.html (accessed 15 June 2010).

Saxer, M. 2005. *Journeys with Tibetan Medicine*. Masters Thesis, University of Zurich, http://anyma.ch/journeys/doc/thesis.pdf (accessed 22 July 2012).

———— 2010. 'Tibetan Medicine and Russian Modernities' in V. Adams, M. Schrempf and S. Craig (eds), *Medicine Between Science and Religion: Explorations on Tibetan Grounds*. New York and Oxford: Berghahn.

———— 2011. 'Herbs and Traders in Transit: Border Regimes and Trans-Himalayan Trade in Tibetan Medicinal Plants', *Asian Medicine* 5 (2009): 317–339.

———— 2012. 'A Goat's Head on a Sheep's Body? Manufacturing Good Practices for Tibetan Medicine', *Medical Anthropology* 31(6): 497–513.

Scheid, V. 2001. 'Shaping Chinese Medicine: Two Case Studies From Contemporary China', in E. Hsu (ed.), *Innovation in Chinese Medicine*. Cambridge: Cambridge University Press.

———— 2002. *Chinese Medicine in Contemporary China: Plurality and Synthesis*. Durham, NC: Duke University Press.

Schrempf, M. 2007. *Soundings in Tibetan Medicine: Anthropological and Historical Perspectives*. Leiden: Brill.

Scott, A. 2004. 'China Threatens to Close Plants Failing GMP Standard', *Chemical Week* 166(17): 26.

Scott, J.C. 1976. *The Moral Economy of the Peasant: Rebellion and Subsistence in Southeast Asia*. New Haven, CT: Yale University Press.

———— 1985. *Weapons of the Weak: Everyday Forms of Peasant Resistance*. New Haven, CT: Yale University Press.

———— 1998. *Seeing Like a State: How Certain Schemes to Improve the Human Condition Have Failed*. New Haven, CT: Yale University Press.

———— 2009. *The Art of Not Being Governed: An Anarchist History of Upland Southeast Asia*. New Haven, CT: Yale University Press.

SDA. 2002. 'Quecksilber in Heilmitteln', *Neue Luzerner Zeitung*, February 8.

See, G. 2008. 'Mapping the Harmonious Society and CSR Link', *Wharton Research Scholars Journal*, http://repository.upenn.edu/wharton research scholars/48 (accessed 7 November 2009).

Serres, M., and B. Latour. 1995. *Conversations on Science, Culture, and Time*. Ann Arbor: University of Michigan Press.

SFDA. 2001. 'Drug Administration Law of the People's Republic of China', *State Food and Drug Administration of the PRC*, Laws and Regulations, http://former.sfda.gov.cn/cmsweb/webportal/W45649037/A48335975.html (accessed 2 June 2011).

———— 2002. 'Good Agricultural Practice for Chinese Crude Drugs (Interim)', *State Food and Drug Administration of the PRC*, Normative Documents, http://former.sfda.gov.cn/cmsweb/webportal/W45649039/A55807078.html (accessed 2 June 2011).

———— 2004. 'Measures for the Administration of Pharmaceutical Trade Licence', *Laws of the PRC*, http://www.asianlii.org/cgi-bin/disp.pl/cn/legis/cen/laws/mftaoptl550/mftaoptl550.html?query=traditional+medicine (accessed 8 July 2009).

———— 2005a. 'SFDA Issues Provisions for Import Crude Drugs (Interim)', *State Food and Drug Administration of the PRC*, What's New, http://eng.sfda.gov.cn/cmsweb/webportal/W43879541/A64005999.html?searchword=%28crude%29 (accessed 11 October 2008).

—— 2005b. 'SFDA Specify the Production Scope of Foreign-invested Manufacturers of Prepared Slices of Chinese Crude Drugs', *State Food and Drug Administration of the PRC*, What's New, http://former.sfda.gov.cn/cmsweb/webportal/W43879541/A64006764.html (accessed 8 July 2009).

—— 2006a. 'Provisions for Drug Insert Sheets and Labels', *State Food and Drug Administration of the PRC*, Normative Documents, http://eng.sfda.gov.cn/cmsweb/webportal/W45649039/A64030242.html (accessed 7 June 2009).

—— 2006b. 'SFDA Specifies Requirements for the Implementation of Provisions for Import Crude Drugs (Interim)', *State Food and Drug Administration of the PRC*, What's New, http://eng.sfda.gov.cn/cmsweb/webportal/W43879541/A64006943.html?searchword=%28crude%29 (accessed 11 October 2008).

—— 2007. 'Provisions for Drug Registration', *State Food and Drug Administration of the PRC*, Normative Documents, http://former.sfda.gov.cn/cmsweb/webportal/W45649039/A64028429.html (accessed 2 June 2011).

—— 2009. 'SFDA Issues Guidelines on the Protection of Traditional Chinese Medicines', *State Food and Drug Administration of the PRC*, What's New, http://eng.sfda.gov.cn/cmsweb/webportal/W43879541/A64029686.html (accessed 21 April 2009).

Shahi, P. 2010. 'Poacher's release may boost wildlife crime', *The Kathmandu Post*, April 18. http://www.ekantipur.com/the-kathmandu-post/2010/04/18/top-stories/Poachers-release-may-boost-wildlife-crime/207337/ (accessed 2 July 2010).

Shakabpa, T.W.D. 1984. *Tibet: A Political History*. New York: Potala Publications.

Shakya, T. 1999. *The Dragon in the Land of Snows: A History of Modern Tibet Since 1947*. London: Pimlico.

Shepherd, R. 2006. 'UNESCO and the Politics of Cultural Heritage in Tibet', *Journal of Contemporary Asia* 36(2): 243–257.

Shiva, V. 1997. *Biopiracy: The Plunder of Nature and Knowledge*. Boston: South End Press.

—— 2001. *Protect or Plunder? Understanding Intellectual Property Rights*. New York: Zed Books.

Shue, V. 1995. 'State Sprawl: The Regulatory State and Social Life in a Small Chinese City' in D. S. Davis, R. Kraus, et al. (eds), *Urban Spaces in Contemporary China: The Potential for Autonomy and Community in Post-Mao China*. Cambridge: Woodrow Wilson Center Press and Cambridge University Press.

—— 2006. 'The Quality of Mercy: Confucian Charity and the Mixed Metaphors of Modernity in Tianjin', *Modern China* 32(4): 411–452.

Sigley, G. 2006. 'Chinese Governmentalities: Government, Governance and the Socialist Market Economy', *Economy and Society* 35(4): 487–508.

Silano, M. , M. De Vincenzi, A. De Vincenzi and V. Silano. 2004. 'The New European Legislation on Traditional Herbal Medicines: Main Features and Perspectives', *Fitoterapia* 75(2): 107–116.

Sinclair, U. 1906. *The Jungle.* New York: Doubleday, Page & Co.

Sinopharm. 2009. 'New Guidelines on the Protection of Traditional Chinese Medicine Encourages Innovation', *Sinopharm,* http://www.sinopharm.com/news_7906.html (accessed 21 May 2009).

SIPO. 2009. 'What Kind of Invention Cannot Be Patented in China?', *State Intellectual Property Office of the PRC,* Frequently Asked Questions, www.sipo.gov.cn/sipo_English/FAQ/200904/t20090408_449725.html (accessed 19 December 2009).

Society for Critical Exchange. 1993. 'Bellagio Declaration', *Society for Critical Exchange,* http://www.cwru.edu/affil/sce/BellagioDec.html (accessed 17 May 2010).

SPC. 2005. *Pharmacopoeia of the People's Republic of China.* Beijing: People's Medical Publishing House, for the State Pharmacopoeia Commission.

Strathern, M. 2000. 'The Tyranny of Transparency', *British Educational Research Journal* 26(3): 309–321.

Strøm, A.K. 1997. 'Between Tibet and the West: On Traditionality, Modernity and the Development of Monastic Institutions in the Tibetan Diaspora', in J. Korom (ed.), *Tibetan Culture in the Diaspora.* Vienna: Verlag der Österreichischen Akademie der Wissenschaften.

Su, G. 2003. 'Protection and Development of the Traditional Medicine in China', *China Biodiversity-related IP Information Network,* www.biodiv-ip.gov.cn/english/rdxx_e/t20040113_24258.htm (accessed 19 December 2009).

Swain, M.B. 1990. 'Commoditizing Ethnicity in Southwest China', *Cultural Survival Quarterly* 14(1): 26–30.

Tashi Tsering. 2005. 'Designing Modernization to Promote Traditional Tibetan Medicine', *Trin-Gyi-Pho-Nya: Tibet's Environment and Development Digest* 2(6) http://www.tibetjustice.org/tringyiphonya/num9.html#tibetmed (accessed 4 October 2007).

Taylor, K. 2005. *Chinese Medicine in Early Communist China, 1945–63: A Medicine of Revolution.* London: Routledge Curzon.

Therborn, G. 1995. 'Routes to/through Modernity', in M. Featherstone, S. Lash and R. Robertson (eds), *Global Modernities.* London: Sage.

Thompson, E.P. 1964. *The Making of the English Working Class.* New York: Vintage Books.

——— 1971. 'The Moral Economy of the English Crowd in the Eighteenth Century', *Past and Present* 50: 76–136.

——— 1991. *Customs in Common.* New York: New Press.

Timmermans, S., and M. Berg. 2003. *The Gold Standard: The Challenge of Evidence-based Medicine and Standardization in Health Care.* Philadelphia: Temple University Press.

TIN. 2004. 'Tibetan Medicine in Contemporary Tibet'. London: Tibet Information Network.

Todorov, V. 1995. *Red Square, Black Square: Organon for Revolutionary Imagination.* Albany: State University of New York Press.

Tsai, L.L. 2008. 'Understanding the Falsification of Village Income Statistics', *China Quarterly* 196: 805–826.

Tsering Drolma. 2007. 'The Status Quo of Tibetan Traditional Medicine and Thoughts on Its Development', *China Tibet Information Center*, http://eng.tibet.cn/culture/tis/t20071212_291002.htm (accessed 11 September 2008).

Tsultrim Tsering Gyaltsen. 2005. 'Response to Tashi Tsering's Editorial "Designing Modernization to Promote Traditional Tibetan Medicine" in *Trin-Gyi-Pho-Nya* Vol. 2, No. 6', *Trin-Gyi-Pho-Nya: Tibet's Environment and Development Digest* 3(1), http://www.tibetjustice.org/tringyiphonya/num10.html (accessed 4 October 2007).

Tu, W. 1996. 'Confucian Traditions in East Asian Modernity', *Bulletin of the American Academy of Arts and Sciences* 50(2): 12–39.

TYC. 2009. 'Tibetan Youth Congress to Observe the Year 2009 (Tibetan Year 2136 of Earth Ox) As Black Year', *Tibetan Youth Congress*, press release, http://www.tibetanyouthcongress.com/download/Press_Release_Losar_09.pdf (accessed 28 June 2010).

UNESCO. 1993. 'Lhasa, Case No. 707', *World Heritage List*.

——— 2003. 'Convention for the Safeguarding of the Intangible Cultural Heritage', http://unesdoc.unesco.org/images/0013/001325/132540e.pdf (accessed 1 July 2009).

United Nations. 1993. 'Convention on Biological Diversity (with Annexes)', www.cbd.int/convention/convention.shtml (accessed 12 December 2009).

van der Geest, S., and S.R. Whyte. 1989. 'The Charm of Medicines: Metaphors and Metonyms', *Medical Anthropology Quarterly* 3(4): 345–367.

van der Geest, S., S.R. Whyte and A. Hardon. 1996. 'The Anthropology of Pharmaceuticals: A Biographical Approach', *Annual Review of Anthropology* 25: 153–178.

Walach, H., T. Falkenberg, F. Vinjar, G. Lewith and W.B. Jonas. 2006. 'Circular Instead of Hierarchical: Methodological Principles for the Evaluation of Complex Interventions', *BMC Medical Research Methodology* 6(29): 1–9, http://www.biomedcentral.com/1471-2288/6/29 (accessed 12 June 2007).

Waldram, J.B. 2000. 'The Efficacy of Traditional Medicine: Current Theoretical and Methodological Issues', *Medical Anthropology Quarterly* 14(4): 603–625.

Wang, G., J. L. Innes, J. Lei, S. Dai and S. W. Wu. 2007. 'China's Forestry Reforms', *Science* 318(5856): 1556.

Wang, K. 2007. 'Shaolin Abbot: Buddhism Contributes to a Harmonious Society', http://china.org.cn/english/2007lh/202397.htm (accessed 11 November 2009).

Wang, Y. 2008. 'Public Diplomacy and the Rise of Chinese Soft Power', *Annals of the American Academy of Political and Social Science* 616: 257–273.

Weber, M. 1947. *The Theory of Economic and Social Organization*, trans. and ed. T. Parsons. New York: Oxford University Press.

——— 1962[1951]. *The Religion of China: Confucianism and Taoism*. New York: Free Press,.

——— 1986[1904]. 'Die Protestantische Ethik und der Geist des Kapitalismus' in *Gesammelte Aufsätze Zur Religionssoziologie I*, Tübingen: Mohr..

———— 2002[1919]. 'Wissenschaft als Beruf' in *Schriften 1894–1922*, ed. D. Kaesler. Stuttgart: Kröner.

White, S.D. 2010. 'The Political Economy of Ethnicity in Yunnan's Lijiang Basin', *Asia Pacific Journal of Anthropology* 11(2): 142–158.

WHO. 2002. 'WHO Traditional Medicine Strategy 2002–2005'. Geneva: World Health Organization.

———— 2003. 'WHO Guidelines on Good Agricultural and Collection Practices (GACP) for Medicinal Plants', Geneva: World Health Organization.

———— 2004. 'WHO Guidelines on Safety Monitoring of Herbal Medicines in Pharmacovigilance Systems'. Geneva: World Health Organization.

———— 2005a. 'National Policy on Traditional Medicine and Regulation of Herbal Medicines: Report of a WHO Global Survey'. Geneva: World Health Organization.

———— 2005b. 'Supplement Guidelines on Good Manufacturing Practices (GMP): Validation', *World Health Organization*, http://www.who.int/medicines/services/expertcommittees/pharmprep/Validation_QAS_055_Rev2-combined.pdf (accessed 16 September 2008).

———— 2006a. 'Good Manufacturing Practices: Updated Supplementary Guidelines for the Manufacture of Herbal Medicines (Final Draft)', *World Health Organization*, Working Document, http://www.who.int/medicines/services/expertcommittees/pharmprep/QAS04_050Rev3_GMPHerbal_Final_Sept05.pdf (accessed 22 July 2012).

———— 2006b. 'Traditional Medicine', *World Health Organization*, Agenda Item 14.10, WHO Resolution, 56th World Health Assembly, http://whqlibdoc.who.int/wha/2003/WHA56_31.pdf (accessed 22 July 2012).

———— 2007. 'WHO Guidelines on Good Manufacturing Practices (GMP) for Herbal Medicines', *World Health Organization*, http://apps.who.int/medicinedocs/index/assoc/s14215e/s14215e.pdf (accessed 2 July 2010).

Winkler, D. 2008a. 'The Mushrooming Fungi Market in Tibet – Exemplified by Cordyceps Sinensis and Tricholoma Matsutake', *Journal of the International Association of Tibetan Studies* 4: 1–46.

———— 2008b. 'Yartsa Gunbu (Cordyceps Sinensis) and the Fungal Commodification of the Rural Economy in Tibet AR', *Economic Botany* 62(3): 291-305.

———— 2010. 'Caterpillar Fungus (Ophiocordyceps Sinensis) Production and Sustainability on the Tibetan Plateau and in the Himalayas', *Chinese Journal of Grassland* 32(supplement): 96–108.

Winteler, C. 2002. 'Schwermetall in tibetischen Pillen', *Tages-Anzeiger*, February 7.

Wittrock, B. 2000. 'Modernity: One, None, or Many? European Origins and Modernity As a Global Condition', *Daedalus* 129(1): 31–60.

Woeser. 2009. 'I Took to the Streets, and What I Want Is Freedom and Rights', *Invisible Tibet – Woeser's Blog*, http://woeser.middle-way.net/2009/02/blog-post_3129.html (accessed 22 July 2012).

Wolfgang, L. 1995. 'Patents on Native Technology Challenged', *Science* 269(5230): 1506.

Wong, E. 2009. 'Dalai Lama Says China Has Turned Tibet Into a "Hell on Earth", *New York Times*, March 10.

Wong, R.B. 1999. 'Review: Seeing Like a State, by James Scott', *Political Science Quarterly* 114(2): 340–342.

WTO. 1994. 'Trade-related Aspects of Intellectual Property Rights (TRIPS Agreement)', *World Trade Organization*, Annex 1C of the Marrakesh Agreement, http://www.wto.org/english/docs_e/legal_e/27-trips pdf (accessed 8 January 2010).

Wylie, T. 1959. 'A Standard System of Tibetan Transcription', *Harvard Journal of Asiatic Studies* 22:261–267.

Xie, P.F. 2003. 'The Bamboo-beating Dance in Hainan, China: Authenticity and Commodification', *Journal of Sustainable Tourism* 11(1): 5–16.

Xinhua. 2005. 'Building Harmonious Society Important Task for CPC: President Hu', *People's Daily Online*, http://english.people.com.cn/200502/20/eng20050220_174036.html (accessed 11 November 2009).

———— 2006a. 'China Publishes Its Resolution on Building a Harmonious Society', *China News and Report*, http://china.org.cn/english/report/189591.htm (accessed 11 November 2009).

———— 2006b. 'Wu Jianmin: "Harmonious World" Helps Rebut "China Threat"', http://china.org.cn/english/international/162349.htm (accessed 11 November 2009).

———— 2007. 'President: Harmony, Stability Prerequisite for Tibet Development', http://china.org.cn/english/2007lh/201629.htm (accessed 11 November 2009).

———— 2008. 'Traditional Tibetan Medicine Sees New Boom in Talent, RandD', http://news.xinhuanet.com/english/2008-07/12/content_8534361.htm (accessed 29 July 2008).

———— 2009. 'Tibetan Studies Show New Year Is Not Black', *Xinhua News*, http://www. nyconsulate.prchina.org/eng/zt/xzwt/t538193.htm# (accessed 20 February 2009).

Yang, M.M. 1988. 'The Modernity of Power in the Chinese Socialist Order', *Cultural Anthropology* 3(4): 408–427.

———— 1989. 'The Gift Economy and State Power in China', *Comparative Studies in Society and History* 31(1): 25–54.

———— 1994. *Gifts, Favors, and Banquets: The Art of Social Relationships in China*. Ithaca, NY: Cornell University Press.

———— 2002. 'The Resilience of Guanxi and Its New Deployments: A Critique of Some New Guanxi Scholarship ',*China Quarterly* 170: 459–476.

Yeh, E. 2007. 'Exile Meets Homeland: Politics, Performance, and Authenticity in the Tibetan Diaspora', *Environment and Planning D: Society and Space* 25(4): 648–667.

———— 2008. 'Modernity, Memory, and Agricultural Modernisation in Central Tibet, 1950–1980', in R. Barnett and R. Schwartz (eds), *Tibetan Modernities: Notes From the Field on Cultural and Social Change*. Leiden: Brill.

Yi, Y. 2003. 'Modern Medicines to Make Use of Tibetan Traditions', *China Daily*, 9 September, http://www.chinadaily.com.cn/en/doc/2003-09/23/content_266435.htm (accessed 8 January 2010).

You, J. 1998. *China's Enterprise Reform. Changing State*. London and New York: Routledge.

Yuthog (Yuthog Yonten Gonpo the Younger). 2005. *G.yu Thog Snying Thig* [Yuthog Heart Essence]. Beijing: Mi rigs dpe skrun khang.

Zhang, Q. 2007. 'Recent Developments in China's IP Laws and Regulations Concerning Pharmaceuticals', *China Intellectual Property*, http://www.chinaipmagazine.com/en/journal-show.asp?id=171 (accessed 19 December 2009).

✣ Index